Spehlmann's EEG Primer

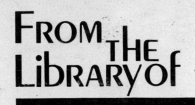

Spehlmann's EEG Primer

Second Revised and Enlarged Edition

BRUCE J. FISCH, M.D.

*Director, Epilepsy Monitoring Unit
and Quantitative EEG Analysis Laboratory,
The Neurological Institute of New York,
Columbia University College of Physicians
and Surgeons, New York, NY, USA*

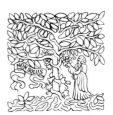

1991
ELSEVIER

Amsterdam - New York - Oxford

ISBN − hardbound: 0-444-812423
 − paperback: 0-444-814205

First edition: 1981   Fourth printing: 1987   Seventh printing: 1988
Second printing: 1982   Fifth printing: 1987   Eighth printing: 1990
Third printing: 1985   Sixth printing: 1988   Second edition: 1991

This book is printed on acid-free paper.

Published by: Sole distributors for the USA and Canada:
Elsevier Science Publishers B.V. (Biomedical Division) Elsevier Science Publishing Company Inc.
P.O. Box 211   655 Avenue of the Americas
1000 AE Amsterdam   New York, NY 10010
(The Netherlands)   (U.S.A.)

Printed in The Netherlands

This book is dedicated to Susan, Ian and Paul.

Library of Congress Cataloging-in-Publication Data

Fisch, Bruce J.
    Spehlmann's EEG primer. -- 2nd ed., rev. and enl. / Bruce J.
Fisch.
        p. cm.
    Rev. ed. of: EEG primer / R. Spehlmann. c1991.
    Includes bibliographical references and index.
    ISBN 0-444-81242-3 (hardbound : alk. paper). -- ISBN 0-444-81420-5
(pbk. : alk. paper)
    1. Electroencephalography. I. Spehlmann, Rainer, 1931- EEG
primer. II. Title: EEG primer.
    [DNLM: 1. Electroencephalography. WL 150 F528s]
RC386.6.E43S64 1991
616.8 047547--dc20
DNLM/DLC
for Library of Congress

Preface to the Second Edition

This second edition of the *EEG Primer* has been renamed Spehlmann's EEG Primer in honor of the late Dr. Rainer Spehlmann. Dr. Spehlmann will be remembered by his colleagues and students for his contributions to neuroscience and for his dedication to the advancement of clinical neurophysiology. Those who knew him well will remember him affectionately as a kind, soft-spoken and modest person.

Spehlmann's EEG Primer is intended to introduce the fudamentals of EEG recording and interpretation in a clear and concise fashion. It is a primer in the sense that the text focuses on well established techniques and clinical correlations; those which are either controversial or not clinically relevant are not discussed. Information that is essential for physicians seeking special certification in clinical neurophysiology has been included in the revised text and newly created appendix. The addition of the American EEG Society Guidelines in EEG, the International Classification of Epileptic Seizures, and the glossary of terms of the International Federation of Societies for EEG and Clinical Neurophysiology, as well as a more extensive index, should also help to make this edition a useful laboratory reference.

As with the first edition, *Spehlmann's EEG Primer* is intended to be used in conjunction with direct experience in the EEG laboratory. EEG interpretation can only be learned by reading under the supervision of an experienced electroencephalographer. For this instruction the reader should seek out an individual with special qualification and interest in EEG.

Since the *EEG Primer* was first published in 1981, computerized EEG analysis and topographic display systems have become commonplace. Certain aspects of computerized signal analysis (such as montage reformatting, the temporal analysis of epileptiform spikes, and electrographic seizure detection) have proved to be clinically important developments. Unfortunately, routine topographic mapping has not as yet. Nevertheless, since topographic mapping is in widespread use, and because topographic maps are even more likely to be misinterpreted than are routine recordings, clinical electroencephalographers need to have some familiarity with this technology. For these reasons, an expanded chapter on special recording techniques now includes an introduction to topographic mapping and computerized EEG analysis.

A preface can serve many purpose, but perhaps the most important is to thank those who generously contributed their time and effort. In this regard I am especially grateful to my good fried and colleague Dr. Timothy Pedley for his support and thoughtful advice on a variety of topics. I also thank Dr. Donald Klass who, along with Drs. Frank Sharbrough, Barbara Westmoreland, and Jack Grabow at the Mayo Clinic, introduced me to the field of EEG and provided valuable advice during the revision of this edition. Finally, I am grateful to Dr. Jerome Engel whose recommendations helped make this work possible.

B.F. Fisch

Contents

Preface to the Second Edition   *vii*

Part A: Technical background

Introduction   *3*

1   *The source of the EEG*   *7*

   1.1   The generator of the EEG   7
   1.2   Rhythmical EEG activity   13
   1.3   Recording of electrical potentials with scalp electrodes   16

2   *Recording electrodes*   *21*

   2.1   Electrode shapes and application methods   21
   2.2   Electrical properties of recording electrodes   27
   2.3   Electrode placement   31

3   *The EEG machine: Parts and functions*   *39*

   3.1   The input board   40
   3.2   Input selector switches   41
   3.3   Calibration   42
   3.4   The amplifiers   43
   3.5   Filters   51
   3.6   Writing units   60

4	*Recording strategy*		67
	4.1	Multichannel recordings	67
	4.2	Specific montages	76
	4.3	Electrode combinations for monitoring extracerebral activity	80

5	*The product of the recording: The clinical EEG record*		87
	5.1	General technical standards	88
	5.2	Standards for pediatric recordings	96
	5.3	Standards for recordings in cases of suspected cerebral death	99
	5.4	Telephone transmission	103

6	*Artifacts*		107
	6.1	Artifacts from the patient	107
	6.2	Interference	119
	6.3	Artifacts arising from recording electrodes and equipment	121

7	*Other methods of recording and analysis*		127
	7.1	Computer assisted signal analysis	127
	7.2	Analog to digital conversion	128
	7.3	EEG signal storage	131
	7.4	Special methods of computerized signal analysis	133
	7.5	Ambulatory EEG cassette recording	150
	7.6	EEG recording with simultaneous video monitoring	151

Part B: The normal EEG

8	*Definition of the normal EEG, relation to brain function*		159
	8.1	Definition of the normal EEG	159
	8.2	A normal EEG does not always mean normal brain function	161
	8.3	An abnormal EEG does not necessarily mean abnormal brain function	161

9   *Descriptors of EEG activity*   *163*

9.1	Wave form	163
9.2	Repetition	166
9.3	Frequency	167
9.4	Amplitude	168
9.5	Distribution	169
9.6	Phase relation	170
9.7	Timing	171
9.8	Persistence	172
9.9	Reactivity	173

10   *The normal EEG from premature age to the age of 19 years*   *175*

10.1	Neonatal EEG	175
10.2	Infants from full term to 3 months of age	191
10.3	Infants from 3 months to 12 months of age	194
10.4	Infants, children and adolescents from 1 to 19 years of age	200
10.5	Major abnormalities during the neonatal period and infancy	205

11   *The normal EEG of wakeful resting adults of 20–60 years of age*   *213*

11.1	The alpha rhythm	213
11.2	Beta activity	219
11.3	Mu rhythm	222
11.4	Lambda waves	223
11.5	Vertex sharp transients (V waves)	223
11.6	Kappa rhythm	224
11.7	Normal posterior theta rhythms	224
11.8	The low voltage EEG	225
11.9	Major abnormalities	225

12   *The normal sleep EEG of adults over 20 years*   *229*

12.1	Elements of normal sleep activity	229
12.2	Sleep stages	231
12.3	Sleep cycles	237
12.4	Major abnormalities	238

13   *The normal EEG of adults over 60 years of age*   *243*

    13.1   The alpha rhythm   243
    13.2   Beta rhythm   245
    13.3   Sporadic generalized slow waves   246
    13.4   Intermittent temporal slow waves   246
    13.5   Sleep   247
    13.6   Major abnormalities   249

14   *Activation procedures*   *251*

    14.1   Hyperventilation   251
    14.2   Sleep   255
    14.3   Photic stimulation   257
    14.4   Other stimuli   262
    14.5   Pentylene tetrazol, bemegride and other convulsant drugs   264

Part C: The abnormal EEG

15   *Abnormal EEG patterns, correlation with underlying cerebral lesions and*
    neurological diseases   *271*

    15.1   Definition of the abnormal EEG   271
    15.2   Correlation between abnormal EEG patterns, general cerebral pathology
            and specific neurological diseases   272
    15.3   The diagnostic value of the EEG   276

16   *Classification of seizures*   *281*

    16.1   Definitions   281
    16.2a   Classification of seizures — General   283
    16.2b   Classification of seizures — Specific   290

17   *Localized epileptiform patterns*   *299*

    17.1   Description of patterns   300
    17.2   Clinical significance of focal epileptiform activity   307

17.3   Other EEG abnormalities associated with focal epileptiform activity   311
17.4   Mechanisms underlying focal epileptiform activity   314
17.5   Specific disorders causing focal epileptiform activity   316

18   *Generalized epileptiform patterns*   *329*

18.1   Description of patterns   330
18.2   Clinical significance of generalized epileptiform activity   339
18.3   Other EEG abnormalities associated with generalized epileptiform activity   345
18.4   Mechanisms underlying generalized epileptiform activity   346
18.5   Specific disorders causing generalized epileptiform activity   348

19   *Special epileptiform patterns*   *355*

19.1   Neonatal seizures   355
19.2   The infantile and juvenile patterns of hypsarrhythmia, slow spike-and-wave discharges and multifocal independent spikes   363
19.3   Periodic complexes   370
19.4   Ictal pattern without spikes and sharp waves   381
19.5   Epileptiform patterns withour proven relation to seizures ('pseudoepileptogenic patterns')   384

20   *Local slow waves*   *403*

20.1   Description of pattern   403
20.2   Clinical significance of focal slow waves   406
20.3   Other EEG abnormalities associated with focal slow waves   409
20.4   Mechanisms causing focal slow waves   413
20.5   Specific disorders causing focal slow waves   413

21   *Generalized asynchronous slow waves*   *421*

21.1   Description of pattern   421
21.2   General clinical significance of generalized asynchronous slow waves   426
21.3   Other EEG abnormalities associated with generalized asynchronous slow waves   427
21.4   Mechanisms causing generalized asynchronous slow waves   427
21.5   Specific disorders causing generalized asynchronous slow waves   428

22　*Bilaterally synchronous slow waves*　　*441*

22.1 Description of pattern　　443
22.2 Clinical significance of bisynchronous slow waves　　447
22.3 Other EEG abnormalities associated with bisynchronous slow waves　　449
22.4 Mechanisms causing bisynchronous slow waves　　450
22.5 Specific disorders causing bilaterally synchronous slow waves　　450

23　*Localized and lateralized changes of amplitude: Asymmetries*　　*459*

23.1 Description of pattern　　459
23.2 Clinical significance of asymmetries　　463
23.3 Other abnormalities associated with asymmetries　　464
23.4 Mechanisms causing local changes of amplitude　　465
23.5 Specific disorders causing asymmetries of amplitude　　466
23.6 Asymmetries of alpha, beta, mu and other rhythms　　472

24　*Generalized changes of amplitude: Symmetrically high and low amplitude*　　*477*

24.1 Description of patterns　　479
24.2 Clinical significance of high and low amplitude　　481
24.3 Other EEG abnormalities associated with high and low amplitude　　482
24.4 Mechanisms causing generalized changes of amplitude　　482
24.5 Specific disorders causing a generalized decrease of amplitude of all types of activity　　483
24.6 Generalized decrease or absence of alpha rhythm　　488
24.7 Generalized increase of beta rhythm　　489
24.8 Changes of amplitude of sleep patterns　　490

25　*Deviation from normal patterns*　　*493*

25.1 Abnormal frequency of the alpha rhythm　　493
25.2 Abnormal reactivity of the alpha rhythm　　499
25.3 Rhythmical activity of theta, alpha and beta frequency in coma and during seizures　　501
25.4 Abnormal timing and incidence of sleep patterns　　505
25.5 Immature patterns　　506

26   *The EEG report*   509

26.1 Description of the record   509
26.2 EEG summary   513
26.3 Clinical correlation   514

Appendix I

A glossary of terms most commonly used by clinical electroencephalographers   519

Appendix II

American EEG Society Recording Guidelines   537
Guideline One: Miniumum technical requirements for performing clinical electro-
encephalography   537
Guideline Two: Minimum technical standards for pediatric electroencephalography   546
Guideline Three: Miniumum technical standards for EEG recording in suspected cerebral
death   554
Guideline Four: Standards of practice in clinical electroencephalography   563
Guideline Five: Recommended job descriptions for electroencephalographic technologists 565
Guideline Six: Recommendations for telephone transmission of EEGs   569
Guideline Seven: A proposal for standard montages to be used in clinical EEG   573
Guideline Eight: Guidelines for writing EEG reports   583

Appendix III

Clinical and electroencephalographic classification of epileptic seizures: Definition of terms 591

Appendix IV

Guidelines for standard electrode position nomenclature
as proposed by The American EEG Society   607

Subject Index   613

Part A
Technical background

Introduction

The steps involved in recording an EEG are illustrated in Figure 0.1 and described in Chapters 1 to 7 comprising Part A of this text.

(1) *The Source* of the EEG are electrical potentials generated by nerve cells in the cerebral cortex in response to various kinds of input, including that from pacemakers of rhythmical activity in the depth of the brain. These fluctuating potentials summate and penetrate to the scalp where they can be recorded as the scalp EEG.

(2) *Recording electrodes* usually consist of small metal cups or discs which are attached to the scalp so that they make good mechanical and electrical contact. They cover the surface of the head at regular intervals.

(3) *The EEG machine* receives electrical input from the scalp electrodes which are connected to an input board. The cable of the input board terminates at the input selector switches which are used to select a pair of electrodes, or a calibration voltage, as the input of each recording channel. The input is connected to differential amplifiers which increase the size of the electrical potential differences between the two electrodes and reject interference simultaneously affecting both electrodes. High and low frequency filters are used to reduce the size of very slow and very fast potential changes and to emphasize clinically important electrical activity in the medium frequency range. A 60 Hz filter can eliminate the most common electrical interference in EEG recordings, namely that from power lines, if it cannot be eliminated by other means. The amplified electrical potentials are used to drive an ink pen, or other writing devices, up and down on chart paper which is pulled along at a constant speed.

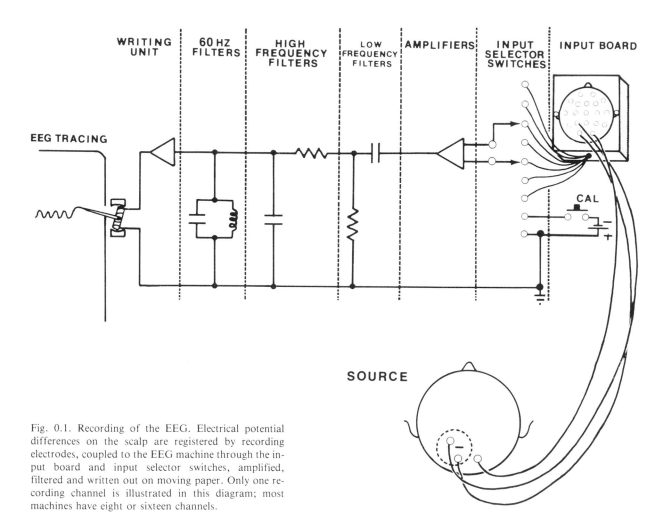

WRITING UNIT 60 HZ FILTERS HIGH FREQUENCY FILTERS LOW FREQUENCY FILTERS AMPLIFIERS INPUT SELECTOR SWITCHES INPUT BOARD

EEG TRACING

CAL

SOURCE

Fig. 0.1. Recording of the EEG. Electrical potential differences on the scalp are registered by recording electrodes, coupled to the EEG machine through the input board and input selector switches, amplified, filtered and written out on moving paper. Only one recording channel is illustrated in this diagram; most machines have eight or sixteen channels.

4

(4) *Recording strategy* uses several different combinations of electrodes, or montages, to display the potential changes from all parts of the head and to localize the origin of abnormal potential changes.

(5) *The product* of the recording, namely the clinical EEG record, must satisfy a number of technical requirements to be acceptable. Requirements for routine clinical recordings differ from those for recordings from infants and small children, for all-night sleep recordings, for recordings in cases of suspected cerebral death and for recordings transmitted by telephone.

(6) *Artifacts* are pen deflections that are not due to cerebral activity and may come from such extracerebral activity as eye movements, heart beat and muscle contraction or from electrical interference, malfunctioning recording electrodes, or defects of the EEG machine. They must be eliminated or clearly explained to avoid confusion with cerebral activity.

(7) *Other methods of recording and analyzing the EEG*, including digital signal analysis and topographic mapping, are used to answer questions which cannot be answered by the conventional method of examining the pages of a routine recording.

The source of the EEG

1

SUMMARY

(1.1)   *The EEG* is generated almost exclusively by inhibitory and excitatory postsynaptic potentials of cortical nerve cells. These potentials summate in the cortex and extend through the coverings of the brain to the scalp. By comparison, neuronal action potentials, which have much smaller potential fields and are much shorter in duration (1 msec or less compared to postsynaptic potentials with durations of 15 to more than 200 msec), do not contribute significantly to either routine scalp recordings or to EEG recordings from the cortical surface.

(1.2)   *Rhythmical activity* in the routine scalp recorded EEG represents postsynaptic cortical neuronal potentials which are synchronized by the complex interaction of large populations of cortical cells. Rhythmical EEG activity is thought to arise mainly from the interaction between cortical neurons and organizing impulses from subcortical pacemakers. Surgically isolated cortex, therefore, shows a substantial reduction in rhythmical activity. Desynchronization of rhythmical activity may result from either intrinsic cortical changes or an inhibition of subcortical pacemaker activity.

(1.3)   *Scalp electrodes* record mainly the summated postsynaptic potential changes of neurons in the underlying cortex, favoring slow potential changes generated in large areas near the recording electrode. Scalp electrodes rarely record potentials produced in distant parts of the brain. However, subcortical structures may send synchronizing impulses to cortical neurons and induce widespread synchronous cortical potential changes. Scalp electrode recordings may also show extracerebral potential changes produced either by biological activity such as eye movements, heart beat and scalp muscle activity, or by interference or defects of the recording equipment.

1.1   THE GENERATOR OF THE EEG

The EEG is generated by changes in the electrical charge of the membrane of cortical nerve cells (Fig. 1.1). These neurons, like other nerve cells, have a *resting potential* which is a difference in electrical potential between the interior of the cell and the extracellular space. The resting potential fluctuates as a result of impulses arriving from other neurons at contact points, or synapses, located on the cell body

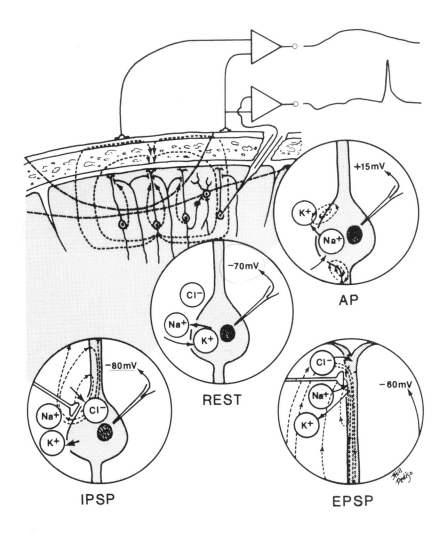

Fig. 1.1. The generation of the EEG by the cerebral cortex. Scalp electrodes record potential differences which are caused by postsynaptic potentials in the membrane of cortical neurons. The closed loops of the lighter dashed lines represent the summation of extracellular currents produced by the postsynaptic potentials; the open segments of heavier dashed lines connect all points having the same voltage level. The two scalp electrodes are at different voltage levels and record this difference, as it changes with time, in the form of a wave which is indicated by the first of the two tracings at the upper right. A simultaneous recording made with a microelectrode from a single cortical neuron is indicated by the second tracing and bears no close relation to the scalp EEG. The round insets show the major ionic and electrical events at single neurons. *REST*: The uneven distribution of ions across the cell membrane, partly maintained by the semipermeable membrane, partly by the active extrusion of sodium ions and intrusion of potassium ions, causes a steady potential difference of 70 mV recordable with an intracellular microelectrode. *IPSP*: An inhibitory postsynaptic potential is caused by activation of an inhibitory synapse on the cell body which transiently increases the permeability of the postsynaptic membrane to potassium and chloride ions and thereby increases the membrane potential, generating electrical current flow of decreasing intensity along the cell membrane. *EPSP*: An excitatory postsynaptic potential, caused by activation of an excitatory synapse on a dendritic process of the neuron, causes a nonselective increase of permeability to ions including sodium ions and thereby transiently decreases the membrane potential locally, generating current flow which tends to depolarize the membrane of the cell body. *AP*: An action potential is initiated at the axon hillock of the cell body by the summation of excitatory postsynaptic potentials which reduce the membrane potential to a level at which the membrane suddenly becomes freely permeable to all ions so that the membrane potential momentarily collapses and reverses; local current flow depolarizes neighboring membrane parts and results in the propagation of an action potential along the membrane of the cell body and axon.

and its processes. Such impulses generate relatively sustained local *postsynaptic potentials* which cause electrical current flow along the membrane of the cell body and dendrites. These changes may reduce the membrane potential to a critical level at which the membrane loses its charge completely, generating an *action potential* of brief duration which is propagated along the axon. The fluctuations in the surface EEG are produced mainly by the temporal and spatial summation of electrical currents caused by the relatively slow postsynaptic potentials with little or no contribution by the brief action potentials.

see Fig 1-1

1.1.1 *The resting potential* of a neuron measures 50–100 mV and is negative on the inside of the cell membrane with respect to the outside. It is the result of (a) passive and (b) active properties of the cell membrane. (a) *The passive properties* are those which do not require metabolic energy. They result from unequal permeability of the membrane to sodium, potassium, chloride and other ions (Fig. 1). Diffusion and electrical charge tend to drive ions in or out of the cell so that they distribute unevenly on both sides of the membrane, sodium and chloride being more concentrated on the outside and potassium being more concentrated on the inside; this uneven distribution causes a steady difference of electrical potential at rest. (b) *Active properties* require metabolic energy to counteract some leakage of ions across the membrane; leaking ions are continuously transported against diffusional and electrical gradients back to concentrations appropriate for resting conditions. Most important is the active transport of sodium out of the cell, coupled with the transport of potassium into the cell. Conditions which disrupt cerebral metabolism, such as anoxia or ischemia, may reduce or abolish this pumping action of the membrane, causing reduction of the membrane potential which can result in increased excitability or complete collapse of neuronal function.

1.1.2 *Postsynaptic potentials* in a neuron are caused by impulses arriving from other neurons via axons which terminate in a specialized contact zone, or synapse, located on the cell body or its processes. The impulse in the afferent neuron causes release of a neurotransmitter substance from its nerve terminal which diffuses across the synaptic cleft to the postsynaptic neuronal membrane patch where it interacts with a specialized receptor. The interaction produces a transient change in permeability to some ion species in the membrane portion near the synapse; this causes a local change in the resting potential or a postsynaptic potential (PSP). An *excitatory post*-synaptic potential (EPSP, Fig. 1.1) is a transient partial reduction in membrane potential which is usually due to an increased local permeability to sodium and other ions, whereas an *inhibitory postsynaptic potential* (IPSP, Fig. 1.1) is a transient increase in membrane potential which is usually the result of a local increase of permeability to potassium or chloride ions. The potential difference between the postsynaptic membrane portion and the other parts of the neuronal membrane causes an electrical current to flow along the neuronal membrane and to change the membrane potential of the cell body. Postsynaptic potentials alter the neuronal membrane potential by several millivolts and last for up to over 100 msec. The potentials generated at synapses on different parts of the cell are thus summated in the membrane potential of the cell body. EPSPs decrease the membrane potential or depolarize the cell and make it more likely to fire an action potential; IPSPs increase the membrane potential or hyperpolarize the cell and make it less likely to fire.

1.1.3 *Action potentials* occur when the neuronal membrane is depolarized beyond a critical level or threshold (Fig. 1.1). This threshold is lowest at the junction of the cell body and the axon, or the axon hillock. A depolarization of the resting potential by about 30 mV at this point triggers a self-limited sequence of events consisting of a brief increase of the membrane permeability to sodium and potassium ions which leads to a sudden collapse, brief reversal and quick restitution of the membrane potential. This electrical change is the action potential; it has an amplitude up to over 100 mV and lasts only about 1 msec. By depolarizing and inducing the same sequence of events in neighboring membrane parts, the action potential spreads as a wave of excitation over the cell membrane; it travels from the axon hillock down to the terminal where the depolarization releases neurotransmitter and causes an EPSP or IPSP in other neurons. The action potential itself causes only a very brief local current which does not penetrate far into the extracellular space.

∴ does not contribute to the EEG signal

1.1.4 *Summation of electrical potential changes in the cortex* occurs mainly at the vertically oriented large pyramidal cells of the cortex. These neurons are especially suited for this role for several reasons. (a) The dendrites of the pyramidal cells extend through nearly all layers of the cortex, guiding the flow of currents generated by postsynaptic potentials at either the cell body in the deep layers of the cortex or at dendrites in the more superficial layers through the entire thickness of the cortex. (b) These neurons are closely packed and oriented parallel to each other, facilitating spatial summation of the currents generated by each neuron. (c) Groups of these neurons receive similar input and respond to it with potential changes of similar direction and timing; the currents generated by these neurons summate in the extracellular space as indicated in Fig. 1.1. Most of the current is limited to the cortex. However, a small fraction penetrates through the meningeal coverings, spinal fluid and skull to the scalp where it causes different parts of the scalp to be at different potential levels. These potential differences, having amplitudes of usually only 10–100 μV, can be recorded between two electrodes and constitute the EEG.

Although the EEG is a result of neuronal potential changes, it is far too complex to be deciphered in terms of the underlying neuronal events. For instance, a potential change recorded at the scalp may be caused by a potential change of the same polarity produced at dendrites near the surface of the cortex, but it may also be caused by a potential change of the opposite polarity occurring at the cell bodies

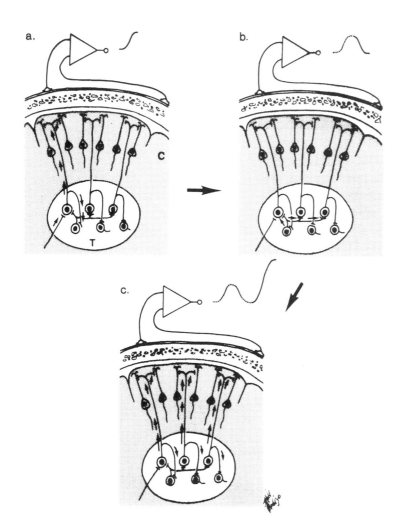

Fig. 1.2. Steps in the production of rhythmical EEG activity in the cortex (C) as proposed by *the facultative pacemaker theory*. (a) A thalamocortical relay neuron (TCR) in the thalamus (T) is excited by an afferent neuron and sends an impulse simultaneously to cortical neurons and to an inhibitory thalamic interneuron. Postsynaptic potentials of cortical neurons generate the first deflection in the cortical EEG. (b) The output of the inhibitory thalamic interneuron suppresses the activity of several TCR neurons. The resultant disappearance of postsynaptic cortical activity represents the end of the first deflection of the cortical EEG. (c) Several TCR interneurons, simultaneously released from inhibition by interneurons, send synchronous impulses to cortical neurons, causing another larger deflection of the cortical EEG. Simultaneous impulses to larger numbers of inhibitory thalamic interneurons initiate the next cycle of rhythmical activity.

in the depth of the cortex. Excitation in one place can therefore not be distinguished from inhibition in another place, and the activity of single neurons or specific groups of neurons can only be speculated about. Thus, although the cellular mechanisms which generate the EEG are now rather clearly known, this knowledge cannot be applied directly to the clinical interpretation of EEGs.

1.2   RHYTHMICAL EEG ACTIVITY

Although one might expect that the complex neuronal activities of the brain would result in irregular EEG waves, the human EEG, awake and at rest, commonly contains rhythmical activity (e.g., the alpha and mu rhythms, 11.1–11.3). Our understanding of the mechanisms responsible for the production of rhythmical EEG activity is based largely on animal experimentation. These experiments have shown that: (1) the repetitive stimulation of nonspecific nuclei of the medial and intralaminar thalamus produces rhythmical cortical activity in a widespread distribution that resembles barbiturate induced rhythmical spindle shaped activity (the so-called *recruiting response*); (2) repetitive stimulation of specific nuclei of the lateral thalamus produces rhythmical cortical activity over more localized areas (the so-called *augmenting response*) corresponding in distribution to the thalamocortical pathways for primary sensory information; (3) following surgical isolation of the cortex from the thalamus rhythmical activity persists in the thalamus whereas little evidence of such activity is recorded at the cortex; and (4) transection of the brainstem below the level of the thalamus has little influence on sleep spindles or barbiturate induced spindle-like activity, but destruction of the thalamus obliterates such activity. These findings have led to the prevailing view that EEG rhythmicity depends largely on thalamic pacemaker cells. — *e.g, sleep spindles*

Subsequent observations led Andersen and Andersson (1968) to propose that the

13

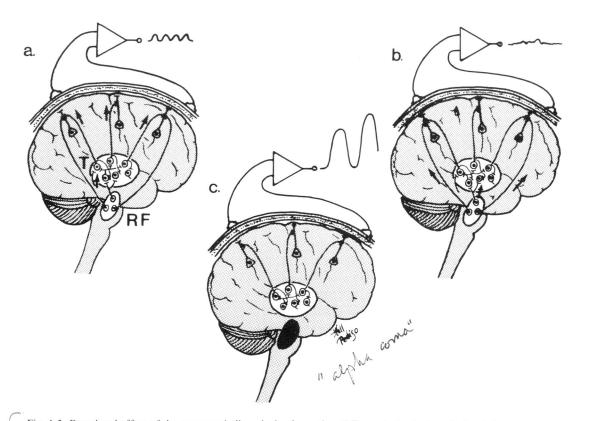

a.

b.

c.

" alpha coma"

Fig. 1.3. Postulated effect of the mesencephalic reticular formation (RF) on rhythmical cortical activity induced by a thalamic pacemaker (T). – a. Rhythmical activity is generated by the pacemaker system in the absence of strong activating impulses from the reticular formation. – b. Activating impulses from the reticular formation to the cortex and the thalamus abolish rhythmical cortical activity. – c. Lesions destroying or inactivating the reticular formation or its rostral connections result in the appearance of rhythmical slow waves, presumably caused by release of synchronizing centers from a tonic desynchronizing input by the reticular formation.

alpha in resting

attention or concentration inhibits alpha

14

thalamic generation of rhythmical EEG activity depends on two main types of thalamic cells: thalamocortical relay (TCR) neurons and thalamic inhibitory interneurons. According to this theory (sometimes refered to as *the facultative pacemaker theory*), TCR cells send fibers to the cortex as well as giving off branches which turn back and end on thalamic inhibitory interneurons (Fig. 1.2a). The firing of one or a few TCR neurons, in addition to affecting a few cortical neurons, excites thalamic inhibitory interneurons via recurrent collateral fibers (Fig. 1.2a). The output of the interneurons inhibits a large number of TCR cells (Fig. 1.2b). At the end of the period of inhibition, the pool of TCR neurons overshoots into excitation, giving off a synchronized volley which is again distributed both to cortical neurons and to inhibitory thalamic interneurons (Fig. 1.2c). The interneurons inhibit an even larger number of TCR neurons, thus generating another cycle of rhythmical discharges. In this way interneurons which have an inhibitory action lasting a tenth of a second could cause periodic and synchronous inhibition and rebound excitation of TCR neurons ten times a second. The projection of those impulses to the cortex at the same rate would thus induce postsynaptic potentials and a 10-Hz rhythmical EEG activity.

More recent work indicates that more complex interactions between the thalamus and the cortex are responsible for EEG rhythmicity. This work has shown that cortical to cortical connections are more abundant than thalamic to cortical connections, and that the rhythmical activity of one cortical area may correlate more closely with the rhythmical activity of another cortical area than with similar activity in the thalamus. The facultative pacemaker concept has also been weakened by the observations that recurrent collateral fibers of many TCR cells are very limited in number and some thalamic nuclei appear to contain few, if any, inhibitory interneurons. Finally, recent computer modelling experiments based on cortical neuronal recordings suggest that although single cortical cell recordings may not show rhythmical activity, EEG rhythmicity may occur as the result of a complex interaction among large numbers of such cortical cells (Traub et al., 1989).

In summary, EEG rhythmicity appears to be dependent on interactions between the cortex and thalamus, both of which have certain structural and functional features that lend themselves to the production of rhythmical activity. Thus, certain rhythmical activities, such as sleep spindles, may be abolished by lesions involving either thalamic structures or cortical structures directly, or by involving only subcortical areas that contain thalamocortical pathways.

The interruption of rhythmical activity, also referred to as desynchronization of the EEG, has been shown to occur with activation of the ascending reticular activating system. This brainstem system receives input from practically all sensory systems and cortical areas and sends its output to the entire cortex through direct connections and through relays in the diencephalon (Fig. 1.3a). It can thereby interrupt the production of rhythmical cortical activity both by directly modifying cortical neuronal function and by influencing the thalamic neurons that participate in the generation of rhythmical activity (Fig. 1.3b). Either an increase or a decrease of the tonic activity of the ascending reticular activating system causes rhythmical cortical activity to disappear: Cortical rhythms in humans may be abolished by either arousal and heightened attention, drowsiness, or sleep. Abnormal rhythmical activity, such as the spindle coma pattern (25.3.5), may also appear as the result of brainstem damage which reduces the desynchronizing action of the reticular formation (Fig. 1.3c).

1.3 RECORDING OF ELECTRICAL POTENTIALS WITH SCALP ELECTRODES

Electrodes on the scalp record mainly the summated electrical changes of the underlying cortex; they may also record some potential changes generated in distant parts of the brain and potential changes produced outside the brain. The amplitude of the recorded potentials depends on the intensity of the electrical source, on its distance and spatial orientation, and on the electrical resistance and capacitance of the structures between the source and the recording electrodes. These factors favor the recording of potential changes which (a) occur near the recording electrodes, (b) are generated in a large area of tissue and (c) rise and fall at slow speed.

1.3.1 *Potentials generated in the underlying cortex* are the major source of the scalp EEG. However, the EEG recorded with scalp electrodes differs from that recorded simultaneously with electrodes placed directly on the underlying cortex ('electrocorticogram', 'ECoG'). The scalp EEG is of lower amplitude and may be distorted in shape. Generally, faster frequencies are attenuated more than slower ones. Very fast and brief potential changes may be lost completely in scalp recordings or may be picked up only over their production site whereas slower potentials may be conducted farther and thus be recorded over greater distances. These distortions depend in part on the electrical properties of structures between cortex and scalp electrodes. The amplitude of the scalp EEG may decrease as a result of either (a) an increase of electrical impedance between the source and the recording electrodes, for instance an increase in the thickness of the skull, which reduces the flow of currents between the source and the recording electrodes, or (b) a decrease in the impedance across the path of these currents, for instance a collection of subdural blood or of cerebrospinal fluid which shunts the currents before they reach the recording electrodes.

Even though the scalp EEG directly reflects mainly local potential changes, it may indirectly reveal abnormalities at distant sites which can give rise to cortical potentials of very similar shape and timing over wide parts of the brain. This mechanism has been called 'projection' or 'bilateral synchrony' and the resulting rhythms have been called 'projected rhythms' or 'rhythmes à distance'. Because the pacemaker for bilaterally synchronous discharges is presumed to be located at the center of the brain, the term 'centrencephalic' has also been used. Although these rhythms may be induced by the action of distant centers, they are generated by the cortex under the recording electrodes, not by distant sites.

1.3.2 *Potentials generated at distant sites* are only rarely recorded by scalp electrodes. This is illustrated by the observation that scalp electrodes over an area of cortex with completely abolished function will generally show complete absence of electrical activity. However, some types of activity of high amplitude, such as slow waves deep in the frontal pole or spikes in the mesial and basal parts of the brain are occasionally conducted electrically through the volume of the interposed tissue and appear in scalp electrodes at considerable distance, superimposed on the EEG representing local cortical activity. Electrical conduction probably also accounts for the appearance of EEG potentials at scalp electrodes over partially or completely removed hemispheres and for the recording of a depth EEG ('DEEG') by electrodes which have been inserted surgically into the brain but may be located at some distance from nerve cells generating EEG potentials.

1.3.3 *Potentials generated by sources other than the brain* are often picked up by scalp electrodes and recorded together with the EEG; such extracerebral potentials are usually called 'artifacts' (6). For instance, muscle fiber activity may be recorded by a scalp electrode located over muscle. Movements of the eyes, tongue and other large and electrically charged structures can generate changing electrical fields, which are recorded by scalp electrodes. Heart muscle contraction can induce potential changes at scalp electrodes similar to the potential changes recorded in the electrocardiogram. Strong sources of alternating current near the recording site may interfere with the recording.

REFERENCES

Abraham, K. and Ajmone Marsan, C. (1958) Patterns of cortical discharges and their relation to routine scalp electroencephalography. Electroenceph. clin. Neurophysiol. 10: 447–461.
Andersen, P. and Andersson, S.A. (1968) Physiological Basis of the Alpha Rhythm. Appleton, New York.

See summary

Andersen, P. and Andersson, S.A. (1974) Section IV. Thalamic origin of cortical rhythmical activity. In: Rémond, A. (Ed.), Handbook of Electroenceph. clin. Neurophysiol., Vol. 2C, Elsevier, Amsterdam, pp. 90–118.

Ball, G.J., Gloor, P. and Thompson, C.J. (1977) Computed unit-EEG correlations and laminar profiles of spindle waves in the electroencephalogram of cats. Electroenceph. clin. Neurophysiol. 43: 330–345.

Buser, P. (1987) Thalamocortical mechanisms underlying synchronized EEG activity. In: Halliday, A.M., Butler, S.R. and Paul, R. (Eds.), A Textbook of Clinical Neurophysiology, Wiley, New York, pp. 595–622.

Cooper, R., Winter, A.L., Crow, H.J. and Walter, W.G. (1965) Comparison of subcortical, cortical and scalp activity using chronically indwelling electrodes in man. Electroenceph. clin. Neurophysiol. 18: 217–228.

Creutzfeldt, O. and Houchin, J. (1974) Section I. Neuronal basis of EEG-waves. In: Rémond, A. (Ed.), Handbook of Electroenceph. clin. Neurophysiol., Vol. 2C, Elsevier, Amsterdam, pp. 5–55.

Gabor, A.J. (1978) Physiological basis of electrical activity of cerebral origin. Quincy, MA: Grass Instrument Co. (available on request).

Gloor, P. (1985) Neuronal generators and the problem of localization in electroencephalography: Application of volume conductor theory to electroencephalography. J. Clin. Neurophysiol. 2: 327–354.

Goldensohn, E.S. (1979) Neurophysiological substrates of EEG activity. In: D. Klass and D. Daly (Eds.), Current Practice of Clinical Neurophysiology, Raven, New York, pp. 421–440.

Kellaway, P., Gol, A. and Proler, M. (1966) Electrical activity of the isolated cerebral hemisphere and isolated thalamus. Exp. Neurol. 14: 281–304.

Leissner, P., Lindholm, L.-E. and Petersén, I. (1970) Alpha amplitude dependence on skull thickness as measured by ultrasound technique. Electroenceph. clin. Neurophysiol. 29: 392–399.

Lopes da Silva, F. (1987) Dynamics of EEGs as signals of neuronal populations: models and theoretical considerations. In: Niedermeyer, E. and Lopes da Silva, F. (Eds.), Electroencephalography: Basic Principles, Clinical Applications and Related Fields, Urban and Schwarzenberg, Baltimore, pp. 15–28.

Pfurtscheller, G. and Cooper, R. (1975) Frequency dependence of the transmission of the EEG from cortex to scalp. Electroenceph. clin. Neurophysiol. 38: 93–96.

Schlag, J. (1974) Section V. Reticular influences on thalamo-cortical activity. In: Rémond, A. (Ed.), Handbook of Electroenceph. clin. Neurophysiol., Vol. 2C, Elsevier, Amsterdam, pp. 119–134.

Speckman, E.-J. and Elger, C.E. (1987) Introduction to the Neurophysiological Basis of the EEG and DC potentials. In: Niedermeyer, E. and Lopes da Silva, F. (Eds.), Electroencephalography: Basic Principles, Clinical Application and Related Fields, Urban and Schwarzenberg, Baltimore, pp. 1–14.

Traub, R.D., Miles, R. and Wong, R.K.S. (1989) Model of the origin of rhythmic population oscillations in the hippocampal slice. Science 243: 1319–1325.

Recording electrodes

2

SUMMARY

Recording electrodes transfer electrical potentials at the recording site to the input of the recording machine.

(2.1) *Electrode types* most commonly used in clinical EEG are metal discs or cups attached to the scalp and other recording sites. Needle electrodes which are inserted into the scalp are no longer recommended for routine clinical use. Nasopharyngeal and sphenoidal electrodes require special insertion procedures and are used in some laboratories in addition to scalp electrodes to record the EEG from the undersurface of the temporal lobe.

(2.2) *Electrical properties* should enable recording electrodes to couple potential changes from the head to the input of the EEG machine without distortion. Electrodes should have a surface made of gold, chlorided silver or other materials which do not interact chemically with the scalp. Electrodes must be applied so as to make electrical contact having impedances between 100 and 5000 Ω. Electrodes with much higher impedances can attenuate the recording and cause 60 Hz artifact; impedances of less than 100 Ω are usually the result of accidental short-circuits between electrodes. Polarization and bias potentials develop at the interface between electrode and tissue and can be minimized by careful technique.

(2.3) *Placement of electrodes* should cover the entire head evenly and be reproducible between subjects and laboratories. This is accomplished with the International 10–20 System. This system uses measurements between bony landmarks on the skull to determine the coordinates for 21 recording electrodes with provisions for additional electrodes as needed. Fewer electrodes may be used in infants.

2.1 ELECTRODE SHAPES AND APPLICATION METHODS

In general, electrodes consist of a conductor connected by a lead wire and plug to the input of the recording machine. Scalp electrodes are applied after determining the precise location and after preparing the scalp to reduce electrical impedance. Metal surface electrodes should be cleansed with a solution of an antiseptic soap

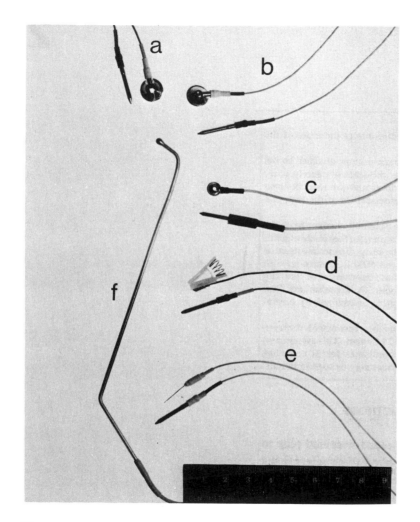

Fig. 2.1. Various types of EEG electrodes, shown with their connector plugs and part of their lead wires. a. Large metal cup electrode with a central hole; b. Large metal cup electrode without hole; c. Small metal cup electrode with central hole; d. Clip electrode; e. Needle electrode; f. Nasopharyngeal electrode.

after each use. Nasopharyngeal electrodes should be autoclaved; penetrating electrodes used on patients with contagious diseases should be discarded after use. Special cleaning procedures must also be used for surface electrodes used on patients at special risk for contagious diseases such as AIDs, viral hepatitis or Creutzfeldt-Jacob disease.

2.1.1 *Metal disc and cup electrodes* usually have diameters of 4–10 mm (Fig. 2.1). Smaller or larger electrodes do not make stable mechanical and electrical contact with the scalp. An insulated lead wire is attached to each electrode. The insulation of each wire has a different color for easy identification of each electrode. Mechanical and electrical problems are reduced if the insulations of the lead wires are attached to each other in the form of a stranded cable from which the leads separate only at the two ends. Before electrodes are applied, the application site is determined by measurements (2.3) and prepared by wiping with alcohol or abrasive electrolyte gels (such as Omni Prep).

Several methods may be used to attach electrodes to the scalp. The collodion technique has the advantage of giving very stable recordings with relatively few artifacts. In this technique, cup electrodes with a central hole are placed onto the prepared scalp site and held in place with a stylus while a few drops of collodion are applied around the edge of the electrode and spread onto the scalp. The spreading and drying of the collodion may be facilitated by a stream of compressed air guided through a tube around the stylus. After the electrode is securely attached, the stylus is removed and the cup is filled with conductive jelly which is injected with a blunt hypodermic needle inserted through the central hole of the cup. If cup electrodes without a central hole are used, they are filled with conductive paste before application to the scalp. Some laboratories place small pieces of gauze soaked with collodion over the electrodes to hold them in place. Electrodes are removed by dissolving the collodion with acetone. Because of the chemicals involved, the collodion method should not be used in areas which have limited ventilation or explosion hazards such as infant isolettes or operating rooms.

Another method of applying electrodes uses a paste which can both hold the electrode in place and provide good electrical contact. After preparation of the scalp site, a piece of this adhesive conductive paste is placed on the scalp and the electrode is pressed into the center of the paste until it makes firm contact. Electrodes with a central hole allow the paste to escape through the hole so that the rim of the cup sits firmly on the scalp. A gauze pad or cotton ball may be placed over the electrode to hold it more securely in place and to delay drying of the paste. This method is fast, but electrodes tend to lose good mechanical and electrical contact more readily than when they are applied with collodion.

Other methods of applying disc or cup electrodes involve the use of: (a) paraffin wax, (b) suction electrodes, or (c) headbands, straps or caps which hold an entire set of electrodes in place. These methods generally give less satisfactory results than the methods described earlier.

Metal disc or cup electrodes may be placed around the eyes, on the chest or other parts of the body to monitor electrical potentials which are generated by eye movements, heart beat, respiration, muscle contraction or body movement and which may contaminate the EEG (4.3). While EEG electrodes may be used to monitor the occurrence of extracerebral activity, they introduce some distortion and special electrodes are required if faithful recordings of such activity are desired.

2.1.2 *Clip electrodes* are sometimes used for recordings from the earlobes. The clips should contain cups or discs made from the same materials as the scalp electrodes to avoid electrical problems caused by recording from dissimilar electrodes.

2.1.3 *Needle electrodes* are sharp wires, usually made of steel or platinum. They are inserted into the superficial layers of the scalp after thorough disinfection of the insertion site. The advantage of fast application is outweighed by the disadvantages of pain, possible infection and unfavorable electrical characteristics. Some laboratories still use these electrodes for emergency recordings from comatose patients, but most electroencephalographers feel they should not be used.

2.1.4 *Nasopharyngeal electrodes* are used in addition to scalp electrodes by some laboratories in patients who are suspected of having epileptiform activity in the basal parts of the temporal lobe but who do not show such activity in scalp recordings.

Nasopharyngeal electrodes are made of a conducting wire embedded in rigid plastic which has a z-shape to fit the path of insertion. The tip is an uninsulated metal ball of 2–5 mm diameter. One electrode is inserted through each nostril, slid backwards along the bottom of the nasal cavity near the midline, and then rotated outward. This places the tip against the roof of the nasopharynx and very close to the skull at the base of the middle cerebral fossa, i.e. close to the tip of the temporal lobe. Because the insertion can cause discomfort, gagging and slight injury to the mucous membranes, it is usually done by a physician.

It is important to recognize that nasopharyngeal electrode recordings occasionally produce artifacts that mimick epileptiform spikes and sharp waves. Thus, epileptiform activity occurring exclusively at the nasopharyngeal electrode should be considered artifact until proven otherwise. The main advantage of nasopharyngeal recordings is to emphasize or clarify activity also recorded at other electrode sites. In this regard, however, it is also important to recognize that certain benign patterns, such as small sharp spikes, may be greatly amplified by nasopharyngeal recordings. This amplification frequently leads readers unfamiliar with nasopharyngeal recordings to mistakenly identify pseudoepileptiform patterns as abnormal epileptiform patterns.

2.1.5 *Sphenoidal electrodes* are used to detect epileptiform activity in the temporal lobes. This electrode consists of a flexible wire with an uninsulated tip which is placed near the sphenoidal wing through a cannula inserted through the temporal and masseter muscles. Electrode placement can be checked by X-ray. The electrodes can be left in place for several days of serial EEG recordings without danger of breaking or injury to the patient. For a more detailed explanation of electrode placement refer to the references at the end of the chapter.

Sphenoidal electrodes are mainly of value for distinguishing between mesial and lateral temporal epileptogenic lesions. They *do not* significantly increase the likelihood of detecting antero-mesial temporal discharges, particularly if surface electrodes are placed near the sphenoidal electrode insertion points, or if so-called true anterior temporal surface electrodes are used (2.3.2).

2.1.6 *Electrocorticographic electrodes* are used during some neurosurgical procedures, usually excision of epileptogenic foci, to record the ECoG from the exposed cortical surface. These electrodes consist of metal balls or saline-soaked cotton wicks which may be mounted on springs and held in place by swivel joints for easy placement.

2.1.7 *Subdural and epidural electrodes* are used to localize epileptiform activity and to map cortical function. They consist of sheets or single column strips of evenly spaced disc electrodes (usually made of platinum or stainless steel) embedded in a thin layer of flexible translucent Silastic. The sheets are inserted through a craniotomy opening, whereas the strips consisting of single rows of electrodes can alternatively be introduced into the epidural or subdural space through a burr hole. Once the electrodes are in place, the underlying cortical activity can be recorded by connecting the electrode leads to the input board of any routine EEG machine. In addition, the subdural electrodes can be used to stimulate the underlying cortex by applying an electrical current to individual electrodes. The results of stimulation, which typically include involuntary movements, sensory manifestations, or dysphasia, are used to map the locations of critical cortical functions so they may be spared during cortical resection.

2.1.8 *Depth electrodes* are used in a few centers, usually to define the targets for surgical destruction. These electrodes consist usually of a bundle of fine wires which terminate with uninsulated tips at different levels and thus allow for recordings from different depths. The insertion of depth electrodes is guided by determining the position of the target in a three-dimensional reference system and by translating the coordinates of this system to the head of the patient using standard landmarks and X-ray control.

2.2 ELECTRICAL PROPERTIES OF RECORDING ELECTRODES

Good recording electrodes should couple the electrical potential changes at the recording site to the input of the recording machine without distortion. To obtain such high fidelity recordings, one must (1) choose recording electrodes of suitable material; (2) measure electrode resistance to ascertain electrical continuity between the two ends of the electrode if in doubt; (3) measure electrode impedance after every electrode application and during the recording to evaluate the electrical contact between electrode and scalp; (4) avoid electrode polarization and bias potentials.

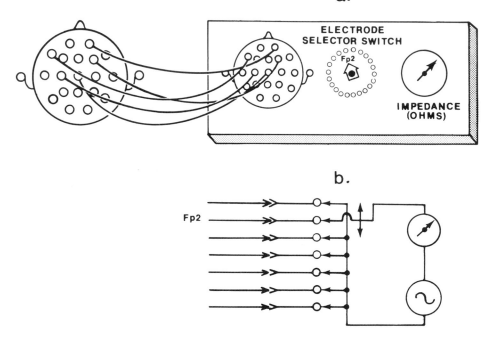

a.

ELECTRODE
SELECTOR SWITCH

Fp2

IMPEDANCE
(OHMS)

b.

Fp2

Fig. 2.2. Measurement of electrode impedance. – a. Diagram of the input board with receptacles for the connectors from scalp electrodes (left), selector switch designating electrode Fp2 for impedance measurement (middle), and impedance meter (right). – b. Electrical circuit used for impedance measurement: A weak alternating current is passed through the impedance meter to the electrode selected for measurement (Fp2) and its contact with the scalp (not shown); the current is returned through a combination of all other scalp electrodes. The impedance of the selected electrode is read from the impedance meter; the impedance of the return path is negligible relative to that of the electrode being tested.

2.2.1 *Electrode materials* should be those which do not interact chemically with the electrolytes of the scalp. Electrodes coated with gold, silver chloride, tin or platinum are satisfactory.

2.2.2 *Electrode resistance*, or opposition to direct current flow, is measured occasionally, namely when a break in the electrical continuity between electrode, lead wire and connector plug is suspected. This measurement is made while the electrode is not attached to the scalp. The two uninsulated ends of the electrode are connected to an ohmmeter which passes a weak direct current through the electrode. The resistance of an intact electrode should measure no more than a few ohms.

2.2.3 *Electrode impedance*, or opposition to alternating current flow, is measured after an electrode has been applied to the recording site to evaluate the contact between electrode and scalp. The impedance of each electrode should be measured routinely before every EEG recording and should be between 100 and 5000 Ω. Electrode impedance is measured with an impedance meter which passes a weak alternating current from the electrode selected for testing through the scalp to all other electrodes connected to the meter (Fig. 2.2). The measured impedance reflects mainly that of the selected electrode, the other electrodes offering multiple return pathways with negligible total impedance.

An alternating current is used for this measurement for two reasons. (a) Alternating current is more representative of the alternating potential changes recorded in the EEG, especially if it alternates at about 10 Hz, a common frequency of EEG potential changes; the opposition to current alternating at this frequency may differ from that to alternating current of other frequencies and, especially from that to direct current. (b) Passage of direct current through an electrode attached to the scalp can electrically polarize the interface between electrode and skin and thereby lead to distortion of subsequent EEG recordings.

Impedance:

100 – 5,000 Ω

Most modern EEG machines have provisions for testing electrode impedance during the recording. This is done by injecting a weak alternating current of constant intensity through a pair of electrodes connected to the input of a recording channel. This causes a pen deflection in that channel with an amplitude proportional to the sum of the impedances of the two electrodes. If the deflection indicated unacceptably high or low impedance, the faulty electrode of the pair must be identified by pairing each electrode with another electrode of acceptable impedance and repeating the current injection.

Both very high and very low impedance are undesirable. Very low impedance acts like a shunt between the recording electrodes and effectively short-circuits the EEG potential differences. It is practically impossible to reduce electrode impedance to less than a few thousand ohms without there being an abnormal pathway of conduction between the electrodes. An electrode showing very low impedance may be making contact with another electrode by an excess of electrolyte jelly or paste, or by saline or sweat forming a conductive bridge between the electrodes on the scalp. Such an electrode should be inspected, cleaned, and reapplied or exchanged if necessary.

Very high impedance is undesirable mainly because connecting an electrode of very high impedance and one of lower impedance to the input of a differential amplifier causes an imbalance which favors the recording of 60 Hz interference* (3.4). Electrodes showing high impedance readings should be checked for good mechanical and electrical contact and the junctions of the lead wire with the metal disc or cup and with the plug terminal should be inspected for possible breaks.

2.2.4 *Electrode polarization and bias potentials* may occur and distort EEG recordings even when mechanical and electrical recording conditions seem good.

---

* Interference has a frequency of 50 Hz in countries using alternating current of that frequency.

Fortunately, the effect of these phenomena on the routine clinical EEG is negligible with modern electrodes, methods of electrode application and recording machines. (1) *Polarization* results from current flow across the interface between electrode and tissue. The current carries positive ions to the more negative part of the junction and negative ions to the more positive part. This ion movement polarizes the electrode so that it favors current flow in one direction and resists flow in the opposite direction and thereby distorts the recording of alternating EEG potentials. Polarization is kept to a minimum by (a) a fairly large contact area between electrode and scalp which keeps current density at any one point low; (b) high impedance of the amplifier inputs which keeps the intensity of the current flowing through the electrodes during the recording low; (c) avoidance of steady current flow, especially that used to measure electrode resistance. With these precautions, it is not necessary to use nonpolarizable electrodes such as chlorided silver electrodes for routine clinical EEG recordings, although such electrodes are necessary for other purposes, especially for faithful recording of very slowly changing or steady potential differences. (2) *Bias potentials* result from the exchange of metal ions and electrolytes in the absence of current flow. They interfere with EEG recordings only when they are not steady. Steady bias potentials are the cause of the blocking of amplifiers which occurs immediately after switching to a new selection of electrodes at the input. The effect of bias potentials can be minimized by using (a) electrodes of pure metals with clean surfaces which reduce ion exchange and (b) electrodes of the same kind at the inputs of each amplifier; this neutralizes electrical differences caused by bias potentials.

2.3 ELECTRODE PLACEMENT

2.3.1 *The International 10–20 System* of electrode placement provides for uniform coverage of the entire scalp. It uses the distances between bony landmarks

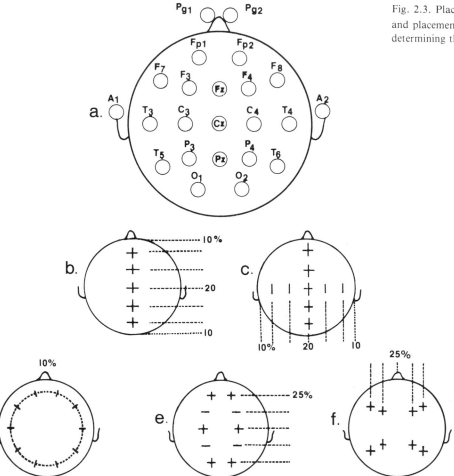

Fig. 2.3. Placement of recording electrodes. – a. Electrode names and placements in the International 10–20 System. – b–f. Steps in determining the electrode placements as described in the text.

of the head to generate a system of lines which run across the head and intersect at intervals of 10 or 20% of their total length. Electrodes are placed at the intersections. The use of the 10–20 System assures symmetrical, reproducible electrode placements and allows comparison of EEGs from the same patient and from different patients, recorded in the same or different laboratories. The system is flexible: additional electrodes, which may be needed to accurately localize an abnormality, can be incorporated by further subdividing the distances between intersections.

The standard set of electrodes for adults (Fig. 2.3) consists of 21 recording electrodes and one ground electrode. The recording electrodes are named with a letter and a subscript. The letter is an abbreviation of the underlying region: prefrontal or frontopolar (Fp), frontal (F), central (C), parietal (P), occipital (O) and auricular (A). The subscript is either the letter z, indicating zero or midline placement, or a number, indicating lateral placement. Odd numbers refer to electrodes on the left, even numbers refer to electrodes on the right side of the head. The numbers increase with increasing distance from the midline except for numbers of temporal and frontopolar electrodes which increase from front to back. The inferior frontal electrodes F7 and F8 are often called 'anterior temporal' electrodes because they fairly faithfully record activity from the anterior temporal area.

see Fis motages

Exact measurements are needed to precisely determine the placement of each recording electrode. Measurements are best made with a metric measuring tape of cloth or plastic. A grease pencil is used to mark electrode locations and the intermediate measurements needed to determine them. The measurements refer to three bony landmarks of the skull: (1) the inion, or the bony protruberance in the middle of the back of the head, (2) the nasion, or the bridge of the nose directly under the forehead, and (3) the preauricular point, or the depression of bone in front of the ear canal. Measurements are made in a sequence of five steps (Fig. 3.3).

Step 1:   The distance between nasion and inion is measured along the midline.

MODIFIED COMBINATORIAL NOMENCLATURE

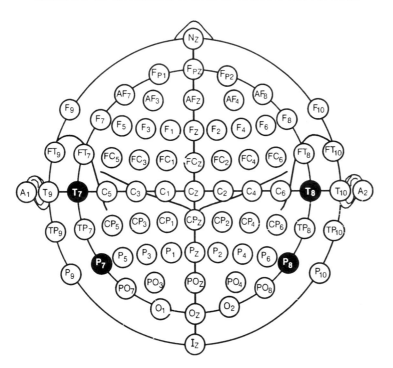

Fig. 2.4. Modified expanded '10–20' system as proposed by the American EEG Society. See also Appendix IV.

Along this line, the frontopolar point, Fp, is marked at 10% above the nasion. Frontal (Fz), central (Cz), parietal (Pz) and occipital (O) points are marked at intervals of 20% of the entire distance leaving 10% for the interval between O and inion. The midline points Fp and O are used only for intermediate measurements but receive no electrode and therefore carry no subscript.

Step 2: The distance between the two preauricular points across Cz is measured. Along this line, the transverse position for the central points C3 and C4 and the temporal points T3 and T4 are marked 20 and 40% respectively from the midline.

Step 3: The circumference of the head is measured from the occipital point (O) through the temporal points T3 and T4 and the frontopolar points Fp. The longitudinal measurement for Fp1 is located on that circumference , 5% of the total length of the circumference to the left of Fp. The longitudinal measurements for F7, T3, T5, O1, O2, T6, T4, F8, Fp2 are at distances of 10% of the circumference.

Step 4: The longitudinal distance from Fp1 and Fp2 through C3 and C4 to O1 and O2 is measured on each side. The midpoints of these distances give the longitudinal coordinates of C3 and C4. The midpoints between Fp1 and C3 on the left, and Fp2 and C4 on the right give the longitudinal coordinates for F3 and F4. The midpoints between C3 and O1 on the left, and C4 and O2 on the right give the longitudinal coordinates for P3 and P4.

Step 5: Measurements from F7 to F8 through Fz define the transverse coordinates for F3 midway between F3 and Fz, and for F4 midway between Fz and F8; measurements from T5 to T6 through Pz define the transverse coordinates for P3 midway between T5 and Pz and for P4 midway between Pz and T6.

Electrodes are placed at Fz, Cz and Pz, at all lateral points designated above, on or near both ears in positions called A_1 and A_2 or on the mandibular angles (4.2.4) in positions called M_1 and M_2, and on the point chosen for the ground electrode, usually in the middle of the head or over one of the mastoids. The use of a smaller number of electrodes in routine EEG is now considered substandard. If needed, additional electrodes may be placed midway between these recording electrodes. In some cases, scalp lesions, skull asymmetries or other abnormalities may make it impossible to place electrodes in the positions of the 10–20 System. In these cases, electrodes should be placed as closely as possible to these positions and as symmetrically as possible on the two sides. The deviations from standard placement should be indicated in a diagram on the EEG record. Other electrode placements may be used for EEG recordings from small infants and for monitoring of extracerebral activity such as eye movements, heart beat, respiratory or other movements (4.3).

2.3.2 *True anterior temporal electrodes.* Because interictal epileptiform activity frequently emanates from the anterior temporal lobe, some laboratories occasionally use additional electrode placements that are closer to the anterior temporal region than F7 and F8. Often these are placed according to the recommendation by Silverman (1960) and are referred to as *true anterior temporal electrodes.* Although these electrodes are often labeled as T1 and T2, according to the International 10–20 System, T1 and T2 would be placed between F7 and T3, and F8 and T4, respectively. The positions for so-called true anterior temporal electrodes are located by first finding an imaginary line between the external auditory canal and the lateral canthus of the eye. The point along that line that is anterior to the external auditory canal by 1/3 the distance of the total line is then located. The electrode is placed 1 cm directly above that point.

2.3.3 *Modified 10–20 system.* The placement of additional electrodes to those routinely employed in the 10–20 system may be indicated to: (1) improve the localization of ictal or interictal epileptiform activity; (2) increase spatial resolution for special studies using computerized EEG signal analysis; or (3) detect highly localized evoked potentials. Recently, the American EEG Society has developed new guidelines for extending the 10–20 system of electrode placement. In order to create a logical nomenclature, four electrodes, T3, T4, T5 and T6 have been renamed T7, T8, P7, and P8, respectively (Fig. 2.4). The American EEG Society guidelines which

36

explain renaming of these electrodes and the placement of the additional electrodes have been reproduced in Appendix IV.

REFERENCES

American EEG Society Guidelines in EEG and Evoked Potentials. Report of the Committee on Infectious Diseases. (1986) J. clin. Neurophysiol. 3 (Suppl. 1): 38–42.

Binnie, C.D. (1987) Recording Techniques: Montages, electrodes, amplifiers and filters. In: A.M. Halliday, S.R. Butler and R. Paul (Eds.), A Textbook of Clinical Neurophysiology, Wiley, Chichester, pp. 3–22.

Binnie, C.D., Rowan, A.J. and Gutter, T.H. (1982) A Manual of Electroencephalographic Technology. University Press, Cambridge.

Binnie, C.D., Marston, D., Polkey, C.E. and Amin, D. (1989) Distribution of temporal spikes in relation to the sphenoidal electrode. Electroenceph. clin. Neurophysiol. 73: 403–409.

Blume, W., Buva, R. and Okazaki, H. (1974) Anatomic correlates of the 10–20 electrode placement system in infants. Electroenceph. clin. Neurophysiol. 36: 303–307.

Broughton, R., Hanley, J., Quanbury, A.O. and Roy, O.Z. (1976) Section I. Electrodes. In: Rémond, A. (Ed.), Handbook of Electroenceph. clin. Neurophysiol., Vol. 3A, Elsevier, Amsterdam, pp. 5–27.

Cooper, R., Osselton, J.W. and Shaw, J.C. (1981) Electrodes. In: EEG Technology. Butterworth, London, pp. 15–29.

Geddes, L.A. (1972) Electrodes and the Measurement of Bioelectric Events. Wiley, New York.

Grings, W.W. (1974) Recording of electrodermal phenomena. In: Thompson, R.F. and Patterson, M.M. (Eds.), Bioelectric Recording Techniques, Vol. 1C, Academic Press, New York and London, pp. 273–296.

Harner, P.F. and Sannit, R. (1974) A Review of the International Ten-Twenty System of Electrode Placement. Grass Instrument Co., Quincy, Mass.

Homan, R.W., Herman, J. and Purdy, P. (1987) Cerebral location of international 10–20 system electrode placement. Electroenceph. clin. Neurophysiol. 66: 376–382.

Ives, J.R. and Gloor, P. (1978) Update: Chronic sphenoidal electrodes. Electroenceph. clin. Neurophysiol. 44: 789–790.

Jasper, H.H. (1958) The ten-twenty electrode system of the International Federation. Electroenceph. clin. Neurophysiol. 10: 371–375.

Lehtinen, L.O.J. and Berstrom, L. (1970) Naso-ethmoidal electrode for recording the electrical activity of the inferior surface of the frontal lobe. Electroenceph. clin. Neurophysiol. 29: 303–305.

Lesser, R.P., Luders, H., Klem, G., Dinner, D.S., Morris, H.H., Hahn, J.F. and Wyllie, E. (1987) Extraoperative cortical functional localization in patients with epilepsy. J. clin. Neurophysiol. 4: 27–54.

Luders, H., Lesser, R.P., Dinner, D.S., Morris, H.H., Wyllie, E. and Godoy, J. (1988) Localization of cortical function: New information from extraoperative monitoring of patients with epilepsy. Epilepsia 29 (Suppl. 2): S56–65.

Mavor, H. and Hellen, M.K. (1964) Nasopharyngeal electrode recording. Am. J. EEG Technol. 4: 43–50.

Picton, T.W. and Hillyard, S.A. (1972) Cephalic skin potentials in electroencephalography. Electroenceph. clin. Neurophysiol. 33: 419–424.

Sannit, T. (1963) The ten-twenty system: Footnotes to measuring technique. Am. J. EEG Technol. 3: 23–30.

Silverman, D. (1960) The anterior temporal electrode and the ten-twenty system. Electroenceph. clin. Neurophysiol. 12: 735–737.

Sperling, M.R. and Engel Jr., J. (1986) Sphenoidal electrodes. J. clin. Neurophysiol. 3: 67–74.

Venables, P.H. and Martin, I. (1967) Skin resistance and skin potential. In: Venables, P.H. and Martin, I. (Eds.). A Manual of Psychophysiological Methods. North-Holland, Amsterdam, pp. 53–102.

Wieser, H.G., Elger, C.E. and Stodieck, S.R.G. (1985) The foramen ovale electrode: a new recording method for the preoperative evaluation of patients suffering from mesio-basal temporal epilepsy. Electroenceph. clin. Neurophysiol. 61: 314–322.

Zablow, L. and Goldensohn, E.S. (1969) A comparison between scalp and needle electrodes for the EEG. Electroenceph. clin. Neurophysiol. 26: 530–533.

Summary

(3.1)   *The input board* is a box which serves to connect the electrodes on the patient's head to the input selector switches of the EEG machine. The terminals of the electrodes are plugged into the receptacles on the input board which are labelled with standard symbols and often arranged in a diagram representing the head. The input board should either contain an impedance meter or provide connections to such a meter. The input board may also contain circuitry which limits the current flow between electrodes.

(3.2)   *Input selector switches* on the EEG machine are used to select two electrodes as the input to each amplifier. The selected electrodes, amplifier and writing unit form a system for detection, amplification and display of potential differences between an electrode pair; this system is called 'channel'. In addition to the individual selector switches for each channel, a hardwired or programable master selector switch is often provided to choose, with the setting of only one switch, a standard combination of electrodes for all channels.

(3.3)   *Calibration pulses* of known voltage are used to measure the amplitude of EEG potentials and to test the functioning of all amplifiers. To verify that the scalp to amplifier interface is working adequately in all channels a *biocalibration* can be performed by connecting the same electrode pair to the inputs of all amplifiers for a brief trial recording.

(3.4)   *Amplifiers* are the major components of each channel of the EEG machine. Each amplifier has two input terminals, connected to the input selector switches. EEG amplifiers increase only the difference of voltage between the input terminals; identical voltages appearing at the two inputs are not amplified but rejected. This differential amplification serves to distinguish cerebral potentials, which are likely to have different amplitude, shape and timing at recording electrodes in different areas of the head, from electrical artifacts, which are likely to be similar at different recording electrodes. EEG amplifiers are constructed so that if input one becomes more negative than input two, the pen deflects upward. If input one becomes more positive than input two then the pen deflects downward. Amplification is usually expressed as sensitivity which relates the voltage of a signal to the height of the pen deflection (microvolts per millimeters of pen deflection). Less often, amplification is described as gain, i.e. the ratio of output voltage to input voltage.

(3.5)   *Filters* selectively reduce the amplitude of voltage changes, or signals, of selected frequencies. A low and a high frequency filter are used to exclude from the EEG very slow and very fast waves and thereby to select the spectrum of frequencies which has the greatest clinical significance. A 60 Hz filter may be used to selectively reduce interference which cannot be controlled by other means. The filters are part of the amplifiers and modify their output before it is connected to the penwriters.

(3.6) *The writing units* are driven by the amplified and filtered potential changes recorded at the scalp. Moving pens or, less often, ink jets or other devices move up and down, writing on chart paper which is moved horizontally at an even speed of usually 3 cm/second.

3.1 THE INPUT BOARD

The connectors at the ends of the electrode lead wires are plugged into receptacles in a small input board or box. Each receptacle is labelled with a symbol which indicates the location of the electrode on the head. To aid in selecting the correct receptacle, the receptacles are often arranged in a diagram representing the head. At least 23 receptacles should be available for the standard recording and ground electrodes. Additional receptacles, if available, may be used for additional electrode placements. The wires from each receptacle run in a cable to the EEG machine where they terminate at the input selector switches. In most EEG machines, the input board either contains an impedance meter or has connections for such a meter so that electrode impedance can be measured without changing electrode connections.

Because electrode lead wires should be no longer than 1 meter to minimize artifacts, the input board is kept near the patient. The cable from the input board to the EEG machine may be much longer since it is electrically shielded and less likely to pick up interference. In laboratories using a shielded recording room for the patient, the input board must stay in that room; if the machine is located outside the shielded room, the cable is fed through an opening in the shielding to the EEG machine.

For the safety of the patient, the input board and its connections to the EEG machine should be built so that no more than 20 μA of current can flow from any one of the electrodes through the patient to ground. Such leakage currents can be kept to a minimum by connecting the patient to the ground of the EEG machine through a ground electrode terminating on the input board. If the EEG machine and the power outlets are properly grounded, this ground electrode is at the same potential as the chassis of the EEG machine and any other grounded piece of metal equipment in the room. To further reduce the chances of accidental current flow through the patient, the patient should be connected to ground through only one electrode. In the ICU or the operating room, patients are often grounded through monitoring equipment, for instance through ECG recording devices. These patients *should not be grounded* through an EEG electrode. However, when the ground electrodes of other monitoring equipment are too far from the patient's head to provide a good reference point for the EEG amplifier inputs to discriminate against 60 Hz and other interference (3.4.1), it may be better to disconnect the patient temporarily from the ground of the monitoring equipment and to ground the patient instead through an EEG electrode for the duration of the EEG recording.

3.2 INPUT SELECTOR SWITCHES

All EEG machines should have individual selector switches for each channel; as a convenience, many machines also have a master selector switch. These switches are used to connect each channel to the calibration signal, one or more recording electrodes or the ground of the amplifier.

3.2.1 *Individual channel selector switches* may consist of mechanical rotary, push button, or slide switches with over 21 contact positions. Alternatively, individual electrodes for each channel may be programmed for each channel using a monitor screen with a moveable cursor.

3.2.2 *A master electrode selector switch*, if available, may be used to connect a specific combination of electrodes to the input terminals of each amplifier. A hard-

41

wired or programmable master switch has only one setting for each combination and can reduce the time spent in selecting individual channel switches; this is useful for routine recordings using standard electrode combinations. Individual channel settings must be available for cases where other combinations of electrodes are needed to demonstrate a particular EEG abnormality.

3.2.3 *Possible selections* are of four types. (1) The calibration position connects the source of the calibration signal to the amplifier input. (2) Any receptacle of the input board, except that of the ground electrode, can be connected to any amplifier input. The same electrode may be selected at the input of more than one amplifier. However, if the same electrode is selected at both inputs of one amplifier, the inputs are short-circuited, and closed and the penwriter displays a flat line. (3) Combinations of two or more electrodes can be selected at one input to an amplifier on many machines. This selection, often called 'average reference electrode', electrically ties together the selected electrodes so that each one contributes equally to the potential fluctuations recorded from their combination. (4) Ground can be selected as an input to an amplifier, connecting that input to the ground of the amplifier and effectively closing the input regardless of whether or not the ground is connected to the patient.

3.3 CALIBRATION

Calibration in clinical EEG has two main purposes: (a) to measure the voltage of the EEG potentials by comparing them with a potential of known voltage; (b) to ascertain whether all channels amplify the same signal in the same way. Both purposes are served by the most commonly used calibration procedure of applying standard voltage pulses simultaneously to the input of all amplifiers. The functioning of the amplifiers can also be compared by using the patient's EEG as a calibration signal.

42

3.3.1 *Calibration pulses.* A negative potential of pre-selected voltage is applied to the input of an amplifier by actuating a calibration switch. This results in a sudden pen deflection. Only the initial deflection represents the amplitude of the calibration voltage; even when the calibration voltage is sustained, the pen gradually drifts back to the baseline as the result of the low frequency filter (3.5.1). When the calibration voltage is turned off after the pen has reached baseline, the pen is suddenly deflected in the opposite direction and to the same amplitude as at the beginning of the calibration pulse. For routine calibration, a series of such deflections is recorded in all channels.

The pen deflections of the calibration pulses serve to determine the voltage of EEG potentials recorded at the same amplifier settings. For instance, an EEG potential deflecting a pen to a height of 14 mm at an amplifier setting at which a calibration pulse of 50 μV produces 7 mm pen deflection has an amplitude of 100 μV. Although the amplitude of the calibration pulses at different amplifier settings can be derived by multiplying the amplitude of the calibration pulses by the change in amplification, it is good practice to calibrate the amplifiers at the end of a recording for all the settings used during a recording.

3.3.2 *Biocalibration.* The patient's EEG may be used to compare the performance of all amplifiers and, more importantly, test the integrity of the entire recording system. To obtain a wide range of relatively high amplitude EEG frequencies for this comparison, a frontopolar electrode and an occipital electrode on the opposite side are usually selected as the input for all amplifiers. The tracings of all pens should be identical.

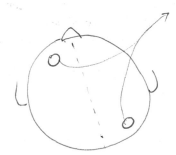

3.4 THE AMPLIFIERS

EEG amplifiers have two main purposes: (1) *Discrimination* is the ability to pick up differences of electrical potential between the electrodes connected to the two inputs

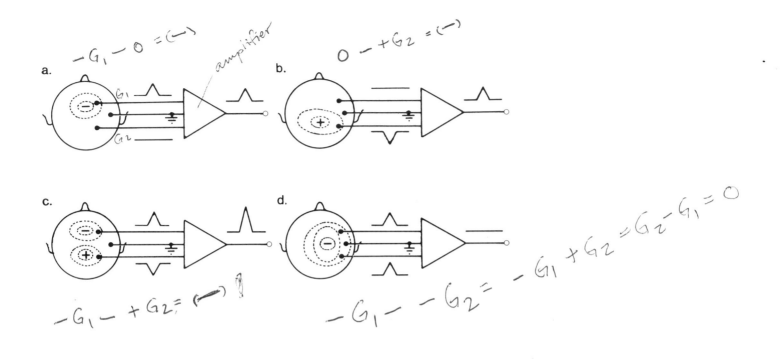

Fig. 3.1. Differential amplification of simple signals, applied to input 1 (top input at the triangular amplifier symbol) and input 2 (bottom input) with respect to an electrical zero level at the ground connection (middle input). Electrical changes at scalp electrodes are indicated by fields on the head diagram; a change towards negative in an electrode is indicated by an upward deflection of the signal above or below the electrode lead; a change towards positive is indicated by a downward deflection. The same polarity convention is used for the signals at the amplifier output which represent pen deflections. – a. A negative signal at input 1 causes an upgoing pen deflection; – b. A positive signal at input 2 is inverted at the ground level and also causes an upgoing pen deflection; – c. Two signals of equal size but opposite polarity appearing simultaneously at both inputs are added to each other and cause a pen deflection twice the size of that caused by each potential alone; – d. Two signals of equal size and the same polarity applied simultaneously to both inputs are subtracted from each other and cause no pen deflection.

while rejecting potentials which are common to the two electrodes (referred to as *common mode rejection*); (2) *Amplification* serves to increase the size of potential differences to a level at which they can drive the pens of the EEG machine and be written out on the paper record.

3.4.1 *Discrimination*. Each amplifier of the EEG machine has two input terminals named 'input 1' and 'input 2' (formerly called 'grid 1' and 'grid 2'). Potential changes, or signals, applied to each terminal are amplified to the same degree but in opposite direction with reference to the ground of the amplifier. This is done by inverting the polarity of the signal applied to input 2 so that it is effectively subtracted from the signal applied to input 1. This mode of operation is called 'differential' or 'balanced' amplification.

The polarity of the output signal of a differential amplifier thus depends not only on the polarity of the input signal but also on the input terminal to which it is applied. EEG machines are wired so that a net negativity at input 1 causes an upward deflection at the output whereas a relative negativity at input 2 causes a downward deflection. Because upward and downward deflections of the pens do not reveal the polarity at either input, up or down deflections should not be called 'negative' or 'positive'.

The results of differential amplification are illustrated by four extreme cases illustrated in Figure 3.1.

(a) A negative signal applied to input 1 causes an upward deflection at the output.

(b) A positive signal applied to input 2 also causes an upward deflection at the output. (relative negativity at input 1)

(c) Two signals of opposite polarity applied simultaneously to each input produce an output which represents the sum of the outputs caused by either signal alone.

(d) Two signals of the same amplitude, polarity and timing applied to both inputs are subtracted from each other and produce no output. Such signals are said to be in 'common mode'.

el más negativo jala

✗ i.e. positivity at input 1

45

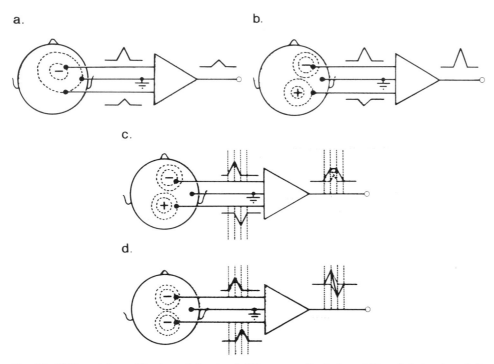

Fig. 3.2. Differential amplification of signals of different amplitude (a and b) and timing (c and d). Symbols are the same as in Fig. 3.1. – a. Simultaneous appearance of a negative potential at input 1 and of a negative potential of half its size at input 2 causes an upgoing pen deflection half the size of that produced by the potential at input 1 alone; – b. Simultaneous appearance of a negative signal at input 1 and of a positive signal of half its size at input 2 causes an upgoing pen deflection of an amplitude one and a half times that produced by the signal at input 1 alone. – c. Appearance of a negative signal at input 1 followed by appearance of a positive signal of the same size at input 2 causes a sustained upgoing pen deflection; – d. Appearance of a negative signal at input 1 followed by a negative signal of the same size at input 2 causes a diphasic pen deflection of a longer total duration and of a faster falling phase than that caused by either signal alone.

46

The four examples in Figure 3.1 show potentials of identical shape, amplitude and timing. Such potentials are not produced by the brain. However, the simple rules illustrated by these examples can also be applied to more complicated conditions such as shown in Figure 3.2. A change of potential affecting both electrodes to a different degree causes an output of an amplitude corresponding exactly with the difference between the potential at both inputs. For instance, if the potential level at input 1 becomes more negative by 100 μV and that at input 2 more negative by 50 μV or more positive by 50 μV, the amplifier input 'sees' a potential difference between the inputs of 50 μV or 150 μV, respectively (Fig. 3.2a and b). Potential changes involving both inputs in sequence may be offset in time and cause a prolonged output; a potential change which appears at input 2 with some delay in regard to a change at input 1 causes the two changes to be added to each other (Fig. 3.2c) or to be subtracted from each other (Fig. 3.2d). In essence, the output represents an amplification of that part of the input signals which is not common to both input terminals.

Obviously, in differential amplification one type of output can be the result of different kinds of input. The methods used to deduce from the output, namely the EEG, the input, namely the polarity, distribution and relative amplitude of the electrical potentials on the scalp, are discussed in the next chapter.

Discrimination means selection of signals which differ at both inputs and rejection of common mode signals. It is expressed as a ratio comparing differential with common mode amplification of an amplifier. This ratio is measured by applying a signal differentially, i.e. between input 1 and input 2, at a gain setting which produces a measurable output, and by then determining the size of the signal needed to produce the same output when the signal is applied in common mode, i.e. between an interconnection of the two inputs and ground; the ratio of the amplitude of the second input signal over that of the first input signal is the discrimination of the amplifier. Good EEG machines have amplifiers with high discrimination, or rejection ratios, of 10,000 or more.

Differential amplification has the main purpose of eliminating electrical potentials which do not come from the brain. Potentials from the brain are usually not evenly distributed over the scalp and therefore cause different potential levels to appear in at least some of the scalp electrodes connected to the amplifier inputs; these differences are amplified and appear in the EEG. In contrast, potentials from outside the brain usually affect all scalp electrodes in the same manner and are therefore rejected or cancelled by the differential amplifier. This is true especially of 60 Hz interference. However, differential amplification does not always distinguish between cerebral activity and artifacts because some artifacts may produce slightly different potentials at some of the scalp electrodes, and some cerebral potentials may be in common mode at most electrodes. This can lead to (1) failure to reject artifacts and (2) cancellation of cerebral activity.

(1) *Failure to reject artifacts* is usually due to either (a) unequal impedance of the recording electrodes or (b) absence of an effective ground connection to the patient.

(a) *Unequal impedance of the recording electrodes* at the two inputs to an amplifier causes potentials of equal amplitude on the scalp to appear with different amplitude at the inputs. This difference in signal amplitude will then be amplified and appear at the output. The most common result of unequal electrode impedance is the appearance at the output of 60 Hz artifact from alternating current sources. The amplitude of the artifact depends on the severity of the impedance imbalance and the strength of the interference signal. The interference is weak in most EEG laboratories, but may be strong when recordings are made in unshielded locations such as patient rooms, intensive care units and operating rooms; minor imbalances of electrode impedances may then become critical. A common cause of impedance imbalance is partial or complete loss of contact between electrode and scalp. This results in an output reflecting only the difference between a single input and the ground of the amplifier. If the amplifier ground electrode has been connected to the patient, the output of the amplifier will then reflect the potential difference between

the ground electrode and the electrode that still has good scalp contact. If the
ground electrode has been placed near the eyes, eye movement artifact will appear
increasingly as the contact of the poorly attached electrode worsens. For this reason,
the ground electrode is usually placed at Fpz so that the presence of abnormally
distributed eye movements can be used by the technician and electroencephalographer to identify defective electrode contacts. Such *ground recordings* usually arise from poor electrode attachment to the scalp. But they may also
be the result of any interruption of electrode contact, including a broken electrode
wire or failure to plug the electrode into the input board.

If the amplifier ground is not connected to the patient, the output represents the
difference between cerebral potential changes and the entirely unrelated potential
level of the amplifier ground. This might be called true monopolar or 'single-ended'
recording and may be of no value if the loss of common mode rejection results in
a recording that is obscured by interference. The term 'monopolar' should therefore
not be used to describe reference montage recordings, since all biological recordings
are between two points located on the subject.

(b) *Absent or ineffective ground connection to the patient* does not preclude
recording of potential differences between input 1 and 2. However, the inputs float
without reference to the potential level at which the amplifier inverts input 2 to
subtract it from input 1. An amplifier with floating input is therefore more likely to
'see' signals which are equal with reference to the patient's head as being different
and to therefore amplify artifacts which would be rejected if the amplifier had an
effective ground connection to the patient's head.

(2) *Rejection of cerebral potentials.* Discrimination cancels cerebral potentials
that are in common mode. EEG potential changes which appear at exactly the same
time and have exactly the same shape and amplitude over all parts of the head would
therefore escape detection in recordings from scalp electrodes and would require
recordings between one electrode over the head and another electrode elsewhere on

the body. Such potential changes probably occur very rarely if at all. More often, even widespread potential changes differ slightly in shape, amplitude and timing at some recording sites over the head.

3.4.2 *Amplification.* The amplifier increases the voltage difference between the inputs so that the voltage of the output can be used to drive the pens of the EEG machine. This amplifying action can be characterized in terms of sensitivity and gain.

Sensitivity is the ratio of input voltage to the pen deflection it produces. Sensitivity is measured in microvolts per millimeter (μV/mm). A commonly used sensitivity is 7 μV/mm. At this sensitivity, a calibration signal of 50 μV causes a pen deflection of about 7 mm. Note that a sensitivity setting of higher numerical value means a lower sensitivity or less amplification: A sensitivity setting of 10 μV/mm will make a calibration signal smaller than a sensitivity setting of 7 μV/mm. Conversely, decreasing the setting from 10 μV/mm to 7 μV/mm increases the sensitivity of the amplifier.

The sensitivity of each channel can be adjusted between high values of 1 or 2 μV/mm and low values of at least 1000 μV/mm. These adjustments are made with switches which increase the sensitivity stepwise by factors of no more than two. A variable control permits equalizing the sensitivity between channels precisely; equalization should be necessary only rarely. In addition to these individual sensitivity controls for each channel, most EEG machines have a master sensitivity switch which controls the sensitivity of all channels.

Because sensitivity can be directly determined by applying a calibration pulse and measuring the pen deflection, sensitivity rather than gain is usually used to describe amplification by EEG machines.

Gain is the ratio of signal voltage obtained at the output of the amplifier to the signal voltage applied at the input. For instance, an amplifier set to give an output

50

voltage of 10 V for an input of 10 μV is said to have a gain of 1 million; this is the usual maximum gain of EEG machines. Gain is sometimes expressed in decibels, the number of decibels amounting to 20 times the logarithm$_{10}$ of the gain. For instance, a gain of 10 equals 20 dB, a gain of 100 equals 40 dB, a gain of 1 million equals 120 dB. In contrast to sensitivity, gain is defined so that it increases with increasing amplification. However, gain is not a useful measure in clinical EEG because the output voltage of the amplifier is not directly measured.

3.5 FILTERS

Filters are used to exclude waves of relatively high or low frequencies from the EEG so that waves in the most important middle range of about 1–30 Hz can be recorded clearly and without distortion. The effect of filters is often illustrated and specified in terms of their actions on electronically generated sine or square waves (Fig. 3.3). It must be stressed that filters affect any component of the EEG to the extent that it raises or falls with a slope corresponding with that of sine waves (Fig. 3.3, right).

Most EEG machines have three kinds of filters. (1) The low frequency filter reduces the amplitude of slow waves. (2) The high frequency filter reduces the amplitude of fast waves. (3) The 60 Hz filter selectively reduces the amplitude of waves of about 60 Hz, the frequency of the most common electrical artifact*. The low frequency filter is alternatively referred to as a *high pass filter*, since it allows the higher frequencies to pass through the amplifier to the penwriter without being attenuated. Similarly, the high frequency filter is sometimes referred to as a *low pass filter*. The 60-Hz filter is sometimes referred to as a narrow frequency band or 'notch' filter because it allows higher and lower frequency waveforms to pass without significant attenuation. Each of these three filter actions is usually provided

* A 50 Hz filter is used in countries using a power line frequency of 50 Hz.

51

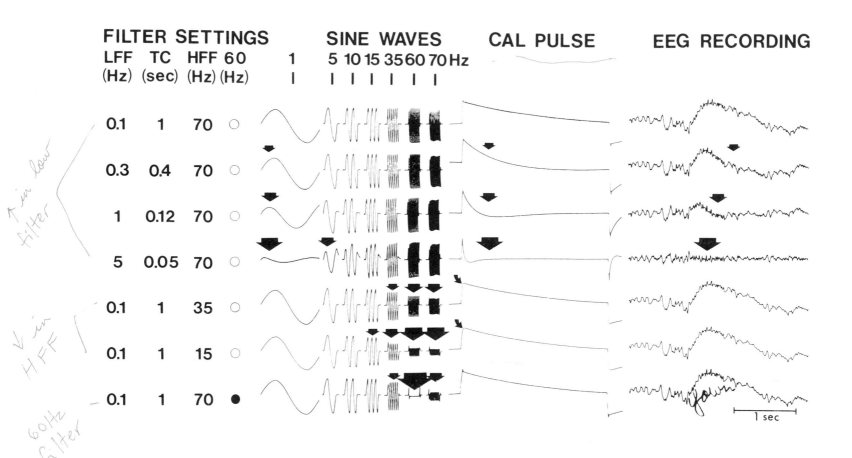

FILTER SETTINGS

LFF (Hz)	TC (sec)	HFF (Hz)	60 (Hz)
0.1	1	70	○
0.3	0.4	70	○
1	0.12	70	○
5	0.05	70	○
0.1	1	35	○
0.1	1	15	○
0.1	1	70	●

SINE WAVES 1 5 10 15 35 60 70 Hz

CAL PULSE

EEG RECORDING

1 sec

by individual channel controls permitting different selections for each channel and by master switches allowing selection of the same settings for all channels.

3.5.1 *The low frequency filter* can be characterized by its effect either on sine waves, giving the 'low filter frequency', or on square pulses, giving the 'time constant'.

Low filter frequency specifies the frequency at which sine waves are reduced in amplitude by a fixed fraction. Figures 3.3 and 3.4 show the effects of different filter settings on sine waves of different frequencies. The first four channels in each figure were recorded with low filter frequencies of 0.1, 0.3, 1 and 5 Hz. The filters reduce the amplitude of sine waves at these frequencies by 20% or 2 dB. Sine waves of lower frequency are reduced more, and even sine waves slightly above the cutoff frequency are reduced some, although by less than 20%. As a result, a sine wave of

---

Fig. 3.3. The effect of different filter settings on sine waves of various frequencies, a calibration pulse and a segment of EEG recording. The same signals are applied to the inputs of all channels; therefore, the differences in the outputs, enhanced by arrows, are due to the different filter settings used in each channel. Filter settings are indicated at the left margin. Low frequency filter settings are given both in terms of low filter frequency (LFF) representing the frequency at which sine waves are reduced by 20% in amplitude, and in terms of the corresponding time constant (TC). High frequency filter settings are indicated in terms of high filter frequency (HFF) representing the frequency at which sine waves are reduced in amplitude by 20%. The 60 Hz filter is used only in the last channel. Channels 1–4 show the effect of increasing the low filter frequency, or of decreasing the time constant: The amplitude of sine waves of low frequency is progressively reduced, the calibration pulse returns to baseline faster, and slow waves are reduced in the EEG. Channels 5 and 6 show the effect of decreasing the high frequency filter: Sine waves of high frequency are reduced in amplitude, the calibration pulse is rounded off at its tip, and fast waves in the EEG are reduced in amplitude and increased in duration as compared with channels 4 and 7, although this effect is less noticeable here than in tracings containing fast activity of higher amplitude (Fig. 6.2., Parts 1 and 2). The last channel shows the effect of the 60 Hz filter: Sine waves of 60 Hz are eliminated and those at 35 and 70 Hz are reduced in amplitude, the calibration pulse shows a barely visible deformation in the rising and falling phase, and the EEG tracing loses the slight amount of superimposed 60 Hz activity which is recognizable as the 'hum' or thickness of the tracing in channel 4 and reduced by the high frequency filter settings used in channels 5 and 6; this effect is better appreciated in tracings containing more 60 Hz artifact (Fig. 6.3, Part 1).

53

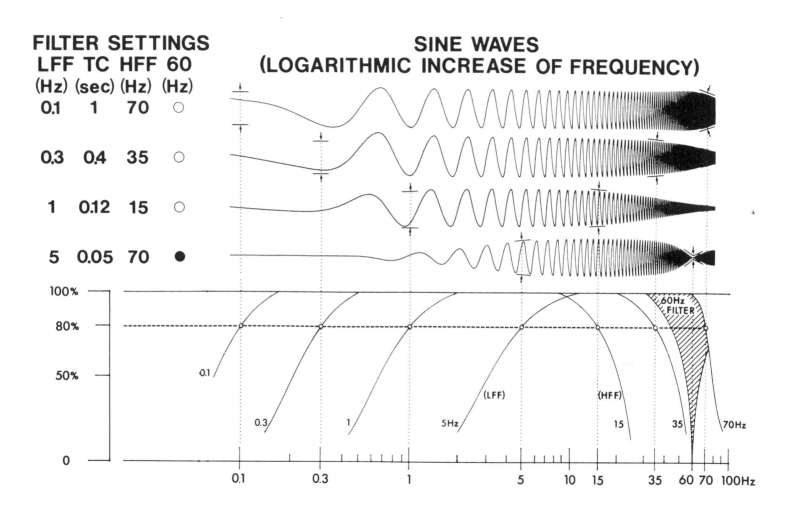

FILTER SETTINGS

LFF (Hz)	TC (sec)	HFF (Hz)	60 (Hz)
0.1	1	70	○
0.3	0.4	35	○
1	0.12	15	○
5	0.05	70	●

**SINE WAVES
(LOGARITHMIC INCREASE OF FREQUENCY)**

0.3 Hz is nearly abolished by a filter setting of 5 Hz, severly reduced by a setting of 1 Hz, and reduced by 20% by a setting of 0.3 Hz; it can be recorded without amplitude distortion only with a filter setting below 0.3 Hz. It may be noted that filters also distort the time relation between waves of frequencies near the cutoff frequency, each filter delaying these waves by different amounts of time.

The relationship between the amplitude and the frequency of sine waves at different filter settings is summarized in the diagram at the bottom of Figure 3.4. Here, each curve on the left side represents one low frequency filter setting and shows the amount of reduction of amplitude of waves having frequencies below the medium range. This figure makes it clear that filters of EEG machines have no sharp cutoff: Waves of frequencies below the low filter frequency are not entirely eliminated, waves slightly above that frequency are not entirely unaffected.

The time constant describes the effect of the low frequency filter on square pulses. The time constant is the time required for the pen to fall to 37% of the peak deflection produced when a steady voltage, such as a calibration pulse, is applied to the input of the amplifier (Fig. 3.5a). The time constant can be easily measured in EEG recordings by drawing a horizontal line at about one-third the height of the calibration signal; the time from the beginning of the calibration pulse to the intersection

Fig. 3.4. The effect of different filter settings on the amplitude of sine waves which have frequencies representative of the spectrum of frequencies recorded in the EEG. *Top*: Sine waves of logarithmically increasing frequency are recorded with filter settings which are indicated at the left margin in the same notation as used for Fig. 3.3. Filter settings for both high and low frequencies are changed between channels 1 to 4 so that the amplitude of slow and fast waves progressively decreases; the 60 Hz filter is used in channel 4. Arrows indicate the frequencies at which the amplitude is reduced by 20%; dotted lines project these values to the graph below. *Bottom*: A graph of filter settings is derived from the recording in the top part and relates the amplitude of sine waves, in percent of total amplification (vertical axis on left), to the wave frequency (horizontal axis with logarithmic scale at bottom). Each curve corresponds with a setting of the low frequency filter (LFF), high frequency filter (HFF) or 60 Hz filter and indicates the reduction in amplitude of sine waves at that setting.

a.

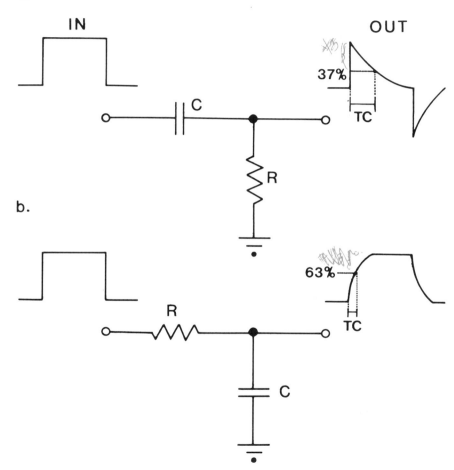

IN

OUT

C

37%

TC

R

b.

63%

TC

R

C

of the horizontal line with the falling phase of the calibration signal is the time constant (Fig. 3.5a). Figure 3.3 shows the effect of different low frequency filter settings on square pulses. These settings are indicated both in terms of low filter frequencies and of time constants on the left side of the figure. Note that an increase in the time constant means that waves of lower frequency are amplified without distortion, i.e. a *long* time constant, or a time constant of *high* numerical value, corresponds with an effect on waves of *low* frequency. The most commonly used time constant settings fall in the range of about 1 to 0.03 sec. — *we use 0.3 ms (about 0.5 Hz)*

The values of time constants and low filter frequency can be interconverted. Thus, the time constant TC in a simple network of resistors and capacitors is related to the low filter frequency by the equation $TC = 1/2 \pi f$ where f is the frequency at which the amplitude is attenuated by 30% or 3 dB. This means that time constants of 1, 0.3, 0.1 and 0.03 sec, used in some EEG machines, correspond with 30% amplitude attenuation of waves of frequencies of 0.16, 0.53, 1.6 and 5.3 Hz. The low frequency settings producing 20% attenuation at 0.1, 0.3, 1 and 5 Hz, used in some other machines, correspond with time constants of 1, 0.4, 0.12 and 0.035 sec.

Limits of low frequency result from the design of EEG machines. Most machines are not designed to record very slow or very long-sustained potential changes. Their inputs do not have direct coupling which is needed to conduct potential changes of zero Hz or direct current (D.C.); instead, they are coupled through capacitors which process alternating signals such as alternating current (A.C.). Direct coupling is not

---

◄ Fig 3.5. Circuits of simple low and high frequency filters made of a capacitor (C) and a resistor (R). – a. Low frequency filter consists of a capacitor in the signal path and a resistor connection to ground. The time constant (TC) of this circuit is defined as the time required for a steady input voltage to drop to 37% of its amplitude at the output and equals the product of R × C. – b. High frequency filter consists of a resistor in the signal path and a capacitor connection to ground. The time constant of this circuit is defined as the time required for the output voltage to rise to 63% of a sudden input voltage and is also equal to the product of R × C.

used in clinical EEG because cerebral activity of very low frequency does probably not contain diagnostic information and is very difficult to record without artifacts due to instability of the electrical properties of skin, electrodes, amplifiers and other machine components.

Electrical construction of filters often uses a capacitor (C) placed in the path of the signal (Fig. 3.5a) which is separated from ground by a resistor (R). The capacitor opposes slow potential changes more than fast ones. The network in Fig. 3.5a is a low frequency filter, or high frequency pass. It has a time constant of $TC = R \times C$ and a low frequency reduction of 3 dB or 30% at a frequency of $f = 1/2\pi R \times C$.

3.5.2 *The high frequency filter* reduces the size of fast waves. Its effect is specified by the frequency of waves which are reduced by a fixed fraction, for instance 30% or 3 dB, or 20% or 2 dB. Figures 3.3 and 3.4 show the effects of high frequency filter settings of 15, 35 and 70 Hz which reduce the amplitude of sine waves at these frequencies by 20% or 2 dB. Sine waves above the cutoff frequencies are reduced more, but sine waves slightly below the cutoff are also reduced, even though by less than 20%. These relations are summarized by the curves on the right side of the diagram at the bottom of Figure 3.4.

The middle part of Figure 3.3 shows the effects of high frequency filters on square waves used for calibration. Square waves contain high frequency components mainly at their peaks. The filtering of high frequencies affects mainly the rise time of the calibration pulses. This effect is barely visible at the normally slow speed of EEG recordings but causes the tips of the calibration pulses to become slightly rounded (curved arrows in Fig. 3.3). This effect becomes more obvious with very low settings of the high frequency filter and very high recording speeds, but measurement of the time constant of the rising phase (TC in Fig. 3.5b) is not practical with the recording methods used in conventional EEG.

High frequency filters must be set to include frequencies faster than those usually considered important in clinical EEG. Although waves of over 35 Hz are of little clinical interest, the use of high frequency filters set at that value can badly distort the EEG. This is especially true of the diagnostically very important fast components contained in spikes and sharp waves; application of high frequency filters can reduce these fast components and thereby transform the spikes and sharp waves into inconspicuous waves. On the other hand, muscle activity, a common contaminant consisting of fast waves, is often not eliminated by filtering as would be desirable, but is instead reduced in amplitude and made to last longer; filtered muscle activity may be more difficult to distinguish from cerebral activity than unfiltered muscle activity (Fig. 6.2).

Limits of high frequency are due to the design of the writing units; the commonly used ink pens cannot be driven to write much faster than 70 Hz without significant distortion.

Electrical construction of high frequency filters often uses a capacitor (C) to shunt high frequencies from the signal path to ground (Fig. 3.5b). The network in Figure 3.5b reduces the amplitude of waves of a frequency of $f = 1/2\pi R \times C$ by 30% or 3 dB.

3.5.3 *The 60 Hz filter* is provided in many EEG machines to eliminate the most common type of electrical artifact, namely interference from devices powered by alternating current. This filter sharply reduces the amplitude of sine waves of 60 Hz*, but it cannot accomplish this without also reducing the amplitude of waves of neighboring frequencies to some extent (Figs. 3.3 and 3.4). Although sine waves of 60 Hz are not usually produced by the brain and could be spared from EEG recordings, the 60 Hz filter should not be used routinely for several reasons. (a) Some EEG components, for instance spikes, may contain slopes corresponding with the 60 Hz

---

* A 50 Hz filter is used in countries using a power line frequency of 50 Hz.

frequency; filtering at 60 Hz, like filtering with high frequency filters, could reduce these components so that they become <u>unrecognizable</u>. (b) 60 Hz interference may indicate a poor electrode contact or an improper input selection which would go undetected and uncorrected if the 60 Hz filter is used indiscriminately. The 60 Hz filter should therefore be used only in the full knowledge of what it may obscure and after all other efforts to eradicate the cause of the interference have been exhausted.

3.6 WRITING UNITS

3.6.1 *The writing devices* serve to convert the fluctuating potential changes at the

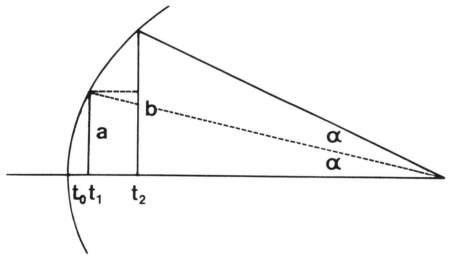

Fig. 3.6. Distortions of the EEG by curvilinear writing movements of pens. The circular movement of the pen around the shaft causes the tracing to deviate from rectangular coordinates both in the horizontal and vertical dimensions. Horizontal error: A pen deflection to the height indicated by line a or b seems to occur at times t_1 and t_2 even though it is synchronous with t_0. Vertical error: The amplitude of b, even though caused by a pen deflection twice that of a, is not twice the amplitude of a.

60

output of the amplifiers into a vertical movement. In most EEG machines, this is accomplished with oscillographs. An oscillograph consists of a galvanometer coil which is mounted in the field of a permanent magnet so that the coil rotates in response to the electrical potential changes coming from the amplifier output. The shaft of the galvanometer coil protrudes above the writing surface and holds the writing device which moves up and down on the EEG paper with excursions corresponding with the amplitude of the electrical potential changes. The most common writing devices are pens consisting of a metal tube filled with ink from an inkwell. Other writing devices use ink jets, carbon paper, and light or heat sensitive paper.

Curvilinear distortion results from the arc-like movement of pens around an axis. The deviation from rectilinear movement causes faulty representation of both vertical and horizontal coordinates (Fig. 3.6). The vertical deflection is neither strictly straight nor strictly proportional to the applied voltage. The horizontal position of a deflected pen depends on the degree of the vertical deflection so that a higher deflection seems to have occurred later in time than a simultaneous deflection of lower amplitude. Both types of distortion increase with the amplitude of the deflection and distort the shape and amplitude of every curvilinear EEG writeout to some degree.

Vertical and horizontal pen alignment should be perfect (Fig. 3.7). The pens must have equal distance from each other and point exactly in the direction of the paper movement. The pens must also be aligned so that a signal appearing in all channels at the same time deflects the pens on the same line on the paper, perpendicular to the paper movement; if one pen protrudes to the left or right of the others, a signal written by that pen will seem to have occurred earlier or later than a signal written at the same time by the other pens.

Faulty pen alignment may be due to the following:

(1) If the horizontal spacing between the pen tips is uneven regardless of whether

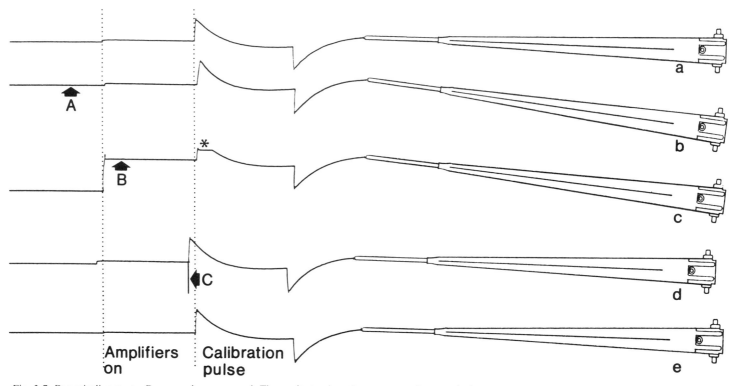

Amplifiers on

Calibration pulse

Fig. 3.7. Pen misalignments. Pens a and e are normal: They write tracings that are properly spaced, show only minimal deflections when the amplifiers are turned on ('Amplifiers on'), and do not distort the calibration pulse; the deflections of these pens fall on the same vertical line (dotted lines); Pen b writes a tracing that is displaced upward both before and after the amplifier output is connected to the pens (arrow A); this is due to a mechanical deviation from the zero line, usually caused by an improper adjustment of the pen on its shaft; Pen c writes a tracing that is displaced upward at the moment when the amplifiers are turned on (arrow B) and clips large signals in that direction (*); this is due to an electrical deviation from the zero line caused by faulty adjustment of the voltage level of the amplifier output; Pen d registers deflections that are displaced to the left (arrow C) and seem to occur earlier than those of the other pens; this horizontal deviation is usually due to improper alignment of the oscillograph or of the pen seat.

or not the pens are connected to the amplifier outputs (Fig. 3.7b), a pen may have been damaged or moved out of its seat; if this is not the case, the pen may have rotated away from its correct position on the galvanometer shaft and should be rotated to the correct position by readjusting its seat on the shaft.

(2) If the horizontal spacing between the pens changes suddenly when they are connected to the amplifier outputs (Fig. 3.7c), the electrical potential level of the output is at fault and should be reset by adjusting the electrical zero potential level of the amplifier outputs. However, minor steps of the baseline may appear during everyday operation and are tolerable if they are not much larger than the width of the ink tracing (Fig. 3.7a and e). Transient pen deflections may appear suddenly when the amplifier inputs are opened immediately after changing the selection of recording electrodes at the input and are usually due to electrode bias potentials (2.2.4).

(3) If the tips of the pens at rest are not aligned in a straight vertical line on the paper (Fig. 3.7d), the pens deviating from this line can be moved left or right into the correct position by adjusting the position of the pen seat or of the oscillator in the EEG machine. Before making this adjustment, one should be sure that the deviation is not due to improper mounting to the pen in its seat on the galvanometer shaft or to bent or damaged pens.

3.6.2 *The paper transport* pulls the paper from a folded stack in a storage bin within the machine, moves it at an even speed under the writing pens and across a surface where the ink dries and the record can be inspected and labelled for at least 60 cm, and deposits it into another storage bin where it is folded again. Modern machines use the internationally recommended paper speed of 3 cm/second and usually have additional faster and slower speeds. EEG paper is often imprinted with vertical lines every 3 cm, corresponding with 1 second at regular speed; these intervals may be subdivided. Many EEG machines have time markers producing a

usual paper speed: 3 cm/sec.

63

pen deflection in an extra channel every 1 second. This should generate intervals of the same length as those printed on the chart paper if the paper is moving at the speed of 3 cm/second.

Physically, the paper transport consists of a motor with gear shift and friction rollers which pull the margin of the paper. The transport mechanism may give rise to various problems.

(a) If the paper slows or stops for a moment during the recording because of a momentary failure of the driving mechanism or because of a momentary resistance of the paper feed, the time base of the recording will be distorted: the pens will deflect up and down with little or no movement to the side and create the impression of very fast and abnormal EEG transients, such as spikes. This artifact can be recognized by the very steep rises and falls of the pen deflections and by the fact that the same phenomenon occurs in all or most channels at the same time (Fig. 6).

(b) When stiff paper with sharp creases is not sufficiently stretched as it is pulled along under the pens, the pens may be bounced up and off the paper at each upward fold. This gives an interrupted, irregular tracing of all pens following each upward fold.

(c) The paper may run not on a straight course or it may track too close to the upper or lower edge. This can be corrected by adjusting the front or rear paper guides and rollers on the machine.

(d) The paper speed may vary due to defects of the friction rollers, gear shift or motor. This distorts the timing of the writeout and makes regular wave shapes appear irregular.

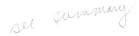

REFERENCES

American EEG Society Guidelines in EEG, 1–7 (Revised 1985). (1986) J. clin. Neurophysiol. 3: 131–168.

Barlow, J.S., Kamp, A., Morton, H.B., Ripoche, A., Shipton, H. and Tchavdarov, D.B. (1978) EEG Instrumentation Standards (revised 1977): Report of the Committee on EEG Instrumentation Standards of the International Federation of Societies for Electroencephalography and Clinical Neurophysiology. Electroenceph. clin. Neurophysiol. 45: 144–150.

Cooper, R., Osselton, J.W. and Shaw, J.C. (1981) EEG Technology. 3rd Ed., Butterworth, London.

Hopps, J.A. (1976) Section V. Shock hazards in electrophysiological recordings. In: Rémond, A. (Ed.), Handbook of Electroenceph. clin. Neurophysiol., Vol. 3A, Elsevier, Amsterdam, pp. 75–79.

McGee, F. (1981) EEG Instrumentation. In: Henry, C.E. (Ed.) Current clinical Neurophysiology, update on EEG and evoked potentials. Elsevier, Amsterdam, pp. 53–64.

Seeba, P.J. (1984) Differential amplifiers and their limitations. Am. J. EEG Technol., 24: 11–23.

Seeba, P.J. (1980) Electrical safety. Am. J. EEG Technol., 20: 1–13.

Tyner, F.S., Knott, J.R. and Mayer Jr., W.B. (1983) Fundamentals of EEG technology. Raven, New York.

Recording strategy

4

SUMMARY

(4.1) *Multichannel recordings* can be used to determine the distribution of potential changes on the scalp when appropriate electrode combinations, or montages, are used. There are mainly two types of montages, each having different advantages and disadvantages. (1) *Bipolar montages* connect pairs of different electrodes to each amplifier, usually selecting adjacent electrodes for successive channels so that each electrode is common to two channels. *Bipolar montages* have the advantage of sharply localizing the peaks of potentials, especially of potentials which occupy small areas, but they also make the morphology and distribution of widespread potentials more difficult to appreciate. (2) *Referential montages* connect input 1 of a group of channels to different scalp electrodes and input 2 of all these channels to the same electrode which thus becomes the reference for each channel. Referential montages can provide an undistorted display of amplitude, configuration and distribution of potentials which occupy a wide area, but can cause problems if the reference electrode itself picks up significant cerebral activity.

(4.2) *Specific montages* are usually designed to compare potentials on both sides of the head and in neighboring areas. The best montages use straight chains of equidistant electrodes along and across the head and display the potentials in an orderly sequence of channels. Several simple bipolar and referential montages should be used for routine recordings in all laboratories; to these may be added locally preferred routine montages and montages developed for specific problems. A list of recommended 18-, 16- and 8-channel montages for routine recordings, for recordings from newborn infants, and for recordings in cases of suspected cerebral death is appended.

(4.3) *Monitoring of extracerebral activity*, for instance of eye movements, heart beat, respiration and muscle activity, is often done to identify artifacts in EEG recordings or to determine sleep stages.

4.1 MULTICHANNEL RECORDINGS

As pointed out in the preceding chapter (3.4.1), the output of a single channel does not reveal the polarity, amplitude and timing of potential changes at input 1 and input 2; recordings from a single channel can therefore not indicate the distribution of potentials on the head. This shortcoming can be overcome by simultaneous recording from more than one channel. Multichannel recording can become a powerful instrument in EEG analysis if appropriate montages are used. The most effective electrode combinations, or montages, use straight chains of electrodes in anterior-posterior or transverse rows.

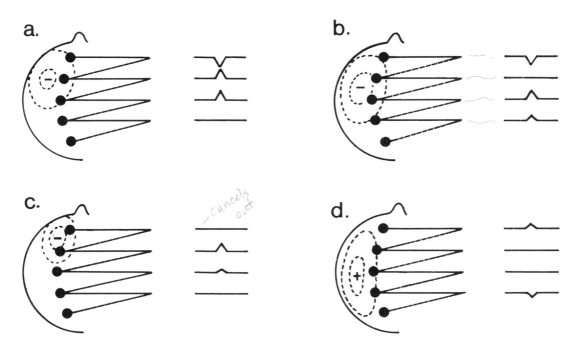

Fig. 4.1. Bipolar montages. a. and b.: Localization of electrical potentials on the scalp by phase reversal; c. and d.: Possible pitfalls of this method.

In general, montages can be divided into two types: bipolar and referential. Although most of the information obtained with one type of montage can be converted into that obtained with the other, each montage has some shortcomings which can be overcome to a degree by the use of the other; both types of montages should therefore be used routinely in every recording.

4.1.1 *Bipolar montages.* *Strategy*: Bipolar montages connect pairs of different electrodes to the inputs of amplifiers. The best bipolar montages link electrodes in anterior–posterior or transverse linear chains of adjacent electrodes (rather than in triangles, diagonal lines, or criss-cross lines) so that an electrode at input 2 of one amplifier is also at input 1 of the next amplifier (Fig. 4.1). In this strategy, the origin of a potential is localized not by the amplitude but by the direction of pen deflections. A potential located at an electrode which is common to two amplifiers in a bipolar linkage causes pen deflections of opposite direction, or 'phase reversal' at the output of these amplifiers. Figure 4.1a shows a bipolar montage recording of a negative potential. The top channel shows a downgoing deflection because it is connected to the electrode near the negative potential through input 2, whereas the next channel, being connected to that electrode through input 1, shows an upgoing deflection. This phase reversal does not indicate a reversal of polarity of the cerebral potential (sometimes referred to as a *true phase reversal*) but only a reversal in the direction of the pen deflection (sometimes referred to as an *instrumental phase reversal*). A positive potential would give a phase reversal in the opposite direction, and cause the pens to deflect apart instead of together.

A potential having a maximum between two recording electrodes (Fig. 4.1b) causes no deflection in the channel connected to these electrodes. However, the potential can be detected because these electrodes are also connected to two other channels which will show a phase reversal (channels 1 and 3 in Fig. 4.1b). In the case of a negative potential, the deflections in these channels are towards each other, in the case of a positive potential, they are away from each other.

69

*they "see" the same potential ∴ it cancels out

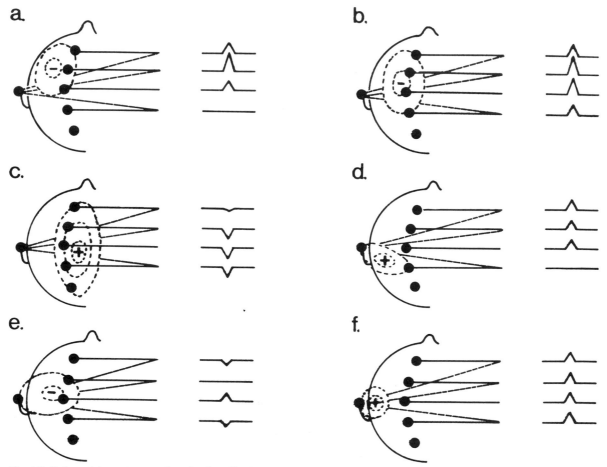

Fig. 4.2. Referential montages. a, b and c: Localization of electrical potentials by amplitude of pen deflections; d, e and f: Possible pitfalls of this method.

Avantages of bipolar recordings: Bipolar linkages sharply distinguish potential changes in neighboring electrodes and thus can localize circumscribed potentials more precisely than referential montages.

Disadvantages: Bipolar montages distort the waveshape and amplitude of potentials which are distributed widely and affect both recording electrodes connected to one channel; in the recording of such a potential, each channel records only that part of the potential which is different at the two electrodes. Potentials between the last two electrodes in a chain may produce confusing pen deflections (Fig. 4.1c), and very widespread potentials may be largely cancelled (Fig. 4.1d).

4.1.2 *Referential montages.* *Strategy*: Referential montages connect inputs 1 of a group of amplifiers to electrodes placed on various parts of the head and inputs 2 of these amplifiers to a common electrode placed in an electrically quiet area; this electrode is called the 'reference electrode'. This method records the potential differences between the various points on the head and the reference electrode. Figure 4.2a shows a referential montage recording the same potential as that recorded with a bipolar montage in Figure 4.1a. In the referential montage, the origin of this potential on the head is recognized by the amplitude: The channel which records the potential of highest amplitude is connected to the electrode nearest the origin of the potential. If the output of two channels is of equal amplitude, the origin of the potential is located an equal distance from each of the two electrodes connected to inputs 1 of these channels (Fig. 4.2b). If several channels have similar output, the potential affects input 1 of all these channels (Fig. 4.2c) to an equal degree. *(large field)*

Advantages: Referential recording can give an undistorted display of the shape of potential changes and is especially useful for recording of potentials which have a wide distribution.

Disadvantages: It is usually impossible to find a reference electrode which is entirely inactive. Potentials at the reference electrode may be large enough to appear

71

in recordings from all channels connected to that electrode. Potentials at such an 'active reference electrode' may produce confusing results and reproduce some of the potential changes usually recorded at the scalp electrodes connected to input 1:

(1) A potential may affect only the reference electrode; for instance a spike in the temporal lobe may appear as a transient positive potential at an ear electrode, a commonly used reference. This will produce an upgoing deflection in all channels connected through input 2 to this electrode (Fig. 4.2f) and appear similar to the potential shown in Figure 4.2b. *(except they are all of similar amplitude)*

(2) A potential located midway between the reference electrode and a scalp electrode may be cancelled in a channel connected to both these electrodes and appear in other channels that are connected to the reference electrode through input 2 (Fig. 4.2d); this is similar to the condition in Figure 4.2a.

(3) A potential may be located between the reference electrode and some scalp electrodes so that it appears as a contribution by input 1 in one channel (channel 3 in Fig. 4.2c), cancels between input 1 and 2 in another channel (channel 2 in Fig. 4.2e) and appears with opposite polarity as a contribution by the reference electrode in input 2 in the other channels (channels 1 and 4, Fig. 4.2c).

It may be difficult to localize the peak of a potential precisely with the referential technique because amplitude, the indicator of a potential peak with this technique, increases with interelectrode distance, i.e. the distance between the scalp and the reference electrode, up to about 10 cm. If the interelectrode distance in different channels of a referential montage varies very much, maximum amplitude may appear not at the electrode nearest the peak but at an electrode located at the greatest distance from the reference electrode.

An average reference electrode may be used as a means to reduce the importance of potential changes introduced by the reference electrode (3.2.3). Although this reference reduces the contribution of potential changes by each electrode in proportion to the number of recording electrodes in the average reference, it may show considerable activity if several electrodes in the reference are affected by the same potential changes.

4.1.3 *Plotting the field* of EEG potentials is not routinely done with pencil and paper, but the steps leading to a picture of the distribution of the contours of potentials in two or three dimensions on the scalp are part of the mental process involved in routine EEG analysis. These plots are based on the idea that the electrode chains laid along and across the head form part of a spatial coordinate system; polarity and amplitude of the potentials at each point are depicted in the vertical direction. The output of all amplifiers at any instant can then be used to plot an electrical field in the form of a picture of mountains and valleys over different parts of the head. The examples of this section use only four channels to define the location of potentials in only one row of electrodes; a three-dimensional picture requires recordings in more than one row of electrodes.

Plots can be made from bipolar and from referential recordings. Figure 4.3a shows the bipolar recording illustrated in Figure 4.1a. The amplitude of each pen deflection is indicated by an arrow to the right of each recording and, because it represents the potential difference between adjacent electrodes, plotted halfway between the recording electrode locations. A line connecting the tips of the arrows outlines the contour of the electrical field in this dimension. Figure 4.3b shows the same potential in a referential recording, also illustrated in Figure 4.2a. The amplitude of each pen deflection, representing the potential difference between each scalp electrode and the reference electrode, is indicated by an arrow to the right of the recordings, and plotted as an elevation above each electrode. The contour of the potential derived from the referential recording is practically identical with the contour obtained from the bipolar recording.

These diagrams show the contour of the field in only one plane. By recording from electrode chains oriented in parallel and at right angles to each other, one can

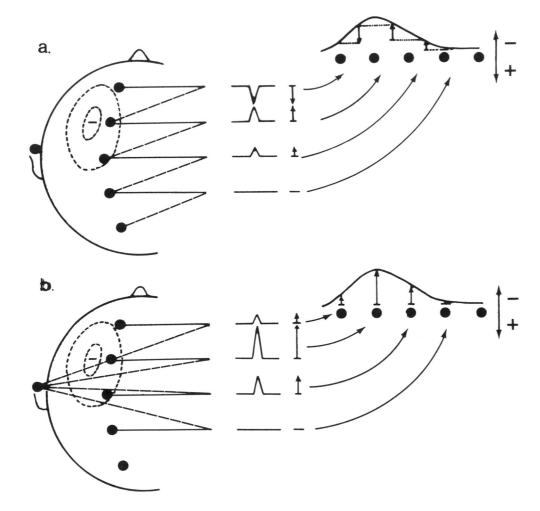

map the distribution of the field in several planes. Points of equal potential levels may be connected with each other and these isopotential lines may be drawn either in a three-dimensional view of peaks and valleys or in a two-dimensional projection of isopotential lines on the surface of the head. Simple two-dimensional views of isopotential lines are used to indicated the distribution of the electrical potentials by the stippled lines in Figures 4.1, 4.2 and 4.3.

The term *dipole* is sometimes used to describe the distribution of EEG activity. Dipoles are electrical sources (or generators) that project positive and negative electrical fields in opposite directions (one end, or pole, is negative and the opposite end is positive). EEG potentials can be viewed as cortical dipoles that have either an approximately vertical, horizontal or diagonal orientation to the surface of the brain. For example, a negative EEG potential may be interpreted as arising from a vertically oriented dipole in the cortex with the negative pole pointing from the cortex of the brain toward the overlying electrode and the positive pole pointing 180° toward the center of the brain. In that case only the negativity is recorded, since the positivity points downward away from the recording electrodes. Alternatively, if two opposite polarity EEG signals occur simultaneously in different locations on the scalp, they may be viewed as the opposite ends of a dipole that has a horizontal or parallel orientation to the scalp. Because *horizontal dipoles* (also referred to as *parallel generators*) are approximately parallel to the surface of the brain, both ends (or poles) are recorded by scalp electrodes.

Fig. 4.3. Plotting the contour line of an electrical field along a chain of electrodes with bipolar (a) and referential (b) montages, both giving the same results. The pen deflections caused by the scalp potential are represented by arrows shown in the middle of the figure; the arrows are used to plot the elevation of the potential above the horizontal electrode chain in the diagram on the right side of the figure. – a. In the bipolar montage, arrows in the diagram are drawn between scalp electrodes and with reference to adjacent arrows; – b. In the referential montage, arrows in the diagram are drawn above scalp electrode locations starting at a common baseline which represents the reference level.

A common example of an EEG activity that often appears as a horizontal dipole is the small sharp spike (also referred to as SSS) or benign epileptiform transients of sleep (BETS; 19.4.4). Small sharp spikes frequently occur with simultaneous opposite polarities located either over opposite hemispheres or in an anterior–posterior direction within a single hemisphere. Epileptiform spikes, such as those occurring in benign Rolandic epilepsy (benign childhood epilepsy with cento-temporal spikes; 17.6.6) or those associated with structural abnormalities in children with cerebral palsy may also appear as horizontal dipoles. It is important to note, however, that the mere appearance of simultaneous and opposite polarity activity at different scalp locations does not necessarily mean that both potentials represent the opposite ends of the same dipole generators. Indeed, for the majority of waveforms it is more likely that the horizontal dipole configuration is either (1) a coincidence, or (2) that different sources are producing opposite polarity activity in a synchronous fashion due to certain functional connections.

4.2 SPECIFIC MONTAGES

Good montages fulfill a few simple requirements.

4.2.1 *The number of channels* available is very important. A machine having a large number of channels can be connected to many electrodes simultaneously to record activity from wide areas of the head; such a machine is more useful than a machine with a smaller number of channels. However, even fairly large machines do not have enough channels to record from all useful electrode combinations at the same time; recordings are therefore made using some electrode combinations followed by recordings using other electrode combinations. This poses no problem in the case of potentials which recur frequently and do not change in distribution and shape, but it causes difficulty in the case of potentials which recur infrequently or vary in distribution and shape; the description of such potentials in all dimensions may require very long recording periods or remain incomplete. The chance to get a complete picture in a reasonably short period of time thus increases with the number of recording channels available.

4.2.2 *Recording strategy* aims at comparing (a) activity in neighboring parts of the head and (b) activity in one area with that in the corresponding area of the other hemisphere. To satisfy both requirements, channels are usually connected to adjacent electrodes, half on one side of the head, and the other half on the other side. The most useful comparisons are made with recordings from chains of equally spaced electrodes connected in bipolar montages of anterior–posterior and transverse electrode linkages and in referential montages.

4.2.3 *Display of activity* is designed to facilitate comparison of activity in various areas. Two types of display are commonly used. (1) *Block montages* display the activity from neighboring parts of one hemisphere in a block of successive channels, and the activity from the corresponding parts of the opposite hemisphere in another block of channels. This method gives a good overview of the general distribution of patterns. (2) *Alternating montages* show activity from one area of one hemisphere in one channel, and the activity from the corresponding area of the opposite hemisphere in the next channel. This method allows very precise comparison between the two sides. Recordings from the front of the head are commonly displayed above recordings from the back.

4.2.4 *Specific montages* vary between laboratories, but standard montages used in most large laboratories usually have some features in common. The American EEG Society has developed 'A proposal for standard montages to be used in clinical electroencephalography' which recommends adoption of a minimum set of

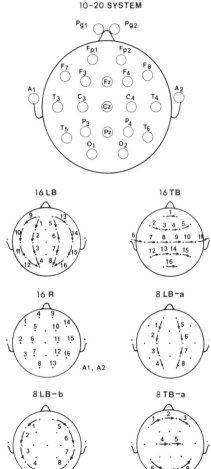

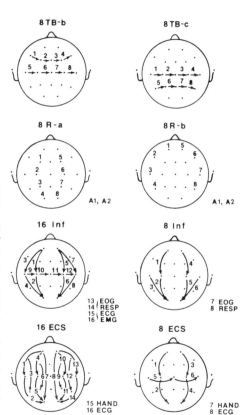

Figs. 4.4 and 4.5. Diagrams of montages for 16-channel and 8-channel EEG machines. All montages use the standard electrode placements of the International 10–20 System. Routine montages use longitudinal bipolar (LB), transverse bipolar (TB) and referential (R) derivations. Recordings of infants (Inf) and recordings made in cases of suspected electrocerebral silence (ECS) combine EEG recordings with monitoring of extracerebral activity (EOG: Electro-oculogram, RESP: respiratory monitor, ECG: heart beat monitor, EMG: surface electromyogram, HAND: hand movement monitor). Each of the small head diagrams represents one montage. The numbers identify the channels. Bipolar montages are indicated by numbers placed near arrows which point from the electrode at input 1 to the electrode at input 2. Referential montages are indicated by numbers placed near the electrode at input 1, input 2 being connected to reference electrodes indicated at the right side of the diagram.

montages for standard use by all clinical EEG laboratories. This set should include (a) *longitudinal bipolar* (LB) montages, i.e. bipolar montages which connect electrodes in anterior–posterior chains; (b) *transverse bipolar* (TB) montages connecting electrodes in chains across the head; and (c) *referential* (R) montages. Additional montages may be used routinely depending on the needs and preferences of each laboratory; special montages should be designed for individual cases with specific problems not solved by routine montages.

The minimum number of routine montages depends on the number of recording channels available. Recordings with machines having 16 or more channels requires only three montages, namely one LB, one TB and one R montage.

The American EEG Society recommends that recordings from the left side of the head be displayed in channels above those recording from the corresponding areas of the right side. The reference electrode may be placed on the earlobe or the mandibular angle. The mandible may be more suitable especially since an ear electrode (a) tends to pick up spikes and other activity from the temporal lobe and (b) provides insufficient interelectrode distances for recordings from temporal electrodes, causing such recordings to have very low amplitude.

Tables 4.1, 4.2, 4.3 and 4.4 contain lists of selected montages recommended by the American EEG Society for routine recordings and for recordings from newborn infants with 18-, 16- and 8-channel machines; alternatives representing slight variations, for instance referential alternating montages instead of referential block montages, are also included in the recommendations of the American EEG Society. The lists also contain montages for 16- and 8-channel recordings in cases of suspected cerebral death or electrocerebral silence. The list is given in two notations. Figures 4.4 and 4.5 show head diagrams using the electrode positions of the 10–20 System. In these figures, bipolar montages are indicated by numbered arrows, each arrow pointing from the electrode at input 1 to the electrode at input 2 of the channel which is indicated by the number of the arrow. Referential montages are indicated by numbers which represent channels and are placed next to the positions of scalp electrodes that are connected to input 1 of these channels while each input 2 is connected to the ipsilateral reference electrode.

4.3 ELECTRODE COMBINATIONS FOR MONITORING OF EXTRACEREBRAL ACTIVITY

The EEG machine may be used to record physiological activity other than the EEG, for instance eye movements, heart beat, respiration and muscle activity. Although

TABLE 4.1

Tables 4.1–4.4. Lists of selected 18-, 16- and 8-channel montages recommended by the American EEG Society. Under the name of each montage the pairs of electrodes which are connected to input 1 and input 2 of the channels are indicated in the column at the left margin

Channel No.	18 LB	18 TB	18 R
1	Fp_1-F_7	F_7-Fp_1	F_7-A_1
2	F_7-T_3	Fp_1-Fp_2	T_3-A_1
3	T_3-T_5	Fp_2-F_8	T_5-A_1
4	T_5-O_1	F_7-F_3	Fp_1-A_1
5	Fp_1-F_3	F_3-F_z	F_3-A_1
6	F_3-C_3	F_z-F_4	C_3-A_1
7	C_3-P_3	F_4-F_8	P_3-A_1
8	P_3-O_1	T_3-C_3	O_1-A_1
9	F_z-C_z	C_3-C_z	F_z-A_1
10	C_z-P_z	C_z-C_4	P_z-A_2
11	Fp_2-F_4	C_4-T_4	Fp_2-A_2
12	F_4-C_4	T_5-P_3	F_4-A_2
13	C_4-P_4	P_3-P_z	C_4-A_2
14	P_4-O_2	P_z-P_4	P_4-A_2
15	Fp_2-F_8	P_4-T_6	O_2-A_2
16	F_8-T_4	T_5-O_1	F_8-A_2
17	T_4-T_6	O_1-O_2	T_4-A_2
18	T_6-O_2	O_2-T_6	T_6-A_2

80

the electrical signals produced by these activities are somewhat distorted in EEG recordings and can be better studied with other methods, they may be included in one or more channels of EEG recording to give an estimate of the occurrence of these activities. One or more of these physiological variables may be recorded intermittently to identify sources of artifacts in the EEG. Two or more of these variables are recorded continuously to identify sleep stages in routine recordings from infants and in special sleep studies in subjects of all ages.

4.3.1 *Eye movements* are usually recorded in two channels; monitoring in one channel is less reliable. If two channels are available, one electrode is placed slightly above and to the side of one eye, say the left eye (E1), and connected to input 1 of

TABLE 4.2

Channel No.	16 LB	16 TB	16 R
1	$Fp_1 - F_3$	$Fp_1 - Fp_2$	$F_7 - A_1$
2	$F_3 - C_3$	$F_7 - F_3$	$T_3 - A_1$
3	$C_3 - P_3$	$F_3 - F_z$	$T_5 - A_1$
4	$P_3 - O_1$	$F_z - F_4$	$Fp_1 - A_1$
5	$Fp_2 - F_4$	$F_4 - F_8$	$F_3 - A_1$
6	$F_4 - C_4$	$A_1 - T_3$	$C_3 - A_1$
7	$C_4 - P_4$	$T_3 - C_3$	$P_3 - A_1$
8	$P_4 - O_2$	$C_3 - C_z$	$O_1 - A_1$
9	$Fp_1 - F_7$	$C_z - C_4$	$Fp_2 - A_2$
10	$F_7 - T_3$	$C_4 - T_4$	$F_4 - A_2$
11	$T_3 - T_5$	$T_4 - A_2$	$C_4 - A_2$
12	$T_5 - O_1$	$T_5 - P_3$	$P_4 - A_2$
13	$Fp_2 - F_8$	$P_3 - P_z$	$O_2 - A_2$
14	$F_8 - T_4$	$P_z - P_4$	$F_8 - A_2$
15	$T_4 - T_6$	$P_4 - T_6$	$T_4 - A_2$
16	$T_6 - O_2$	$O_1 - O_2$	$T_6 - A_2$

the first channel. A second electrode is placed slightly below and to the side of the other eye (E2) and connected to input 1 of the second channel. Input 2 of both channels is connected to a reference electrode on the ear or mastoid on the same side as the first electrode, namely the left side. Most eye movements produce deflections of opposite direction in the two channels whereas cerebral activity produces deflections of the same direction if it comes from both frontal electrodes or from the reference electrode, or deflections in only one channel if it comes from one frontal electrode.

If only one channel is used for monitoring of eye movements, electrodes E1 and E2 are connected to input 1 and input 2 of that channel. The recording will not

TABLE 4.3

Channel No.	8 LB − a	8 LB − b	8 TB − a	
1	$Fp_1 - F_3$	$Fp_1 - F_7$	$F_7 - Fp_1$	
2	$F_3 - C_3$	$F_7 - T_3$	$Fp_1 - Fp_2$	
3	$C_3 - P_3$	$T_3 - T_5$	$Fp_2 - F_8$	
4	$P_3 - O_1$	$T_5 - O_1$	$C_3 - C_z$	
5	$Fp_2 - F_4$	$Fp_2 - F_8$	$C_z - C_4$	
6	$F_4 - C_4$	$F_8 - T_4$	$T_5 - O_1$	
7	$C_4 - P_4$	$T_4 - T_6$	$O_1 - O_2$	
8	$P_4 - O_2$	$T_6 - O_2$	$O_2 - T_6$	

Channel No.	8 TB − b	8 TB − c	8 R − a	8 R − b
1	$F_7 - F_3$	$T_3 - C_3$	$F_3 - A_1$	$Fp_1 - A_1$
2	$F_3 - F_z$	$C_3 - C_z$	$C_3 - A_1$	$F_7 - A_1$
3	$F_z - F_4$	$C_z - C_4$	$P_3 - A_1$	$T_3 - A_1$
4	$F_4 - F_8$	$C_4 - T_4$	$O_1 - A_1$	$T_5 - A_1$
5	$T_3 - C_3$	$T_5 - P_3$	$F_4 - A_2$	$Fp_2 - A_2$
6	$C_3 - C_z$	$P_3 - P_z$	$C_4 - A_2$	$F_8 - A_2$
7	$C_z - C_4$	$P_z - P_4$	$P_4 - A_2$	$T_4 - A_2$
8	$C_4 - T_4$	$P_4 - T_6$	$O_2 - A_2$	$T_6 - A_2$

distinguish between horizontal and vertical eye movements or between eye movements and EEG, but EEG recording is unlikely to interfere at the low sensitivity required to record eye movements from this electrode combination.

4.3.2 *Heart beat* may be monitored by connecting an amplifier to an EEG electrode placed on the neck or the chest and to another electrode at some distance away. If electrodes with long lead wires are available, standard ECG electrode positions on the extremities may be used.

TABLE 4.4

Channel No.	18 Inf	16 Inf	16 ECS	8 ECS
1	Fp_1-C_3	Fp_1-C_3	Fp_1-T_3	Fp_1-C_3
2	C_3-O_1	C_3-O_1	T_3-O_1	C_3-O_1
3	Fp_1-T_3	Fp_1-T_3	F_7-T_5	$Fp_2-C.$
4	T_3-O_1	T_3-O_1	Fp_1-C_3	C_4-O_2
5	Fp_2-C_4	Fp_2-C_4	C_3-O_1	T_3-C_z
6	C_4-O_2	C_4-O_2	F_3-P_3	C_z-T_4
7	Fp_2-T_4	Fp_2-T_4	Fp_1-O_1	Hand
8	T_4-O_2	T_4-O_2	Fp_2-O_2	ECG
9	T_3-C_3	T_3-C_3	F_4-P_4	
10	C_3-C_z	C_3-C_z	Fp_2-C_4	
11	C_z-C_4	C_z-C_4	C_4-O_2	
12	C_4-T_4	C_4-T_4	F_8-T_6	
13	EOG	EOG	Fp_2-T_4	
14	EOG	RESP	T_4-O_2	
15	RESP	ECG	Hand	
16	RESP	EMG	ECG	
17	ECG			
18	EMG			

83

4.3.3 *Respiration* is best monitored by recording respiratory body movements or air flow. Respiratory movement may be recorded with a strain gauge or other transducer attached to the chest or abdomen; a pressure-sensitive balloon in the esophagus may be used to monitor intrathoracic pressure changes. Respiratory air flow can be monitored with thermistors taped under the nostrils or near the mouth or incorporated in a small face mask collecting air flow from both nose and mouth. While EEG electrodes cannot monitor respiration, they may be of some use in identifying respiratory artifact in EEG recordings. For this purpose, EEG electrodes may be placed on parts of the patient or the wires from electrodes attached to the patient may be taped or looped around parts of the respiratory equipment which move with respiration (e.g., the ventilator tubing). This should result in recording of movement artifacts corresponding with inspiration and expiration.

4.3.4 *Muscle activity* can be monitored with EEG electrodes placed over the belly of a muscle. To monitor presence of tonic muscle activity in sleep, a channel may be devoted to a pair of electrodes placed on the neck below the chin at equal distances of at least 1–2 cm from the midline to record from submental muscles. Needle electrodes inserted into a muscle may be used to record local muscle activity which can be displayed on an EEG tracing within the limitations of the high frequency response and the paper speed of the particular EEG machine.

4.3.5 *Movement* caused by tremor, myoclonic or convulsive twitching, or movement occurring in coma or sleep, may be monitored by electrodes placed on the moving body parts; such monitoring is likely to indicate the occurrence of movements, but the type of movement must be described on the chart paper during the recording.

4.3.6 *Blood pressure, galvanic skin response, body temperature, eye position, blood oxygen saturation and other slowly changing or sustained activities* require special electrodes or transducers and can be recorded only with EEG machines and polygraphs equipped with directly coupled amplifiers.

see summary

REFERENCES

American EEG Society Guidelines in EEG, 1–7(Revised 1985). (1986) J. clin. Neurophysiol. 3: 131–168 (see appendix in this volume).

Binnie, C.D. (1987) Recording Techniques: Montages, Electrodes, Amplifiers and Filters. In: Halliday, A.M., Butler, S.R. and Paul, R. (Eds.), A Textbook of Clinical Neurophysiology. Wiley, New York, pp. 3–22.

Brazier, M.A.B. (1951) A study of the electrical fields at the surface of the head. Electroenceph. clin. Neurophysiol. Suppl. 2: 38–52.

Cooper, R., Osselton, J.W. and Shaw, J.C. (1981) EEG Technology. 3rd Ed., Butterworth, London.

Gloor, P. (1985) Neuronal generators and the problem of localization in electroencephalography: Application of volume conductor theory to electroencephalography. J. clin. Neurophysiol. 2: 327–354.

Goldman, D. (1950) The clinical use of the 'average' reference electrode in monopolar recording. Electroenceph. clin. Neurophysiol. 2: 211–214.

Gregory, D.L. and Wong, P.K. (1984) Topographical analysis of the centrotemporal discharges in benign Rolandic epilepsy of childhood. Epilepsia 25: 705–711.

Henderson, C.J., Butler, S.R. and Glass, A. (1975) The localization of equivalent dipoles of EEG sources by the application of electrical field theory. Electroenceph. clin. Neurophysiol. 39: 117–130.

Homan, R.W., Herman, J. and Purdy, P. (1987) Cerebral location of international 10–20 system electrode placement. Electroenceph. clin. Neurophysiol., 66: 376–382.

Katznelson, R.D. (1981) EEG recording electrode placement and aspects of generator location. In: P.L. Nunez (Ed.) Electric Fields of the Brain, Oxford University Press, London, pp. 176–213.

Klass, D.W. (1977) Symposium on EEG montages: Which, when, why and whither. Introduction. Am. J. EEG Technol. 17: 1–3.

Knott, J.R. (1985) Further thoughts on polarity, montages and localization. J. clin. Neurophysiol. 2: 63–75.

Lesser, R.P., Luders, H., Dinner, D.S. and Morris, H. (1985) An introduction to the basic concepts of polarity and localization. J. clin. Neurophysiol. 2: 46–61.

Mac Gillivray, B.B. (1974) Section II. Derivations and montages. In: Rémond, A. (Ed.), Handbook of Electroenceph. clin. Neurophysiol., Vol. 3C, Elsevier, Amsterdam, pp. 22–57.

Magnus, O. (1961) On the technique of location by electroencephalography. Electroenceph. clin. Neurophysiol. Suppl. 19: 1–35.

Niedermeyer, E. (1987) The EEG signal: polarity and field determination. In: Niedermeyer, E. and Lopas da Silva, F. (Eds.), Electroencephalography: Basic Principles, Clinical Applications and Related Fields. Urban and Schwarzenberg, Baltimore, pp. 79–84.

Offner, F.F. (1950) The EEG as potential mapping: The value of the average monopolar reference. Electroenceph. clin. Neurophysiol. 2: 215–216.

Osselton, J.W. (1966) Bipolar, unipolar and average reference recording methods. I. Mainly theoretical considerations. Am. J. EEG Technol. 6: 129–141.

Osselton, J.W. (1969) Bipolar, unipolar and average reference recording methods. II. Mainly practical considerations. Am. J. EEG Technol. 9: 117–133.

Schneider, M. and Gerin, P. (1970) Une méthode de localisation des dipôles cérébraux. Electroenceph. clin. Neurophysiol. 28: 69–78.

Sharbrough, F.W. (1977) The mathematical logic for the design of montages. Am. J. EEG Technol. 17: 73–83.

Tursky, B. (1974) Recording of human eye movements. In: Thompson, R.F. and Patterson, M.M. (Eds.), Bioelectric Recording Techniques, Vol. 1C, Academic Press, New York, pp. 99–135.

The product of the recording: The clinical EEG record

5

SUMMARY

The clinical EEG record should contain a reasonable representation of the normal and abnormal patterns needed for clinical interpretation. To serve this purpose, the recording methods must meet certain general technical requirements. Special requirements are made of recordings from infants and small children, of all-night sleep recordings, of recordings evaluating suspected cerebral death, and of recordings transmitted by telephone. These requirements are described in 'Guidelines in EEG' issued by the American EEG Society.

(5.1) *General technical standards.* At least 21 recording electrodes should be placed according to the International 10–20 System, each with an electrical contact of less than 5000 ohms impedance. The recording should have at least 8 channels. The sensitivity of the amplifiers should initially be set at 5–10 μV/mm and then adjusted as necessary. Filters should be set with the cutoff frequency (30% attenuation) of the low frequency filter at 1 Hz and the high frequency filter at 70 Hz. The record should be calibrated at the beginning and end by calibration pulses, an electrode test, and by a test recording using cerebral activity from the same electrode pair in all channels. Paper speed is usually set at 3 cm/sec. At least 20 minutes of artifact-free recording should be obtained during wakefulness. Wakefulness should *always* be clearly demonstrated by asking alerting questions (e.g., date, calculations) and recording the patient's responses on the record. In addition, recording during hyperventilation, photic stimulation and sleep should be performed when a convulsive disorder is suspected.

The record should be labelled with the patient's name and age, date and time of the recording and other important information. During the recording, notations should be made to indicate the instrument settings, the patient's behavior and any event which could influence the recording or produce artifacts.

(5.2) *Standards for recordings from infants and small children* are the same as the general standards with a few exceptions. A smaller number of electrodes may be used in newborns. Eight-channel machines are insufficient for newborns because recordings should include monitoring of eye movements, respiration, heart beat and muscle activity. Sensitivity and filter settings must be adjusted to display slower and larger potentials than are typical in adult recordings. Recordings in newborns usually require over one hour to include a full cycle of quiet sleep. Labelling of the record must precisely reflect the patient's condition, position and all changes during the recording; the gestational and conceptional ages must be indicated for newborns.

(5.3) *Standards for recordings in cases of suspected cerebral death* are designed to produce a record which unequivocally answers the question whether or not any cortical activity is present. Electrocerebral

impedance < 5,000 ohms / > 100 ohms

paper speed = 3 cm/sec

Filters 1 – 70 Hz

* biocalibration

inactivity (ECI), or electrocerebral silence, is defined as no EEG activity over 2 μV when recording from scalp electrode pairs 10 or more cm apart with inter-electrode impedances under 10,000 ohms, but over 100 ohms. There are 10 minimum technical requirements for recording ECI (as described in section 5.3). Recordings demonstrating the absence of electrocerebral activity should not be called 'flat', 'isoelectric' or 'linear' because, if done properly, they virtually always pick up activity from extracerebral sources. Telephone transmission should not be used for these recordings.

(5.4) *Standards for EEG transmission by telephone* require one fully trained technician and one fully equipped EEG machine at both the transmitting and the receiving sites. The recordings at both sites should be identical and include all notes and comments made during the recording by the transmitting technician. These requirements can be fulfilled with current techniques except for some restrictions on high frequencies and limitations on the high sensitivities required for evaluation of cerebral death.

5.1 GENERAL TECHNICAL STANDARDS

Good clinical EEG recordings must satisfy many technical requirements. The American EEG Society has issued 'Guidelines in EEG and Evoked Potentials' (see reference at end of chapter) which contain minimum technical requirements for performing clinical electroencephalography. Eight of those guidelines apply specifically to EEG practice and have been reproduced in Appendix 1. This chapter summarizes the 5 guidelines that discuss technical aspects of EEG and includes additional information that the editor has found useful.

(1) *Electrode types.*   Silver–silver chloride or gold electrodes are preferred, but adequate recordings can also be obtained with other electrode materials (e.g., tin). One should always, when possible, avoid mixing different kinds of electrodes in the same patient because of the likelihood of increasing electrical interference (due to impedance mismatches). In general, electrodes are best applied with collodian. The main advantages of collodian are that the electrodes remain firmly attached without changing position over time and are functional for long periods of time (hours). At the end of the recording electrodes are removed by dissolving the collodian with acetone. Because the fumes from acetone are potentially noxious, adequate ventila-

tion is important and must always be kept in mind. For example, if a young infant is in an isolette and cannot be at least partially removed from it and placed under warming lights then collodian and acetone should not be used. In such circumstances electrode pastes should be substituted for collodian. Pastes are less desirable for routine use because they do not firmly anchor the electrodes to the head. In addition, paste is suboptimal for recordings lasting more than 30 to 60 minutes since drying of the paste will result in poor electrical contact.

(2) *Electrode placements.*   At least 21 recording electrodes should be used and placed according to the International 10–20 System. Additional electrodes may be placed between the standard electrodes to localize very circumscribed activity. A ground electrode should be added and connected to the ground input of the EEG machine unless the patient is connected to ground through other electrical equipment.

If electrode positions were not measured but only estimated, the terms '10–20 System' or 'modified 10–20 System' should not be used, but the term 'estimated 10–20 System' may be applied. Recordings which do not use the 10–20 System should define the relationship between the electrode placements used and those of the 10–20 System.

(3) *Electrode impedance.*   The impedance of disc electrodes should be checked routinely before every recording (2.2) and should not exceed 5000 ohms. Electrode impedances should not exceed 5000 ohms except in the case of needle electrodes where higher impedances cannot be avoided. Although the EEG Society does not state a particular frequency of alternating current for impedance measurements, a frequency of about 10 Hz is most appropriate. Electrode impedance should also be checked when an unusual EEG pattern suggests the possibility of an artifact.

(4) *Number of recording channels.*   The EEG should be recorded on at least 8 channels at the same time. Sixteen or more channels are preferred because: (1) the likelihood of correctly localizing intermittent abnormalities increases with the

Range: 100 – 5,000 Ω

number of recording channels; and (2) certain recordings (e.g., neonatal recordings) require additional channels for physiological monitoring.

(5) *Montages.* Recordings should routinely include at least one longitudinal bipolar (LB), one transverse bipolar (TB), and one referential (R) montage as recommended by the American EEG Society (4.2.4). Additional montages should also be as simple as possible, easy to describe and easy to interpret. They should use electrodes along straight lines and with equal interelectrode distances. Activity from the front of the head should be displayed at the top of the record, activity from the back at the bottom. In addition, in North America left-sided leads should be placed above right sided leads for either alternating pairs of derivations or blocks of derivations.

(6) *Sensitivity.* The sensitivity at the beginning of a routine recording should be set at 5–10 μV/mm for all channels. A commonly used sensitivity setting is 7 μV/mm which results in a pen deflection of about 7 mm for a calibration pulse of 50 μV. The sensitivity of all channels should be adjusted during the recording so that the full range of the pen deflection is used to its best advantage: The EEG should be shown with good resolution and without driving the pens to the extremes or flattening the tracing.

(7) *Filters.* During the recording, the low frequency filter should be routinely set at 1 Hz and the high frequency filter at 70 Hz. On most EEG machines this corresponds to no more than a 30% (−3dB) attenuation of activity at 1 Hz (i.e., a low frequency filter time constant setting of approximately 0.16 seconds) and 70 Hz. These settings therefore produce an increasing attenuation of activity below 1 Hz or above 70 Hz. They should be changed only to emphasize or clarify unusual EEG patterns. Changing filter settings should be a temporary maneuver, and the technician should write the new filter settings and the reason why they were changed on the record. It is important to be aware that changing filter settings may produce misleading results. For example, slow activity may be removed by setting the low

We use 0.5 – 70

90

frequency filter at a higher frequency. Setting the high frequency filter at a lower frequency than usual may give high frequency artifact (e.g., muscle artifact) the appearance of epileptiform spikes or fast background activity.

(8) *Calibration*. Each record should be calibrated by applying known voltages to all channels at the beginning and the end of the recording. The calibration at the end should include calibration pulses recorded at each of the various combinations of sensitivity and filter settings used in the recording. The calibration pulses should have voltages strong enough to produce pen deflections of 7 mm or more, so that differences of 5% or more between channels can be detected; the pulses should not be so strong that they overdrive the pen deflection. Calibration pulses of different voltage need to be used for different sensitivity settings. If the amplitude, shape, horizontal and vertical alignment of the calibration pulses differs between channels, the cause for these differences must be determined and eliminated.

In addition to the square wave calibration, a biological calibration (also referred to as *biocalibration*) may be performed by recording the same electrode pair in every channel. For this purpose, a frontal and an occipital electrode provide a relatively high amplitude signal by virtue of the long interelectrode distance and will include a variety of activities (eye blinks, the alpha rhythm, etc.). Although this can be helpful for evaluating the pen, filter and amplifier function, it should be recognized that a careful inspection of the square-wave calibration is actually a much more precise way of evaluating these components. Another useful procedure is the performance of an electrode test at the beginning and at the end of each recording. This may alert the technician to any abnormalities of electrode contact that have occurred since the time of application. It also informs the electroencephalographer whether or not the electrodes have been adequately applied and if good contact has been maintained throughout the recording.

(9) *Paper speed*. A speed of 30 mm/sec is recommended internationally and is used routinely in most laboratories. Slower speeds may also be used, for instance

91

in neonatal recordings, or to emphasize slower waveforms. Faster speeds are helpful for evaluating fast events, such as time relationships between similar waves in different channels or 60 Hz artifact.

(10) *Length of the recording.* Each montage should be recorded for at least 2 minutes. The waking record should contain at least 20 minutes of artifact-free recording at rest including brief periods when the eyes are open (11.1.6). This period does not include the time required for hyperventilation, photic stimulation and sleep recordings.

(11) *Hyperventilation.* Overbreathing should be used routinely except when contraindicated by diseases of the heart and lungs, sickle cell disease (or trait), Moya Moya disease, other cerebrovascular diseases associated with borderline cerebral blood perfusion, and acute cerebral disorders. The technician should explain and demonstrate hyperventilation, and note the quality of the patient's effort on the record. The EEG should be recorded during and for at least one minute after hyperventilation or longer if hyperventilation induces abnormalities.

(12) *Photic stimulation.* This activation procedure should be used whenever possible because it can induce diagnostically important abnormalities. It may, on rare occasions, induce seizures (which are almost always generalized); this may happen both in patients with a history of seizures and, extremely rarely, in patients without such a history. However, the development of seizures can usually be avoided if photic stimulation is stopped as soon as seizure activity appears.

Photic stimulation is performed with a stroboscopic lamp producing bright flashes of diffuse light. The lamp is placed approximately 30 cm from the patient's eyes. Flashes are given at varying rates typically including 1, 3, 5, 10, 13, 15, 17, 20 and 25 Hz in trains lasting about 10 seconds. Thorough testing includes periods when the eyes are closed, open, and while they are being opened and closed. The occurrence of each flash is monitored on a separate channel using a synchronizing pulse of the flash generator. The monitor pulse is displayed on an auxiliary channel, if available, or on a recording channel.

(13) *Sleep*.   A period of EEG recording during sleep should be obtained in addition to the 20-min waking baseline recording in patients with suspected or known convulsive disorders. To increase the chance of obtaining a sleep recording, many laboratories ask patients to avoid sleeping the night before the recording.

If sleep does not occur spontaneously, it may be induced with a sedative such as chloral hydrate. Chloral hydrate is preferred because, unlike benzodiazepines or barbiturates, minimum sedating doses usually do not induce excessive beta activity. Since patient sedation has obvious legal implications, when possible, patients should be advised to be accompanied by a responsible adult. After the test patients should also be instructed not to drive or to engage in other potentially dangerous activities.

(14) *Special procedures* which are of risk to the patient should be carried out only for specific indications and then only in the presence of a qualified physician, in an environment with adequate resuscitation equipment, and with the informed consent of the patient, responsible relative or guardian.

(15) *Labelling and editing of the record*.   Proper labelling of the record is of the greatest importance; even a technically perfect EEG is useless without written comments by the technician. The technician must describe (a) the patient's medical characteristics, (b) the patient's behavior during the recording, (c) the montages, and (d) the instrument settings.

(a) *The description of the patient* should be written on the record and include at least the patient's name and age, the date and time of the recording, a list of all current medications, the time of the last meal, the name, amount and time of administration of any sedative taken during or shortly before the recording. Failure to document this information on the record can lead to serious medical and legal problems.

In addition to these minimum requirements, the technician should write down other important information. Cranial defects or abnormalities, scalp lacerations and contusions should be identified in a head diagram explaining the spatial relation between the abnormalities and the recording electrodes, especially where the abnormalities necessitated deviations from the electrode placements of the 10–20 System. The technician may obtain important information from the patient or the patient's chart, and thus complement the information given by the referring physician. Items of special importance are a history and description of seizures, head injuries and significant diseases, the provisional diagnosis, reason for the EEG recording, abnormal laboratory test results, etc. Previous EEG recordings of the same patient should be available at least at the time of the interpretation.

(b) *The description of the patient during the recording.* The technician should indicate the patient's level of alertness, namely awake, drowsy, asleep or comatose, and any change of that level occurring during the recording. Unusual behavior such as restlessness, agitation, confusion, failure to cooperate, abnormal speech, hearing and vision should be noted. The technician should try to recognize every movement of the patient, especially eye movements including eye blinks, eye opening and closing, movements of the face and head, swallowing, chewing, talking, coughing, sneezing, etc.; each movement should be indicated on the record at the time it occurs, especially if it causes an artifact in the recording. If there is any doubt whether an artifact is due to any such movement, the technician should ask the patient to repeat the movement and mark the request and the patient's response on the record. During the waking portion of the recording *the patient should always be asked alerting questions* such as the date and double digit calculations. This is necessary because mild normal background slowing due to drowsiness may occur even during commands to open and close the eyes or during hyperventilation. If the patient is unable to answer aforementioned questions correctly then simpler ones should be asked until a correct response is obtained. If seizure activity is suggested by a movement of the patient or by the appearance of epileptiform activity in the EEG, the technician should test the responsiveness of the patient by asking him how he feels and, if there is no answer, giving him a test word to remember. Later, when

94

the patient is responsive, the technician should ask the patient if he or she remembers what was said. These questions and the answers should be written on the record. If epileptiform activity appears frequently or if it can be triggered by stimulation, the technician may ask the patient to count or to recite a nursery rhyme and note any interruptions by spontaneous or triggered epileptiform activity. A more precise measure of reactivity can be obtained by having the patient push a button in response to an auditory tone activated by the technician. Both the patient's and the technician's button presses are recorded on one of the EEG channels. In this way the technician can quickly test reactivity when unusual or epileptiform patterns occur. Most EEG equipment manufacturers offer auditory response testing devices as an option.

The technician should rate the patient's performance of hyperventilation as good, fair or poor. After hyperventilation, the patient should be asked how he felt during hyperventilation and, especially, whether hyperventilation reproduced or intensified any of his usual symptoms. The patient's response should be written on the chart.

In essence, the technician should continuously monitor the patient's behavior and document every movement and every word spoken during the recording. This is necessary because most artifacts can be positively identified only during the recording by correlating pen deflections with movements or other events. The technician is in the unique position of being able to make the diagnosis of a seizure by demonstrating a loss of responsiveness or documenting other, sometimes subtle, behavioral seizure manifestations during the occurrence of epileptiform activity in the EEG. The reader, if unaware of the patient's behavior, may be unable to identify many artifacts of to diagnose a seizure.

(c) *Description of montages*.　The electrode combinations selected for each channel must be clearly indicated at the beginning of each run. This may be done in one of several ways. (1) Abbreviations of the electrode placements used as input 1 and input 2 may be written in front of the tracing of each channel as in Tables

4.1–4.3. (2) Using a head diagram, the tracing of each channel may be connected to two electrode placements in the diagram; a solid line is commonly used to indicate the electrode connected to input 1, and a broken line is used to indicate the electrode connected to input 2; this method is used for many of the EEG illustrations in this text. (3) Electrode placements in the head diagram may be connected with arrows, each arrow being labelled with the number of the channel it represents and pointing from the electrode at input 1 to the electrode at input 2; this method is used in the illustration of montages in this text (Figs. 4.4 and 4.5). (4) Rubber stamps giving a list of the electrodes or a diagrammatic representation of a montage are used in some laboratories, but they can lead to errors more easily than other, less automatic methods. Montages should not be labelled with code names such as 'montage A' or 'run 1' because the meaning of the code may be unknown to the EEG reader.

(d) *Description of instrument settings.* The settings of master and individual channel switches controlling sensitivity and filters should be indicated at the beginning of each run and during calibration; the voltage of the calibration pulse must be identified. Every change of these settings and of chart speed must be indicated on the record when it is made and the affected channels must be clearly specified.

5.2 STANDARDS FOR PEDIATRIC RECORDINGS

Most of the general technical standards also apply to this age group. However, there are a few exceptions which are summarized in the guidelines of the American EEG Society on 'Minimum technical standards for pediatric electroencephalography' and are detailed below (see also 10.1).

(1) *Electrode types.* Silver–silver chloride electrodes in the shape of a cup with a central hole for injection of conductive jelly (2.2.1) are best. Application with col-

lodion is recommended because children are more likely than adults to move and
produce artifacts. Collodion and acetone should *never* be used in isolettes and other
areas with limited air circulation or explosion hazards; electrodes may be applied
with electrode paste under these circumstances.

(2) *Electrode placements*.   Newborn infants, especially those with small heads,
do not need the full number of electrodes prescribed by the 10–20 System. A
minimum reduced array includes the following electrodes: Fp1, Fp2, C3, Cz, C4,
T3, T4, O1, O2, A1 and A2. If the baby's earlobes are too small, mastoid electrodes
M1 and M2 may be substituted for A1 and A2. Fp3 and Fp4 have been suggested
as alternative placements to Fp1 and Fp2 because they are more anatomically correct; the frontal lobes of neonates and young infants occupy a relatively more
posterior position in relation to Fp1 and Fp2 than in adults. Fp3 and Fp4 are placed
midway between the Fp1 and F3 and Fp2 and F4 positions.

(3) *Number of recording channels*.   Instruments with only 8 channels are
undesirable for recording neonates and young infants (i.e., patients less than 48
weeks conceptual age). Sixteen or more channels are preferred since 4 or more will
be occupied by physiological monitors. Examples of montages are listed in Chapter
4 (Table 4.4).

(4) *Montages*.   Recordings from newborns need continuous monitoring of extracerebral electrical activity to identify alertness and sleep states and to recognize
artifacts and abnormalities of breathing and heart rate. Most important is monitoring of respiration, eye movement, muscle tone (submental EMG monitor), and ECG
(see also 10.1).

(5) *Sensitivity*.   The sensitivity needs to be adjusted more often in infants and
young children; their EEG may have fairly high amplitude so that sensitivity needs
to be reduced to 10 or 15 μV/mm. The sensitivity of channels monitoring extracerebral activity of newborns must be adjusted according to the output; eye
movements and submental EMG should be recorded at 7 and 3 μV/mm respectively.

For the respirogram, the sensitivity should be adjusted as necessary to yield a clear deflection with each respiration.

(6) *Filters.* EEG recordings from infants should use time constants between 0.27 and 0.53 sec, i.e. low filter frequency settings which reduce the amplitude of sine waves of 0.3 to 0.6 Hz by 30% (-3 dB). Eye movements should be monitored with the same filter settings. EMG recordings should be made with higher settings of the low frequency filter (about 5 Hz; time constant 0.03 sec) and with the highest setting of the high frequency filter. Respiration should be monitored with very low settings of the low frequency filter but not with direct coupling.

(7) *Length of the recording.* Newborns require usually over one hour of recording to show both active sleep and a full cycle of quiet sleep. The chances of obtaining such a recording are best when the EEG is scheduled at feeding time and the baby is fed after application of the electrodes. Sedation should not be used to obtain a sleep record in newborns. Shorter recording periods than one hour are acceptable only when the EEG is grossly abnormal; even then, a period of one hour may be required to demonstrate the absence of variability.

Children may produce so many artifacts by moving and other mechanisms that satisfactory waking records of the length recommended for adults cannot be obtained; recordings during sleep may then provide the only useful information. In patients over three months of age, the technician should attempt to obtain recordings during wakefulness when the patient's eyes are open and when they are closed; passive eye closure, accomplished by placing the technician's hand over the patient's eyes, may be used to demonstrate the reactivity of EEG rhythms (11.1.6).

(8) *Photic stimulation.* Flashes of 1–30 Hz should be used during wakefulness if indicated for activation in children. Repetitive photic stimulation is not useful for newborns.

(9) *Labelling and editing the record.* In addition to the requirements described for EEG recordings in general, recordings from infants must state the baby's

gestational age at birth and conceptional age, i.e. gestational age plus time since birth, in weeks, together with the chronological age since birth. Other relevant information, such as levels of blood gases and serum electrolytes, should be noted for the use of the electroencephalographer. Before recording EEGs of infants and young hospital patients, especially those requiring bedside recording, the technician should consult with the nursing staff concerning the patient's condition and any limitations on recording procedures. The patient's condition should be clearly indicated at the beginning of every montage; the position of head and eyelids of infants should be noted. Changes of position and other movements must be monitored as carefully as in adults. Stuporous or comatose patients and patients showing an invariant EEG pattern should be given visual, auditory and somatosensory stimulation. The stimuli and the patient's responses should be indicated on the recording paper at the time of their occurrence; absence of responses must also be noted. Infants should be stimulated only at the end of the recording period to avoid interruption of sleep cycles.

5.3 STANDARDS FOR RECORDINGS IN CASES OF SUSPECTED CEREBRAL DEATH

The EEG is an important tool in the evaluation of cerebral death, a diagnosis often considered in victims of severe cerebral damage characterized by coma, absent or insufficient spontaneous respiration and absent brain stem reflexes. This diagnosis requires, amongst other criteria, repeated demonstrations of the absence of electrocerebral activity of over 2 μV in amplitude. For adults and older children, electrocerebral inactivity (ECI) found in one recording is considered highly reliable for the determination of cortical death, unless the recording was made in the presence of either: (1) drugs depressing the central nervous system, (2) significant hypothermia, or (3) circulatory shock. However, younger children, especially those under one year of age, can survive longer periods of ECI without cerebral death. In such cases two recordings separated by a 24-h interval should be performed. ECI is defined by the American EEG Society as *no EEG activity over 2 μV when recording from scalp electrode pairs 10 or more cm apart with inter-electrode impedances under 10,000 ohms, but over 100 ohms.*

Recording techniques in cases of suspected cerebral death must be designed to search for any trace of cerebral activity and take special precautions to avoid the possibility that failure to record EEG activity is due to faulty methods or equipment rather than to absent cerebral activity. The American EEG Society has issued guidelines of 'Minimum technical standards for EEG recording in suspected cerebral death'; the guidelines are summarized and discussed here.

(1) *Electrode placements.* *At least 8 scalp electrodes should be used* and placed in the frontopolar (Fp1, Fp2), central (C3, C4), temporal (T3, T4) and occipital (O1, O2) positions on both sides. Additional electrodes may be placed in the frontal areas (F3, F4), at the vertex (Cz) and on the earlobes (A1, A2), mastoids, mandibular angles or noncephalic reference points. A ground electrode should be added but not connected if other electrical equipment is attached to the patient (3.1). It is preferable whenever possible to employ a full set of recording electrodes (i.e., all 21 electrodes of the routine 10–20 system). Thus, the full set of recording electrodes should be applied at the start of the recording and an initial recording employing all of them is recommended.

(2) *Electrode impedance.* *Inter-electrode impedances should be under 10,000 ohms and over 100 ohms.* In addition, the impedance of all electrodes should be similar to reduce the chance of artifacts caused by an imbalance of amplifier inputs.

(3) *Testing the integrity of the recording system.* If a recording at high sensitivity and wide interelectrode distances shows no electrocerebral activity, it is necessary to demonstrate that this is not due to a fault of the recording system. The recording of calibration pulses does not entirely exclude this possibility because it

tests the recording system only between the inputs of the amplifiers and the penwriters whereas the fault may lie between the electrodes and the amplifier input. To test this part of the recording system, each electrode should be touched gently with a pencil or cotton swab during the recording; the electrode touched and the moment of touching should be indicated on the chart. Touching an electrode should create an artifact in the recording channels connected to that electrode. This artifact verifies that (a) the electrode is capable of recording, and (b) the correct electrode is selected for that channel.

(4) *Interelectrode distances.* *Interelectrode distances of at least 10 cm should be used* because recording with shorter distances may attenuate amplitude. Referential montages may use the Cz electrode as the reference for long interelectrode distances. Ear reference recording nearly always contains too much ECG artifact to be useful. More than one montage should be used depending on how many recording channels are available; examples of useful 16-channel and 8-channel montages are illustrated in Chapter 4 (4.2.4). If occipital leads are difficult to attach or pick up too much movement artifact induced by artificial respiration, the combinations F7-T5, F3-P3, Fz-Pz, F4-P4 and F8-T6 may give better results.

(5) *Sensitivity.* A sensitivity of at least 2 μV/mm, or a higher sensitivity such as 1 μV/mm, should be used *for at least 30 minutes* (see below). This is very important because activity of 2 μV, i.e. the critical amplitude for electrocerebral silence, cannot be clearly distinguished at lower sensitivities. If possible a sensitivity setting of 1.5 or 1 μV/mm will allow the electroencephalographer to make a more confident assessment of low amplitude, and particularly slow frequency, activity.

(6) *Filters.* Filter settings should not attenuate any electrocerebral activity, especially very slow waves which are likely to occur in deep coma. Attempts should be made to record with low frequency filters set no higher than 1 Hz and with high frequency filters set no lower than 30 Hz. The 60 Hz filter should be used as needed.

(7) *Additional monitoring techniques should be employed when necessary.*

Because of the high sensitivity and wide interelectrode distances, recordings in suspected cerebral death are very likely to pick up artifacts. Possible sources of artifacts should be monitored (4.3). As a minimum, heart beat and movement should be included in the recordings (4.2.4).

(8) *Stimulation of the patient.* The reactivity of the EEG of comatose patients should be tested by stimulation with sudden loud sounds and by stimuli which produce pain in wakeful persons, for instance pinching of the skin. Flashes of bright light may also be used. The type and the moment of stimulation and the behavioral reaction of the patient, including the absence of a reaction, should be noted on the chart. The tracing may show different types of reactions: Transient EEG activity may be induced in some patients who have no spontaneous EEG activity or extra-cerebral responses may be elicited (e.g., frontal potentials representing the retinal response to light flashes).

(a) *Artifacts arising from heart beat* are very common and consist of ECG components, pulse waves and ballistic movements transmitted to the head and electrode wires.

(b) *Movement* of the patient may cause artifact which can be monitored with two electrodes on the back of the right hand, separated by 6–7 cm.

(c) *Respiratory artifact*, if impossible to eliminate by positioning of the patient and equipment, should be monitored during at least part of the recording. Stopping the respirator momentarily may help to identify respiratory artifact that cannot be eliminated.

(d) Electrical interference may be evaluated by connecting a resistor of 10,000 Ω between the inputs of one amplifier and placing it near the patient. This 'dummy patient' is representative of the electrical impedances of the EEG electrodes on the patient and can indicate the amount and type of interference from sources other than the patient.

(e) *Muscle artifact* may obscure the tracing. If it cannot be eliminated by

102

repositioning of the patient or massaging the muscles near the contaminated recording electrode, a neuromuscular blocking agent such as pancuronium bromide (Pavulon) or succinylcholine (Anectine) may be used under the supervision of a physician.

(f) *Determining the presence of low amplitude rhythmical artifact* can sometimes be made easier by overlaying two pages of the EEG and aligning identical channels in front of a bright light or against a white sheet of paper. One page of EEG can then be moved relative to the other to inspect for the presence of superimposable repetitive waveforms.

(9) *Recordings should be made only by a qualified technologist.* Recordings in cases of possible cerebral death should be made only by technicians who have had supervised instruction and recording experience in intensive care units and who work under the direct supervision of a qualified electroencephalographer.

(10) *Repeat recordings.* If technical or other problems leave any uncertainty about the diagnosis of electrocerebral silence, the entire recording should be repeated after a few hours.

5.4 TELEPHONE TRANSMISSION

Recommendations for telephone transmission of EEGs have been included in the guidelines of the American EEG Society and in the report of the Committee on EEG Instrumentation Standards of the International Federation of Societies for EEG and Clinical Neurophysiology. The recommendations generally stipulate that technical standards of EEG recording should not be lowered by telephone transmission. This requires two fully trained technicians and two complete EEG recording machines. The machines should be connected so that the EEG at the transmitting site is completely and faithfully duplicated at the receiving site; at present, this requirement cannot be entirely fulfilled because currently used conventional telephone systems limit transmission of high frequencies for an 8-channel EEG to about 50 Hz and may introduce artifacts into recordings of low amplitude. However, these limitations may be acceptable in most cases. Specific recommendations for telephone transmission are listed below.

(1) *Technicians* at both the transmitting and receiving laboratories should be fully trained and qualified EEG technicians. In addition, they should be familiar with telephone transmission techniques and, if possible, with each other's laboratories.

(2) *Duplicate EEG records* should be produced. Recording a copy at the transmitting site is required so that the transmitting technician can correlate ongoing EEG activity with the patient's behavior and identify and eliminate artifacts. The requirement for a copy at the transmitting site may be eliminated in the future if acceptable alternative methods of monitoring the EEG at the transmitting site become available.

The comments of the transmitting technician, especially those which are vital for the identification of artifacts, should be transmitted simultaneously with the EEG to the receiving site. This can be done by signals in a standard code which temporarily replace the EEG recorded in one channel. Such a signalling system may be supplemented by intermittent voice communications between transmitting and receiving sites. A fail-safe code should be included to indicate technical problems, especially the loss of signal at the receiving site during transmission.

(3) *Fidelity of the recording*: The tracing at the transmitting and receiving sites should be identical. As mentioned above, this is currently possible for recordings not including frequencies over 50 Hz and not consisting of very low amplitude activity.

(4) *Cerebral death* cannot be evaluated appropriately by recordings transmitted over the telephone because artifacts from telephone networks may appear and obscure or mimick electrocerebral activity of low amplitude.

see summary *see appendix II p. 537*

REFERENCES

American EEG Society Guidelines in EEG and Evoked Potentials. (1986) J. clin. Neurophysiol. Vol. 3 (Suppl. 1): 1–148.

Alvarez, L.A., Moshe, S.L., Belman, A.L., Maytal, J., Resnick, T.J. and Keilson, M. (1988) EEG and brain death determination in children. Neurology 38: 227–230.

Ashwal, S. and Schneider, S. (1979) Failure of electroencephalography to diagnose brain death in comatose children. Ann. Neurol. 6: 512–517.

Bennett, D.R., Hughes, J.R., Korein, J., Merlis, J.K. and Suter, C. (1976) An Atlas of Electroencephalography in Coma and Cerebral Death. Raven Press, New York.

Chatrian, G.E. (1986) Electrophysiologic evaluation of brain death: a critical appraisal. In: Aminoff, M.J. (Ed.), Electrodiagnosis in clinical neurology. Churchill-Livingstone, New York, pp. 669–736.

Green, J.B. and Lauber, A. (1972) Return of EEG activity after electrocerebral silence: Two case reports. J. Neurol. Neurosurg. Psychiat. 35: 103–107.

Guidelines for the determination of brain death in children. Report of the Task Force. (1987) Neurology 37: 1077–1078.

Hanley, J.W. (1981) A step-by-step approach to neonatal EEG. Am. J. EEG Technol. 21: 1–13.

International Federation of Societies for Electroencephalography and Clinical Neurophysiology: Recommendations for the Practice of Clinical Neurophysiology (1983). Elsevier, Amsterdam.

Klem, G.H. (1979) Some problems of bedside EEG recording. Am. J. EEG Technol. 19: 19–29.

Mizrahi, E.M. (1986) Neonatal Electroencephalography: Clinical features of the newborn, techniques of recording, and characteristics of the normal EEG. Am. J. EEG Tech. 26: 81–103.

Rechtschaffen, A. and Kales, A. (1968) A Manual of Standardized Terminology, Techniques and Scoring System for Sleep Stages of Human Subjects, U.S. Government Printing Office, Washington.

Saunders, M.G. (1979) Minimum technical requirements for performing clinical electroencephalography: Illustrative examples of principles on which some of the technical guidelines of the American EEG Society are based. In: D.W. Klass and D.D. Daly (Eds.), Current Practice of Clinical Electroencephalography, Raven Press, New York, pp. 7–26.

Werner, S.S., Stockard, J.E. and Bickford, R.G. (1977) Atlas of Neonatal Electroencephalography, Raven Press, New York.

Artifacts

6

SUMMARY

Artifacts are recorded signals that are non-cerebral in origin. They may be divided into one of two categories depending on their origin: *physiological artifacts* or *non-physiological artifacts*.

(6.1) *Physiological artifacts* arise from a variety of body activities that are either due to (1) *movements*: movements of the head, body, or scalp (e.g., pulsations of the scalp arteries, scalp muscle movement), (2) *bioelectrical potentials*: from moving electrical potentials within the body (such as those produced by eye, tongue and pharyngeal muscle movement), or electrical potentials generated by the scalp muscles, heart or sweat glands, or (3) *skin resistance changes*: due to sweat gland activity, perspiration and vasomotor activity.

(6.2) and (6.3) *Non-physiological artifacts* arise from two main sources: (1) *external electrical interference* from other power sources such as power lines or electrical equipment, and (2) *internal electrical malfunctioning of the recording system*, arising from recording electrodes, electrode positioning, cables, amplifiers, pen motors or the paper drive.

6.1 ARTIFACTS FROM THE PATIENT

One of the most common reasons for misinterpreting the EEG is the failure to correctly identify non-cerebral potentials. Although artifacts can often be recognized by their characteristic shape and distribution, in many cases a positive identification can only be made by the technologist during the recording. It is therefore extremely important that the technologist be skilled in the identification and elimination of artifacts. The patient and record must be closely observed throughout the recording and notations made whenever artifacts occur.

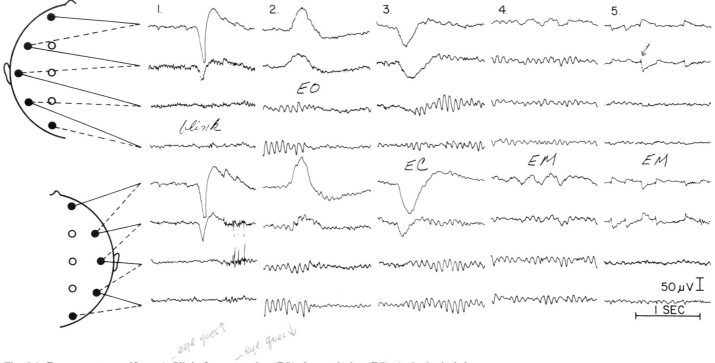

Fig. 6.1. Eye movement artifacts. 1. Blink, 2. eye opening (EO), 3. eye closing (EC), 4. rhythmical slow eye movements (EM), 5. saccadic eye movements (EM) preceded by spicules due to contraction of lateral eye muscles. Tracings show the technician's notations made during the recording to identify the cause of the artifacts.

6.1.1 *Blinking and other eye movements.* These movements cause potential changes which are picked up mainly by frontal electrodes, although they may extend into central and temporal electrodes. A simple but useful way of understanding eye movement artifacts is to picture the front of the eye as a positive charge that either moves towards or away from the recording electrodes. The electrodes that record the largest potential change with vertical eye movements are Fp1 and Fp2 because they are placed directly above the eye. The electrodes that record the largest potential change with horizontal (lateral) eye movements are F7 and F8 because they are approximately lateral to the eyes. In a typical longitudinal bipolar montage an upward vertical eye movement (e.g., eye closure, eye blink) will produce a downward deflection in Fp1-F3 or Fp1-F7 because the positively charged cornea is moving towards Fp1 making it increasingly more positive (Fig. 6.1, 6.3). If the eyes move to the left, in a lateral direction, then F7 will record the greatest increase in positivity and F8 will record the greatest negativity (in this case the negativity recorded by F8 is caused by a loss of positivity as the cornea moves away from it). Therefore the pen will deflect up in Fp1-F7 and down in F7-T3. The opposite will occur in Fp2-F8 and F8-T4. Notice that lateral eye movements make the aforementioned pairs of channels point in opposite directions (Fig. 6.1.5).

Rapid eye movements may cause jagged artifacts (Fig. 12.2). Muscle artifact may appear along with eye movements. Lateral eye movements may be preceded by a single sharp muscle potential sometimes referred to as a *lateral rectus spike*. Rarely, a lateral rectus spike in combination with the eye movement artifact may mimic abnormal epileptiform spike and wave activity.

Eye movement artifacts have long been believed to be due to movement of the eyeball which carries a steady electrical charge, the cornea being about 100 mV positive with respect to the retina. However, it seems that movement of this corneoretinal dipole is not necessary to produce blink artifacts: movements of the lids across the eyeball appear sufficient. Moreover, some eye movement artifacts can be

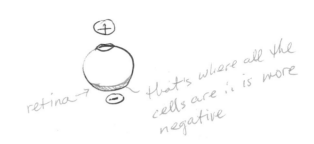

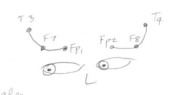

109

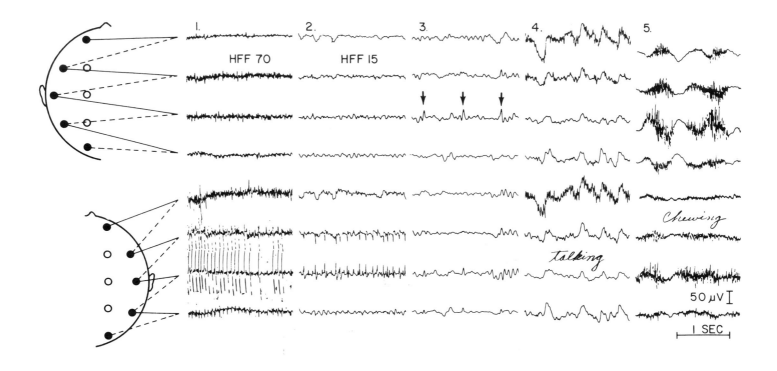

Fig. 6.2. Common artifacts generated by extracerebral physiological activity. 1. Continuous muscle artifact in all channels with superimposed intermittent muscle artifact of high amplitude in channels 6 and 7; the recording is made with a high frequency filter setting of 70 Hz; 2. Continuation of the recording shown in part 1., but with a high frequency filter setting of 15 Hz; 3. Heart beat artifacts (arrows); 4. Artifacts due to talking and frontal muscle contraction; 5. Compound artifact caused by chewing movements and associated muscle artifact.

recorded even after removal of the eye including cornea and retina, suggesting that movement of residual membranes deep in the orbit can cause artifacts.

Eye movement artifacts in the EEG can usually be identified by their frontal distribution, their symmetry on the two sides and their characteristic shape. However, several exceptions to these rules may make identification of eye movements difficult. The frontal origin of eye movement artifacts may remain unclear in referential montages, particularly those using ear electrodes which may be contaminated by eye movements. Repetitive eye movements may mimick cerebral rhythms; slowly repetitive eye movements may closely resemble bilaterally synchronous frontal slow waves, and repetitive eye movements associated with lid flutter during eye closure may cause frontal rhythms of about 10 Hz. As a general rule, it is best to assume that activity in the alpha frequency range localized to the frontopolar head regions is eye movement artifact until proven otherwise.

Asymmetric eye movements usually occur under one of the following circumstances: (1) decreased movement of the eye or eyelid of one eye, (2) absence of an eye or destruction of the retina of one eye, (3) asymmetric electrode placement, or (4) a frontal skull defect. In the case of a missing part or breach of the frontal bone, the eye movement artifact is lower in amplitude *ipsilateral* to the skull defect. This is thought to occur by virtue of a shunting of the eye potential through the skull. — se liquea

Eye movement artifacts can be identified during the recording by observing the patient and correlating eye blinks and movements with pen deflections. Even eye movements during eye closure can usually be seen through the eyelids. These movements can be further identified by their disappearance when the patient complies with the instruction to keep his eyes closed and still. If unable to do this, the patient may be told to place his fingertips on his eyes, or the technician may hold the eyelids and at the same time monitor eye movements felt through the eyelids. Taping cotton balls over the eyes may stop eye movements but obscures observation of eye movements and precludes recording the effect of eye opening and closing on the EEG. If eye movements cannot be stopped and cannot be distinguished from frontal slow waves in the EEG, eye movements may be monitored by electrodes placed near the eyes and linked so that eye movements can be distinguished from cerebral activity (4.3.1). Recordings from these linkages should be displayed simultaneously with, and next to, the recordings of frontal slow waves. Comparison of these recordings usually allows clear distinction between eye movement artifact and cerebral slow waves.

6.1.2 *Muscle artifact.* Muscle activity causes very short potentials which usually recur. If they recur as discrete potentials with the same shape and in the same distribution (Fig. 6.2), they may resemble cerebral spike discharges except that most cerebral spikes are of much longer duration than muscle action potentials. If they recur in rapid bursts of discharges (Fig. 6.2), they usually consist of several different types of potentials which merge and obscure the recording of cerebral activity. Muscle artifacts from scalp and face muscles occur mainly in the frontal and temporal regions but may be recorded by electrodes nearly anywhere on the head. Reducing the settings of the high frequency filter will reduce the amplitude of these fast potentials, but will also change their form (3.5.2) so that single muscle potentials may look more like spikes, and repetitive potentials may look like cerebral fast waves (Fig. 6.2).

Muscle artifact, even if not related to recognizable movement by the patient, is usually easily identified by its shape and repetition. It can be reduced and often eliminated by asking the patient to relax, drop the jaw or open the mouth slightly, or change position. Artifact from a single electrode can sometimes be stopped by gently pushing on that electrode, by stroking or massaging the skin near the electrode, or by reapplying the electrode. Reducing high frequency filter settings is only of limited value because of the aforementioned distortion.

112

A few specific conditions cause special electrographic patterns. Repetitive movements such as chewing, blinking or tremor may give rise to a combination of fast muscle and slow movement artifacts which may resemble cerebral discharges, especially if the combinations repeat with similar shape. Such rhythmical combinations may occur in tremor of Parkinson's disease, photomyoclonic responses, and other nonepileptic myoclonic contractions. On the other hand, seizures may lead to muscle activity so that a recording electrode picks up mixtures of cerebral seizure activity and muscle activity caused by the seizure. Bursts of muscle potentials of one kind may be followed by bursts of muscle potentials of a different amplitude and shape in the rare facial myokymia which is often associated with brain stem lesions causing no other EEG signs.

6.1.3 *Movement artifact.* Movements of the head and body or of the electrode wires can cause artifacts even if all electrodes make good mechanical and electrical contact. Movement artifacts are often erratic and not repetitive unless the movement is rhythmical as, for instance, in tremor, chewing and sucking (Fig. 6.2), breathing, or head movements with each heart beat caused by the force of the blood rushing into the head (also referred to as cardioballistographic artifact).

Movement artifacts are usually easily recognized during the recording by their association with visible movements and should be identified meticulously by indicating the moment and kind of movement on the chart. Many movement artifacts can be abolished by asking the subject to stop moving. In persons who do not comply, for instance in restless or confused patients, infants and children, patients having seizures, tremors or other movement disorders, the movements must be reduced as far as possible.

The main difficulty for the electroencephalographer occurs when the technologist has failed to document in writing on the record the occurrence of movements producing artifacts. Unfortunately, asking the technologist to try to recall if specific waveforms were associated with body movements is almost always a useless exercise. In addition to carefully observing the patient, the recording, and making frequent notations regarding movements, movements may be recorded and sometimes identified with special monitors (e.g., accelerometers). In addition, the ECG channel sometimes serves as an effective monitor for detecting gross body tremors and other movements.

6.1.4 *Electrocardiogram.* Potential changes generated by the heart are picked up in the EEG mainly in recordings with wide interelectrode distances, especially in linkages across the head and to the left ear, and in subjects with short necks. The artifact may appear in all channels using a common reference, or only in one or a few channels. Small artifacts reflect mainly the R-wave of the electrocardiogram (Fig. 6.2). Larger artifacts may reflect additional components of the electrocardiogram. Very large artifacts are often produced by interference from a cardiac pacemaker (Fig. 6.3). The R wave usually appears maximally over the left posterior head regions as a positive sharply contoured waveform and, with lower amplitude, over the right anterior head region as a negative waveform. This is because the main cardiac vector producing the R wave is positive and directed diagonally from right to left and from anterior to posterior. Thus, in a longitudinal bipolar montage the ECG artifact, if present, appears as an upward deflection in T3-T5 and a downward deflection in T5-O1 (i.e., positivity at T5). If the head is turned, then the electrodes situated on the left and posterior with regard to the torso will still record the maximum positivity. The ECG artifact often changes amplitude and distribution as the patient breathes because breathing changes the position of the heart with respect to the head. Premature ventricular contractions are usually maximal over the posterior head regions but are greater in amplitude and duration than the normally conducted heart beat. *Their intermittent occurrence in the absence of an ECG monitor may give the impression of abnormal posterior sharp waves or rhythmic delta activity.*

114

In contrast to most other artifacts, the heart beat artifact cannot usually be eliminated by corrective actions during the recording. It is rarely the only manifestation of a bad electrode contact and can therefore not usually be abolished by improving the contact or replacing the electrode. Referential recordings combining both ears as a reference tend to show less heart beat artifact than referential recordings to one ear. In approximately 80% of individuals a non-cephalic reference montage using a balanced neck to chest electrode pair as the reference will produce a recording free of ECG artifact. This consists of one electrode on the neck and one on the sternum, connected through a variable resistor which may be adjusted to null the ECG components affecting both these electrodes. If there is any doubt whether sharp waves are due to the heart beat artifact or to cerebral activity, the technician should record the heart beat in one channel and compare it with the timing of the suspected sharp waves (4.3.2).

If the heart beat has not been monitored during the recording and the EEG reader has difficulty in distinguishing heart beat artifact from cerebral activity, it is useful to measure the interval between suspected heartbeat artifacts and apply this measure to subsequent suspicious events to determine whether they have equal intervals and therefore are likely due to heartbeat, or fall into the interval between events and are less likely of cardiac origin. However, this method may fail in extrasystoles and other cardiac arrhythmias, especially those altering the shape of the heartbeat artifact.

6.1.5 *Pulse wave artifact.* Periodic waves of smooth or triangular shape may be picked up by an electrode on or near a scalp artery as the result of pulse waves producing slight changes of the electrical contact between electrode and scalp. This is more likely to happen with electrodes in the frontal and temporal areas than with electrodes in the posterior head regions.

This artifact is recognized by its usually regular recurrence. If the heartbeat

p. 480 (see also p. 65 K(+D))

artifact is picked up in the same recording, it precedes the pulse wave artifact by a constant interval (Fig. 24.2). If necessary, the pulse wave artifact may be identified by simultaneous recording of the heartbeat. If it is eliminated by reapplication of the electrode at some distance from the pulsating artery, the new electrode position should be indicated on the chart.

6.1.6 *Skin potential.* There are 2 important artifacts that arise from skin changes. *Perspiration artifact* consists of slow waveforms that are usually greater than 2 sec in duration. Perspiration alone causes slow shifts of the electrical baseline by changing the impedance or contact between the electrode and the skin. In addition, sweat gland activity produces slowly changing electrical potentials that are recorded by the electrodes. Less often rhythmic potentials are produced, particularly if stainless steel or unchlorided silver electrodes have been used. Perspiration artifact almost always appears in more than one channel, but may be lateralized or asymmetric. Therefore, very slow localized waveforms (greater than 2 sec in duration) should never be considered unequivocal evidence of an underlying cerebral dysfunction unless accompanied by other changes such as slowing in the theta frequency range, or amplitude changes in the alpha and beta range. The simultaneous occurrence of perspiration artifact and generalized background slowing should always raise the question of hypoglycemia. Perspiration artifact can be reduced by cooling the patient and drying the scalp with a fan or alcohol.

The second less common artifact produced by the skin is the *galvanic skin response* (GSR), or *psychogalvanic skin response*. The GSR consists of slow waves, each with a duration of 0.5–1 sec (1–2 Hz), that last 1.5–2 sec with 2–3 prominent phases (Fig. 6.4). It represents an autonomic response produced by the sweat glands and changes in skin conductance in response to a sensory stimulus or psychic event. The GSR may be particularly difficult to identify correctly, particularly if it occurs in only one or two channels. It can be monitored by recording between one electrode

fig 8 - p. 49 Klass + Daly

116

placed on the palm (an area with abundant sweat glands) and one placed on the dorsum of the same hand. A lower gain and longer time constant are used than in routine EEG recording.

6.1.7 *Movements of the tongue and other oropharyngeal structures.* These movements may produce intermittent or repetitive slow waves in a wide distribution, often with a maximum in the middle of the head. Tongue movement causes a 'glossokinetic' artifact because the tip of the tongue has a negative electrical charge with respect to the root. Tongue movement explains part of the artifacts generated by speaking, swallowing, chewing, sucking, coughing and hiccoughing; movements of other structures probably contribute to these artifacts (Fig. 6.2) and account for those seen with sobbing. Artifacts from temporal, facial and scalp muscles may be mixed with the movement artifact. Palatal myoclonus causes rhythmical muscle artifacts at rates of about 100–200 per minute which are best seen in referential montages to an ear electrode and persist in sleep (Fig. 6.5).

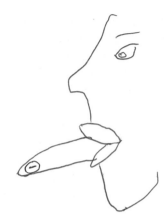

Many of these artifacts may be identified during the recording if they are associated with visible movements and if they disappear when these movements stop. However, the identification of a glossokinetic artifact may be difficult if, for example, the mouth remains closed during tongue movements, or if it occurs with an asymmetric distribution (Fig. 6.6). Therefore, it is recommended that patients be routinely asked during the recording to repeat words which elicit tongue movements, such as 'lilt' or 'Tom Thumb' (Fig. 6.6).

6.1.8 *Dental restorations with dissimilar metals.* Spike-like artifacts may be produced by dental fillings with dissimilar metals whenever the metal pieces are moved against each other, for instance in chewing, swallowing or speaking.

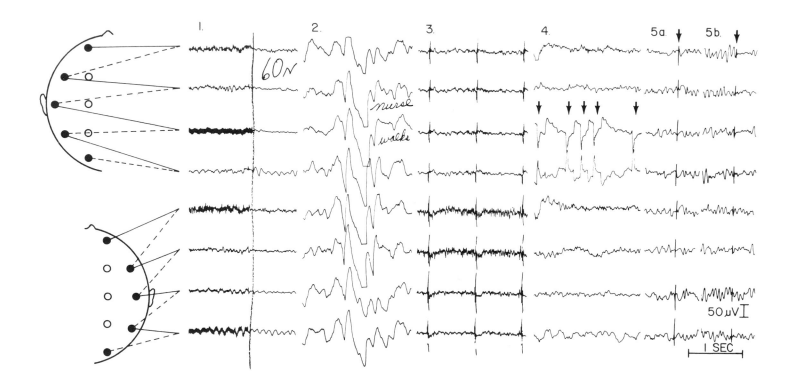

Fig. 6.3. Nonbiological artifacts. 1. 60 Hz interference before and after turning on the 60 Hz filter (60∿);
2. Artifacts induced by a nurse walking near the patient; 3. Cardiac pacemaker artifacts; 4. 'Electrode popping' artifacts (arrows) from the left posterior temporal electrode making poor contact; 5a. and 5b. 'Paper stop' artifacts (arrows) due to intermittent failure of paper drive.

The most common artifact due to electrical interference comes from power lines and equipment. It has a frequency of 60 Hz in North America and of 50 Hz in many other countries. A slight amount of this interference is unavoidable wherever alternating current is used. While this background interference may be picked up by faulty electrodes and may appear in one or a few channels, inordinately strong interference can cause artifacts even with good recording electrodes and equipment; these artifacts are then likely to appear in all channels of all recordings made in the same recording room (Fig. 6.3). The artifacts may be introduced either electrostatically by unshielded power cables and regardless of current flow, or electromagnetically by strong currents flowing through cables and equipment such as transformers and electromotors. Electrostatic interference can be reduced by shielding the offending power cables and by using a shielded room for the recording; electromagnetic interference can be reduced by proper wiring of the power cables. Other types of interference include signals from nearby television stations, radio paging, telephone ringing, cardiac pacemakers (Fig. 6.3), or any movement of a charged body near the recording electrodes; electrostatic artifacts may be produced by a person walking through the recording room (Fig. 6.3) or by drops falling in an intravenous drip. However, modern EEG machines have such high discrimination and input impedance that they reject all but the most powerful sources of interference from the environment. In setting up a laboratory, it is therefore not necessary to shield the recording room unless a trial recording from a patient or a 10,000 Ω resistor, placed at the prospective recording site, shows strong interference.

When recordings are made in an environment with much interference such as an intensive care unit or an operating room, the patient's head and the connections to the EEG machine should be kept as far from power cables as possible. Any swaying

* p.41 K+D

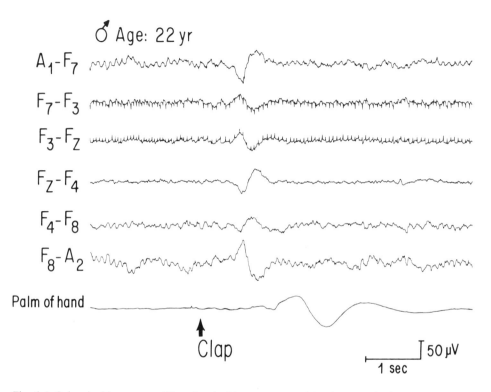

Fig. 6.4. Galvanic skin response. The galvanic skin response resulting from an alerting maneuver appears first over the scalp and then the palm due in part to the longer conduction time of autonomic pathways to the hand. This artifact may also occur with an asymmetric distribution. Courtesy B.F. Westmoreland, Mayo Clinic.

of electrode wires and movement of tubing or of other charged objects should be minimized. Equipment other than the EEG machine should be unplugged if feasible; even the respirator may be stopped for short periods to obtain artifact-free recordings or to determine the cause of interference.

6.3 ARTIFACTS ARISING FROM RECORDING ELECTRODES AND EQUIPMENT

6.3.1 *Artifacts arising from electrodes, electrode terminal board, input cable and selector switches.* Most artifacts in this category are distinguished from cerebral activity in that they differ radically from previously recorded activity, do not blend with other simultaneously recorded activity but seem to be superimposed on it, and appear only in channels connected to one electrode. However, not all of these artifacts are easily recognized. Although some of them have characteristic shapes, others lack such features and may resemble cerebral activity. A common artifact is 'electrode popping' which is due to a sudden change of electrode contact causing pen deflections which rise or fall abruptly and may mimick spike discharges (Fig. 6.3). Other electrode artifacts rise and fall more slowly and may resemble cerebral slow waves.

Identification and correction of artifacts in the distribution of one electrode requires checking electrical and mechanical continuity. Because the artifact is often due to faulty contact between the electrode and the scalp, the first step is to look at that junction: The electrode may be partly or completely detached, the lead wire may be broken, or the conductive paste or jelly may have dried up. As a next step, electrical impedance should be measured (2.2.3); if it is high, the electrode should be refilled with conductive jelly or paste, reapplied, or replaced if it is defective. If the artifact persists, the receptacle jack or the wiring of the input terminal board may be at fault; this can be investigated by changing the connections between electrodes and

121

Bipolar montage

A₂-A₁

A₁-T₃

T₃-C₃

C₃-C₄

C₄-T₄

T₄-A₂

♂ Age: 45 Yr (H.L.)

⊢——⊣ ⊤ 20 µv
  1 sec

Referential montage

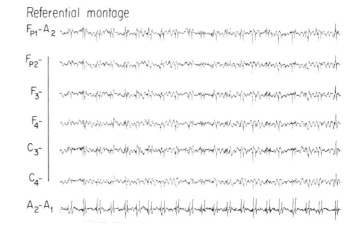

F_P1-A₂

F_P2-

F₃-

F₄-

C₃-

C₄-

A₂-A₁

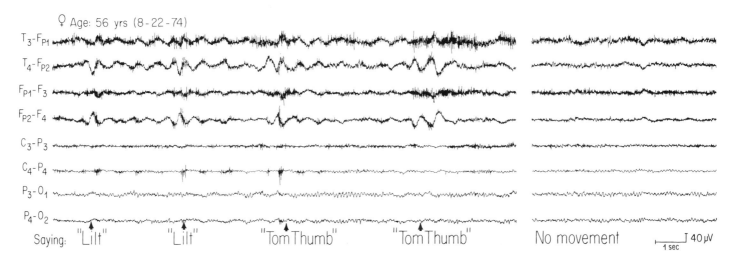

♀ Age: 56 yrs (8-22-74)

T₃-F_P1

T₄-F_P2

F_P1-F₃

F_P2-F₄

C₃-P₃

C₄-P₄

P₃-O₁

P₄-O₂

Saying: "Lilt"   "Lilt"   "Tom Thumb"   "Tom Thumb"   No movement

⊢——⊣ ⊤ 40 µV
  1 sec

122

receptacles of the faulty channel so that the electrodes and the receptacles of that channel are presented in different channels: The electrodes of the faulty channel are connected to receptacles giving good recordings when connected to other electrodes, and electrodes not giving artifacts when connected to other receptacles are connected to receptacles of the faulty channel. If the artifact changes channels corresponding with the electrodes from the faulty channel, one of these electrodes is at fault and can be identified by connecting the two electrodes to different channels and observing in which channel the artifact then appears. However, if the artifact remains at one receptacle, the input board or subsequent components of the recording channel may be at fault. In practice, the technician at this point or earlier will examine a piece of recording made while the inputs are closed. If the artifact persists under this condition, it arises from the recording machine and should be investigated accordingly (6.3.2). However, if the artifact is present only when the input is open, and if an electrode fault has been excluded, the source of the artifact may be further determined by replacing the input board and input cable if replacements are available, and by checking the input terminals and selector switches if they are accessible.

Fig. 6.5. Palatal myoclonus. Each involuntary movement of the pharynx and palate are marked by the fast paired deflections. The 10–20 electrode derivations that typically show this artifact best are those referenced to A1 and A2. This is clearly illustrated by the prominence of the artifact in the referential montage compared to the bipolar montage. Courtesy Dr. B.F. Westmoreland, Mayo Clinic.

Fig. 6.6. Glossokinetic potentials. Glossokinetic potentials evoked for demonstration purposes by asking the patient to repeat the words 'Lilt' and 'Tom Thumb'. In longitudinal bipolar montages the artifact usually appears maximally in the anterior and posterior derivations. In some cases, as shown here, the artifact may have an asymmetric distribution. Courtesy Dr. D.W. Klass, Mayo Clinic.

6.3.2 *Artifacts arising from the recording machine.* Like artifacts from the electrodes, artifacts from the machine may often be recognized by the sudden appearance of waveforms very different from cerebral activity. The source of the artifacts can often be traced to one functional component of the machine. Trouble-shooting is facilitated by two features of modern EEG machines. (a) Many components have indicator lights and electrical contact points with prescribed voltage readings which can be checked easily. (b) Components of individual channels are made of modules which can be exchanged. Artifacts due to faults of components that are common to all channels often cause lack of power or 60 Hz interference. Power failure may be caused by a faulty outlet or a blown fuse in the EEG machine. If a replacement fuse also blows, the power supply may be at fault. Sixty hertz interference in all channels may be due to (a) a powerful source of interference in the recording room (6.2), (b) a faulty or absent connection of the subject with the ground of the EEG machine (3.4.1), (c) defects in the power supply or other parts of the machine.

Artifacts caused by components of individual channels appear only at the output of the defective channels and persist independently of the input selection. The causes of these problems can be traced by exchanging modular components of one channel with the corresponding components of another channel. For instance if 60 Hz artifact in one channel suggests a problem in its amplifier, this can be investigated by exchanging the amplifier for an amplifier of another channel not showing that artifact.

REFERENCES

Barlow, J.S. (1986) Artifact processing (rejection and minimization) in EEG data processing. In: F.H. Lopes da Silva, W. Storm van Leeuwen and A. Remond (Eds.), Clinical Applications of Computer Analysis of EEG and other Neurophysiological Signals, Handbook of EEG (revised series), Elsevier, Amsterdam, pp. 15–64.

Beaussart, M. and Guiev, J.D. (1977) Section III. Artefacts. In: Rémond, A. (Ed.), Handbook of Electroenceph. clin. Neurophysiol., Vol. 11A, Elsevier, Amsterdam, pp. 80–96.

Bennett, D.R., Hughes, J.R., Korein, J., Merlis, J.K. and Suter, C. (1976) Atlas of electroencephalography in coma and cerebral death, Raven, New York.

Brittenham, D. (1974) Recognition and reduction of physiological artifacts. Am. J. EEG Technol. 14: 158–165.

Espinosa, R.E., Klass, D.W. and Maloney, J.D. (1978) Contribution of the electroencephalogram in monitoring cardiac dysrhythmias. Mayo Clin. Proc. 53: 119–122.

Gordon, M. (1980) Artifacts created by imbalanced electrode impedance. Am. J. EEG Technol. 20: 149–160.

Kamp, A. and Lopes da Silva, F. (1987) Polygraphy. In: Niedermeyer, E. and Lopes da Silva, F. (Eds.), Electroencephalography: Basic Principles, Clinical Applications, and Related Fields. Urban and Schwarzenberg, Baltimore, pp. 681–686.

Mac Gillivray, B.B. (1974) Section IV. Artefacts, faults, and fault-finding. In: Rémond, A. (Ed.), Handbook of Electroenceph. clin. Neurophysiol., Vol. 3C, Elsevier, Amsterdam, pp. 88–102.

Pasik, P., Pasik, T. and Bender, M.B. (1965) Recovery of the electro-oculogram after total ablation of the retina in monkeys. Electroenceph. clin. Neurophysiol. 19: 291–297.

Redding, F.K., Wandel, V. and Nasser, C. (1969) Intravenous infusion drop artifacts. Electroenceph. clin. Neurophysiol. 26: 318–320.

Saunders, M.G. (1979) Artifacts: Activity of Noncerebral Origin in the EEG. In: Klass, D.W. and Daly, D.D. (Eds.), Current Practice of Clinical Electroencephalography, Raven, New York, pp. 37–68.

Stephenson, W.A. and Gibbs, F.A. (1951) A balanced non-cephalic reference electrode. Electroenceph. clin. Neurophysiol. 3: 237–240.

Tyner, F.S., Knott, J.R. and Mayer Jr., W.B. (1983) Fundamentals of EEG Technology, Raven, New York, pp. 280–311.

Westmoreland, B.F., Espinosa, R.E. and Klass, D.W. (1973) Significant prosopo-glossopharyngeal movements affecting the electroencephalogram. Am. J. EEG Technol. 13: 59–70.

Other methods of recording and analysis

7

SUMMARY

(7.1) *Computer-assisted EEG signal analysis* allows for a more precise and reproducible examination of certain EEG features than can be accomplished by routine visual inspection. However, aside from evoked potential recording and certain data reduction applications, its role in clinical practice is currently limited. As yet, in routine clinical practice, visual inspection by a qualified electroencephalographer is still the most efficient and informative method of EEG interpretation.

(7.2) *Analog to digital conversion.* Since computers analyze digital data, it is important to understand how the routinely recorded analog EEG signal is converted to a digital signal. The device which performs this conversion is referred to as an analog to digital converter (ADC). The digitized signal may be displayed on an oscilloscope, computer monitor, or printed on paper. A digital to analog converter (DAC) is used to convert the digital signal back into an analog form.

(7.3) *Signal storage.* Magnetic tape (cassette or reel to reel) is used to store the analog EEG signal. Optical disc, fixed or removable hard disc, floppy disc and magnetic tape (cartridge, reel to reel or videotape cassette) are used to store digitized EEG signals.

(7.4) *Computerized signal analysis* is currently used to: (1) quantitate EEG background activity; (2) create topographic displays of EEG activity; (3) detect epileptiform activity; (4) monitor selected EEG features in the ICU and OR; (5) retrospectively filter or reconstruct EEG activity into different montages; and (6) perform signal averaging and artifact rejection for evoked potential analysis.

(7.5) *Ambulatory EEG recording* is routinely performed by recording up to sixteen channels of analog EEG on a cassette-recording system worn by the patient. The EEG recording is reviewed on an oscilloscope and selected epochs may be printed on paper for further inspection.

(7.6) *EEG recording with simultaneous video monitoring* is performed to correlate clinical and electrographic events, often as part of the presurgical evaluation for the treatment of epilepsy. The EEG signal can be acquired by *radiotelemetry* (using a radio transmitter worn by the patient) or by *cable telemetry* (via a lightweight cable directly attached to the patient).

7.1 COMPUTER ASSISTED SIGNAL ANALYSIS

Computer-assisted EEG analysis is used to either quantitate or detect selected EEG features. *Quantitative EEG analysis* refers to the transformation of a particular EEG feature into a numerical value. A typical example of quantitative EEG analysis would be the calculation of a single numerical value that represents the amount of all activity in the 8–13 Hz frequency range recorded over a certain period of time. Such values may then be used for statistical comparisons or for other forms of EEG display, such as topographic mapping. Although most methods of quantitative EEG analysis give very precise and reproducible results, it is important to recognize that virtually all methods are approximations and therefore contain a certain degree of error. Automated *feature extraction* refers to the use of the computer to recognize or isolate a selected EEG activity. An example of automated feature extraction is the computerized detection of electrographic seizure activity.

Quantitative EEG analysis is currently being investigated as a method for detecting clinically relevant changes that are not revealed by routine visual inspection. Despite a number of reports suggesting that computer analysis is helpful for differential diagnosis, verification of such findings by independent investigators has not been forthcoming. Currently, computerized analysis is best viewed as an extension of the routine EEG. It cannot be overemphasized that clinicians attempting to apply these techniques in clinical practice should be experienced electroencephalographers who have a thorough understanding of the signal analysis methods being applied.

7.2 ANALOG TO DIGITAL CONVERSION

Before a signal can be processed by a digital computer it must first be transformed from a continuous *analog* signal into a series of discrete, unconnected data points referred to as a *digital* signal. This function is performed by a device known as an *analog to digital converter* (ADC). The ADC consists of an array of computer chips mounted on a circuit board that has inputs to receive the amplified EEG signal. There are three key features of the ADC that determine how accurately the analog signal will be reproduced in digital form: (1) the sampling rate of the ADC, (2) the voltage range of the ADC, and (3) the number of amplitude levels the ADC can resolve.

The number of digital points used per second to describe the analog signal is referred to as the *sampling rate*. If, for example, the ADC has a sampling rate of 100 Hz, the analog signal will be represented by 100 points each separated by 1/100 of a second. However, the sampling rate must be at least twice that of the fastest frequency in the original signal to truly represent the frequency content of the analog signal. This is sometimes referred to as the *sampling theorem* or *Nyquist theorem*. Thus, if the highest frequency in a signal is 100 Hz, then the ADC must sample it at a rate of at least 200 Hz. If a digital signal is to be displayed for visual inspection, then it is helpful if the sampling rate is at least more than 6 times the fastest frequency in the analog signal. Otherwise the morphology of the signal may have a rough, angular appearance that may make interpretation difficult.

If the A to D converter samples the analog signal at a rate less than twice the fastest frequency in the signal, frequencies that are not present in the analog signal will appear in the digitized signal. This is referred to as undersampling, or *aliasing*. A simple, but dramatic, example of aliasing occurs whenever a waveform is sampled at a rate equal to its frequency, as in a 50 Hz sine wave sampled at 50 Hz. In such a case, each sampling point will fall on the same relative position of the waveform (for instance each top peak of a series of sine waves). If a line is then drawn connecting each of the sampled points, the result is a flat line, seen by the computer as a 0-Hz signal. As the sampling rate increases, a faster and faster, but still false (aliased), digitized signal will be recorded until the sampling rate finally reaches twice the frequency of fastest waveform in the analog signal. *Oversampling* a signal (i.e., sampling at greater than twice the highest frequency of the analog signal) is important if the signal is to be displayed for visual inspection, because it will produce an increasingly smoother appearing waveform. Aliasing can be avoided by either: (1)

increasing the sampling rate of the ADC; or (2) filtering the analog signal with a high frequency analog filter (i.e., a low pass analog filter) to remove all activity with a frequency faster than 1/2 the sampling rate of the ADC.

The amplitudes of digitized signals are *quantized*, or assigned to discrete non-overlapping amplitude levels by the ADC. The number of amplitude levels that the ADC has available is often expressed in terms of *bits*, where each bit is a power of two. For example, an 8 bit ADC has 2^8, or 256 amplitude levels that can be used to describe the signal. The ADC's amplitude resolution is dependent on both its voltage range and the maximum number of bits of discrimination available. Amplitude changes will be registered by the computer only if the signal changes enough to reach the next amplitude level (or bit) of the ADC. For example, if the ADC has 8 levels (or 3 bits; $2^3 = 8$) of amplitude discrimination and its voltage range is set at +400 to −400 μVs, then there will be 8 amplitude levels each separated by 100 μVs (since there are 8 levels spread over 800 μVs; +400 to −400 μVs). If the signal varies between 0 and +99 μVs, no amplitude variation is detected because each level of amplitude discrimination is 100 μVs wide. In contrast, if the signal varies over a much smaller range between +99 and +101 μVs, then an amplitude change is registered with each variation above or below 100 μVs since the signal is crossing the amplitude boundary (between the 0−100 and the 101−200 μV levels). Thus, ADC's with fewer bits make it more likely that relatively large changes will go undetected, and very small amplitude changes may be overrepresented. In the example cited above, digital amplitude resolution can be improved by either; (1) setting the entire voltage range of the A to D converter to +101 to −101 μVs, thereby allowing all eight levels to be distributed in this range (i.e., each amplitude level would then have a range of 25 μVs; 200/8); or (2) using an ADC with a larger number of bits so that more amplitude levels are available over the existing range. ADCs used for EEG and evoked potential analysis should have at least 12-bit amplitude discrimination. The voltage range seen by the ADC is actually in terms of volts (not microvolts), since the analog EEG signal has already been amplified by the EEG machine (usually in the range of +5 to −5 volts) prior to analog to digital conversion.

Digitized signals are converted back into analog signals by *digital to analog converters* (DAC). Like the ADCs, the DACs consist of computer chips mounted on a circuit board. The DAC board is plugged into the computer and then connected to a display device by cable. The EEG signal can then be viewed on an oscilloscope, printed on a plotting device, or played out through a conventional EEG machine penwriters onto paper. To actually reproduce the original signal, the DAC in essence connects the digital signal points. The greater the oversampling of the original analog signal by the ADC, the smoother the appearance of the signal produced by the DAC. The less the signal was oversampled by the ADC, the more it will have a rough, but continuous, staircase appearance, with each step of the staircase being defined by each data point. To give the signal an even smoother appearance, the steplike waveform contour can be removed by passing the signal through a low pass (high frequency) analog filter. More complex methods, using digital interpolation and digital filtering prior to analog filtering are also employed.

7.3 EEG SIGNAL STORAGE

EEG signal storage can be accomplished in several ways. For analog signal storage, the amplified EEG signal can be recorded on magnetic tape. The digitized signal can be stored using a number of devices including optical discs, hard discs, floppy discs, videotape and magnetic tape (cartridge, reel to reel, or videotape cassette). With the exception of ambulatory cassette recording, analog storage has been largely replaced by digital storage. This is because digital storage offers: (1) dramatically reduced costs when recording many channels simultaneously, (2) the avoidance of signal

131

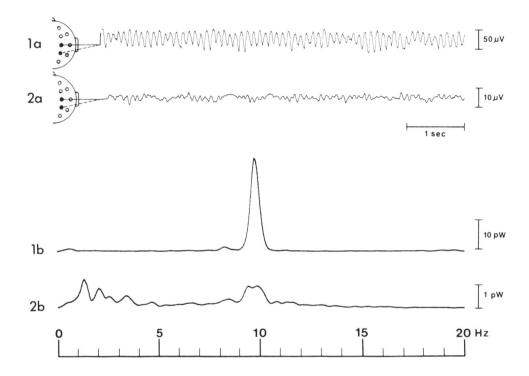

Fig. 7.1. Power spectra of normal (1) and abnormal (2) EEGs. The top two tracings (a) show strips of the paper tracing recorded between the right central and parietal electrode in a normal subject (1a) and a patient (2a). The bottom section shows power spectra (b) computed from about 13 seconds of the same recordings. The power spectrum of the normal subject (1b) shows activity mainly at 10 Hz, representing the 10 Hz waves seen in 1a; the power spectrum from the patient in 2b shows activity at about 1–4 Hz and at 10 Hz, reflecting the combination of slow waves and 10 Hz waves in 2a. Vertical calibration is in picowatts (pW).

noise caused by analog tape recorders, (3) more precise timing of the digitally recorded signal, (4) direct and rapid computer access to the signal for subsequent analysis, (5) reduced storage space needs (e.g., optical discs compared to reels of magnetic tape), and (6) the ability to 'type' in additional identifying information at the key board.

7.4 SPECIAL METHODS OF COMPUTERIZED SIGNAL ANALYSIS

Special methods of computerized signal analysis are used to: (1) convert certain features of the EEG background activity into numerical values (quantitative EEG analysis); (2) create special displays of certain evoked potential or EEG features (e.g., topographic mapping); (3) perform automated analysis (e.g., detect interictal or ictal electrographic changes); (4) monitor certain EEG features over variable periods of time (e.g., ICU or OR monitoring); (5) reexamine the same EEG signal using different montages or filter settings; (6) perform signal averaging for evoked potential recording; and (7) evaluate the similarity between signals.

7.4.1 *Quantitative EEG analysis.* Quantitative EEG analysis consists of transforming a selected feature of the EEG into a numerical value. This is a very precise way of examining the EEG signal which eliminates potential inter- and intra-reader variability. It also makes EEG features available for statistical analysis, and allows for a variety of EEG display techniques. Many methods have been devised for quantifying the EEG and a discussion of each of them is beyond the scope of this text. Because spectral analysis, based on the fast Fourier transform (FFT), is applied more frequently than any other method, it is discussed here in further detail.

   In order to quantitate the frequency components of the EEG signal, methods have been devised which transfer the EEG signal from the *time domain* into the *frequency domain*. The *time domain* refers to signals described in terms of *amplitude vs. time*, as we are used to seeing EEG signals. The *frequency domain* refers to signals described in terms of *amplitude* (or phase) *vs. frequency*. In Fig. 7.1, the original EEG signals displayed in 1a and 2a (i.e., in the time domain), have been transformed into the frequency domain (1b and 2b). Thus, 1b and 2b show the relative intensities of different frequencies present in signals 1a and 2a. In this case, the frequencies analyzed were 0–20 Hz.

It is important to recognize that analyzing a signal in the frequency domain (Fig. 7.1) means that its original morphology can no longer be seen. The advantages of this critical sacrifice of data are that: (1) a great deal of data can be summarized by a few descriptors; (2) selected features in the signal can be examined quantitatively; and (3) the relationships between signals can be revealed more precisely than by visual inspection (see also 7.4.7).

The mathematical manipulation commonly used to make the conversion from the time to the frequency domain, and the one used in Fig. 7.1, is known as the *fast Fourier transform* (FFT). The FFT is based on the fact that any signal can be described as a combination of sine and cosine waves of various phases, frequencies and amplitudes. Accordingly, the FFT generates a number of numerical coefficients that represent the sine and cosine waves present in the original signal in terms of frequency, amplitude, and phase. By using all of the Fourier sine and cosine values, or coefficients, the signal can be reconstructed from the frequency domain back into its original form in the time domain.

A common approach to analyzing the FFT so that the signal can be viewed in terms of frequency vs. intensity consists of squaring the Fourier coefficients to create what is referred to as the *power spectrum* (as shown in 7.1, 1b and 2b). It is, however, important to recognize that the power spectrum contains far less data than the original EEG. This makes the storage of spectral information much more efficient than EEG data storage. Unfortunately, the original EEG signal cannot be

134

reconstructed from the power spectrum (it does not contain phase information). In addition, the squaring of coefficients changes the amplitude relationships of the various frequency components. For example, if the distances of two lines measuring 2 and 4 meters are squared, then both become longer, but their relative difference in length becomes twice as great as it was originally. The amplitude relationships of the various frequency components of the EEG are similarly altered by power spectral analysis. This effect can be overcome by deriving the equivalent of the square root of the power spectrum, thereby creating an *amplitude spectrum*. Not surprisingly, the amplitude relationships displayed in the amplitude spectrum compare more directly with routine visual EEG analysis than do power spectrum amplitude measures.

Certain spectral features of the EEG signal may be examined once the amplitude or power spectrum has been derived. These commonly include: (1) *absolute band amplitude, or power*; (2) *relative band amplitude, or power*; (3) *the spectral edge frequency*; (4) *mean peak frequency*; and (5) *the absolute peak frequency*. Each of these values may, in turn, be statistically analyzed or plotted on a topographic display according to electrode position.

The *absolute band* value corresponds approximately to the area under the curve of the spectrum between the two frequencies that define the bandwidth. The *relative band* value refers to one absolute band value divided by another. In the example of a topographic map of relative bands shown in Fig. 7.2, the 0–4 Hz band is divided by the 0–20 Hz band and the corresponding value at each electrode site is plotted according to a gray scale displayed to the right of the map. As with absolute band values, the upper and lower limits of each band must be stated. Relative band values are often used because: (1) errors created by differences in amplifier gain between channels are minimized; and (2) the effects of amplitude differences of noncerebral origin (such as those due to varying skull thickness or asymmetrical interelectrode distances) are minimized.

135

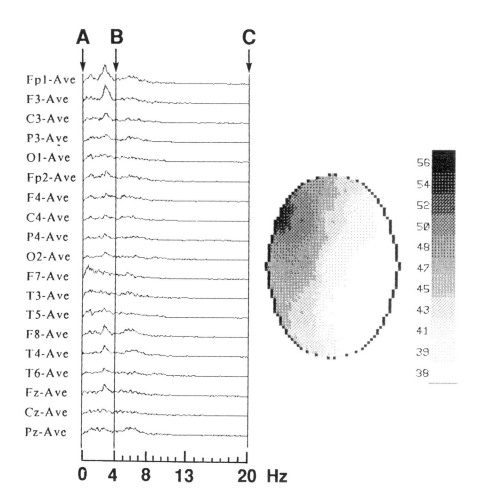

Fig. 7.2. The amplitude spectrum and topographic map of relative delta activity during light sleep. The EEG was recorded using a linked ear reference montage and subsequently reconstructed into a common average reference montage (7.4.5). Four 8-sec epochs of 'artifact free' EEG were selected using a monitor screen and the spectrum of each epoch was computed in each channel. The four spectra in each channel were then averaged to yield the final spectral plots for each channel as shown on the left side of the figure. The absolute band value (the approximate area under the spectral plot) between 0 and 4 Hz (A and B) was divided by the absolute band value between 0 and 20 Hz (A and C) and multiplied times 100 to yield the final relative percentage 0–4-Hz band. The values of the relative band values on the topographic map are shown on the percentage gray scale at the far right. The routine recording demonstrated left anterior temporal background slowing and occasional epileptiform spikes that increased during sleep.

The *spectral edge frequency* refers to the frequency below which a pre-selected percentage of the total frequency range absolute band value lies. For example, if the spectral edge frequency is set at 90%, then the computer will determine the frequency below which 90% of the area under the entire spectral curve is contained. The spectral edge frequency has been used as a gross indicator showing trends in the EEG over time. The median peak frequency can be determined by simply calculating the spectral edge frequency at 50%. Alternatively, a mean peak frequency (also referred to as the *centroid*) equivalent to the center of gravity of the area under the spectral plot may be used.

The *absolute peak frequency* refers to the peak value in a selected band of the frequency spectrum. A frequency band is selected at the keyboard and the computer calculates the greatest spectral amplitude peak in that frequency band. Absolute peak frequency measures have been used to compare the alpha frequency between homotopic derivations, between individuals, and within individuals over time or in response to medications. These studies suggest that differences of as little as 0.3 or 0.4 Hz may be abnormal when comparing left and right occipital derivations with certain montages. In contrast, using routine visual analysis a peak alpha rhythm frequency asymmetry of less than 1 Hz is extremely difficult to appreciate and differences of less than 0.5 Hz cannot be seen. Unfortunately, clearly dominant spectral peak frequencies in the alpha frequency band may be poorly defined in both normal and abnormal individuals (particularly when increasingly longer EEG epoch lengths are analyzed), making the routine use of absolute peak frequency measures difficult.

As noted above, a major limitation of spectral analysis is the loss of the waveform morphology once the EEG has been transformed into the frequency domain. Since any duration of EEG can be transformed into a single frequency spectrum it is important to note that a particular band value gives no indication of how many times a particular waveform has occurred. Thus, the same spectral band value could result from either continuous low amplitude waveforms or from intermittent high amplitude waveforms in the same frequency range. Because the morphology and repetition of waveforms cannot be appreciated in the frequency domain, it is critical that the unprocessed EEG be viewed and interpreted by an experienced electroencephalographer. Otherwise most of the clinically useful information contained in the EEG will be lost. If quantitative EEG analysis is to be used for clinical purposes, then it is also important that an experienced electroencephalographer selects the segments for quantitative analysis. This is done to avoid artifact contamination and to facilitate the interpretation of the results. The selection of EEG segments for processing is typically done by reviewing the EEG on a computer monitor display.

Short EEG epoch FFT analysis (less than 2.5 sec in duration) is often used to increase the likelihood that there will be artifact free data available for analysis. In this way some segments of artifact-free EEG can usually be obtained, even in poorly cooperative patients. Once the individual EEG epochs have been transformed to the frequency domain, their separate frequency spectra can be averaged together to form a final spectrum more representative of a longer time span; a process known as *spectral averaging*. Spectral averaging decreases the influence of any infrequent activity (cerebral or artifactual) and may reduce variability when comparisons are made with subsequent recordings. However, spectral averaging also has inherent limitations. It is based on the assumption that, as in evoked potential recording (see 7.4.6), there is some feature of the signal that persists with little or no change from epoch to epoch. Unfortunately, the EEG is relatively stationary over only short periods of time (typically 20–40 sec with behavioral control) and this variability depends largely on maintaining the behavioral state of the individual being recorded. Therefore, if spectral averaging is to be performed, it is preferable to try to average spectral EEG epochs in which the patient is in approximately the same state. This can be accomplished in a variety of ways. One approach used in our laboratory is to ask the subject to quietly count the number of tones presented during a recording session of several minutes duration. At the end of the session the subject is asked how many tones were presented to verify that relative wakefulness was maintained during the recording.

It is also noteworthy that the averaging of short FFT epochs of EEG is a compromise solution to the problem of artifact contamination. Shorter EEG epochs produce poorer frequency resolution with FFT analysis. This occurs because the frequency resolution of an FFT is directly related to EEG epoch length; the harmonics of the slowest waveform that can be fully described by the epoch length determine spectral frequency resolution. For example, if a 2-sec epoch is selected, the slowest waveform that can be described is 1/2 Hz (i.e., a 2-sec wavelength), and only frequency differences within the EEG of 1/2 Hz or greater can be resolved. In such a case, a difference between 1/2 Hz and 3/4 Hz activity cannot be detected. But if a 4-sec epoch is selected, then differences of as little as 1/4 Hz can be resolved. If one is interested in distinguishing between absolute peak frequencies that differ by 0.1 Hz, then epoch lengths of at least 10 sec (to resolve 1/10-Hz differences) are needed. Other approaches to signal analysis besides the FFT, such as the autoregressive model, are better suited for assessing peak frequency using extremely short epoch lengths.

7.4.2 *Topographic mapping.* Special displays of EEG and evoked potential activity have been developed to emphasize either the trends in EEG activity over time (7.4.4) or the distribution of activity over the scalp. The display of the distribution of scalp recorded activity is referred to as *topographic mapping* (TM). Topographic maps are used to emphasize the spatial relationships of selected EEG or evoked potential features. Whereas TM only converts one type of visual analysis (routine EEG reading) into another (the topographic map), the TM function can be enhanced by mapping statistical values derived from quantitative comparisons. TM used in this way combines statistical and visual analysis and represents an interim step in the development of quantitative analysis techniques.

139

TM may be used for the display of: (1) EEG voltage distributions at a particular point in time (*time domain mapping*); (2) EEG background features derived from frequency analysis (*frequency domain mapping*); and (3) statistical comparisons (*statistical mapping*). Examples from the first category include evoked potentials (EP) and averaged epileptiform spikes. Spike averaging may reveal the presence of widespread field distributions that cannot otherwise be appreciated. Whether spike averaging will contribute to the anatomical localization of epileptogenic foci awaits further investigation. As with spike averaging, EP mapping has been used mainly to illustrate, rather than elucidate, field distributions. Although absolute EP amplitude measures are clinically less useful than peak latencies, EP spatial distributions have not been as extensively studied.

Amplitude measurements for time domain TM are determined according to deviations from the electrical zero baseline set by the analog to digital converter. In actual practice the baseline for the data point being mapped is almost always different from the electrical zero baseline used by the computer. Often the waveform is superimposed on a slower waveform arising from cerebral or non-cerebral activity. This effect can be reduced by digitally filtering out waveforms above and below the frequency of the waveform of interest. In the case of evoked potentials, the signal baseline may also be altered by stimulus artifact. Even more difficult to identify are baseline distortions that arise from amplifier drift (amplifier offset) and changes in resting potentials generated at the scalp-electrode interface. These effects can all lead to TM displays with misleadingly high or low amplitude values that vary in degree from channel to channel. Time domain TM is, therefore, technically difficult and currently provides limited information of clinical relevance.

Frequency domain TM of background activity is usually accomplished by plotting one of several features (7.4.1) derived from a spectral average. Fig. 7.2 shows a typical example of a topographic map of the relative band value of the 0–4 Hz absolute band value divided by the 1–20 Hz absolute band value. Four 8-sec EEG

140

segments were selected during light sleep. Only those epochs without apparent artifact were chosen for analysis. The spectra from all four 8-sec epochs were averaged together to form the final averaged spectra for each of the channels, as shown on the left of the figure. Each band value is plotted at each electrode site according to the percentage scale to the right of the map.

It is important to recognize that the only 'real' values on topographic maps are those that represent the actual channel values. In the example shown in Fig. 7.2 there are only 19 points on the entire map that are real values. All the rest are estimated or interpolated between the real values to make the map more visually pleasing. This is, however, analogous to a situation in which only the location of one point near the top of a mountain and three or four points near the base are known. It cannot be assumed that connecting those points with straight lines correctly demonstrates the shape of the mountain. The only way to improve the spatial resolution of maps is to increase the number of recording electrodes (i.e., actual data points). A second important feature of maps that must be kept in mind is that, as in routine EEG recording, there is no such thing as an inactive reference, and the best approximation of one, a noncephalic reference montage, is difficult to implement in spectral analysis because of EKG artifact. Thus, the activity displayed never reveals the true topography of the EEG. It is therefore probably best to analyze TM, as in routine practice, with more than one montage. Unfortunately, topographic studies have rarely been performed with more than one montage.

Until reliable statistical methods and normal limits for mapped values are established, routine clinical applications for frequency domain TM are limited to the role of informing the electroencephalographer that reinspection of the routine EEG may be necessary. Electrographic evidence for a cerebral dysfunction should not be based on frequency domain TM in the absence of routine EEG findings.

141

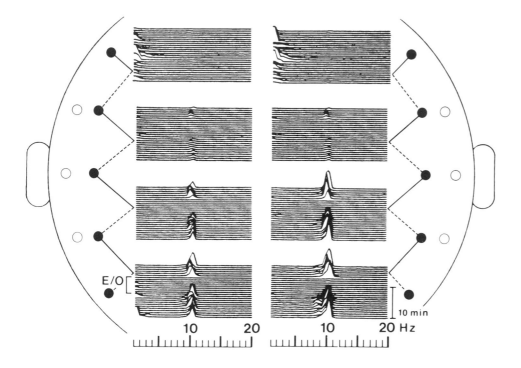

Fig. 7.3. Compressed spectral array of a normal EEG. Each of the eight blocks of tracings represents power spectra computed from simultaneous EEG recordings derived between the electrodes indicate on the head diagrams at the sides of the illustration. Each line in the blocks represents one power spectrum plotted for a recording period of about 35 seconds; successive spectra are stacked vertically. The posterior head regions show power mainly at about 10 Hz which disappears with eye opening (E/O) midway in the recording and reappears after the eyes are closed. The power in the low frequency range in the frontal regions is due to eye movement artifacts.

142

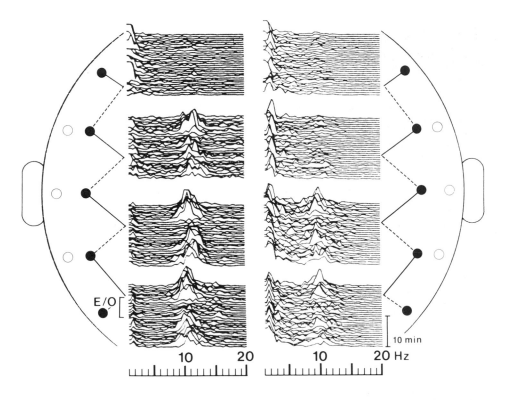

Fig. 7.4. Compressed spectral array of an abnormal EEG. Power spectra are plotted with the same method as used in Fig. 7.2. The spectra from the right posterior head regions differ from those from the left side in that they show a considerable amount of power below 8 Hz with a maximum at 1–3 Hz. Power at 10 Hz is reduced on the right side as compared to the left, especially in the fronto-central region. Eye opening (E/O) reduces power at 10 Hz noticeably on the left side but hardly at all on the right.

7.4.3 *Feature extraction.* Automated recognition of EEG activity is used clinically in epilepsy monitoring. The computer is programmed to 'recognize' either interictal epileptiform activity or electrographic seizures and then to store these events in a separate file for subsequent printing or display. At present, programs that have been developed for this purpose lack specificity, particularly those used to detect interictal epileptiform activity. However, they are sensitive, i.e., real epileptiform activity is usually detected but non-epileptiform activity is also identified as epileptiform. The main advantage of automated feature extraction is that it provides the electroencephalographer with a powerful tool for reducing the amount of EEG recording that needs to be reviewed or stored for further analysis.

7.4.4 *Operating room and intensive care unit monitoring.* Quantitative EEG analysis is being used increasingly to monitor cerebral function in the operating room and intensive care unit. In the OR the scalp recorded EEG is useful for monitoring the level of general anesthesia and for detecting ischemia during carotid endarterectomy. Although this kind of monitoring can also be accomplished easily and reliably by routine visual EEG inspection, different methods of computerized analysis have been implemented. One well-known method consists of stacking successive power or amplitude spectral plots. This is referred to as a *compressed spectral array*. As shown in Figs. 7.3 and 7.4, gross changes which occur over time can be readily detected. Alternatively, a more precise evaluation of individual spectral features, such as the spectral edge frequency, can be plotted as a function of frequency (y axis) vs. time (x axis).

In comparison to OR monitoring, the application of quantitative EEG analysis in the ICU setting has been limited by; (1) the difficulties of maintaining the integrity of an EEG recording system over long periods of time; and (2) the detection and elimination of artifacts. Unlike the OR, EEG monitoring in the ICU is usually performed over long periods of time without an EEG technologist in attendance. Quan-

144

titative EEG analysis in such a situation is ideal because the EEG can be compressed into displays of selected spectral features plotted over long durations of time for quick review. However, without the original EEG, or an on-site technologist, the correct interpretation of artifacts is problematic.

For routine monitoring applications, automated artifact detection is currently used to remove signals which; (1) contain excessive 60-cycle contamination; (2) exceed a preset voltage range; or (3) present as a flat line. Whether or not such limited methods of artifact detection will suffice over long periods of time is currently under investigation. An alternative approach for following spectral trends over long periods of time consists of digitally recording the EEG approximately 1–3 min out of every 30 min, reviewing the 1–3-min segments on a monitor for the presence of artifacts, and then plotting spectral features from only those segments which are known to be artifact free by direct visual inspection. In this way persistent trends which develop over a period of hours may be reliably detected.

7.4.5 *Montage reformatting and digital filtering.*   One of the important advantages of computer-assisted EEG analysis is that the same segment of EEG can be reconstructed into different montages. Montage reformatting is easily understood if it is recalled that the EEG signal from each channel is simply the subtraction of the activity in the electrode in input 2 from the electrode in input 1. For example, the signal from Fp1-A1 is formed by subtracting the activity of A1 from Fp1. If a recording has been obtained from Fp1-A1 and F3-A1, then Fp1-F3 can be calculated by subtracting F3-A1 from Fp1-A1 as follows: $(Fp1-A1) - (F3-A1) = Fp1 - A1 - F3 + A1 = Fp1 - F3$. Notice that as long as all the electrodes that are to be combined can somehow be referred to the same reference electrode it is a simple matter to reconstruct any combination of montages, including the common average reference and Laplacian (source derivation) montages. However, if the original montage does not contain a particular electrode, then a new montage cannot be derived that contains that electrode.

145

Digital filtering allows the electroencephalographer to examine a particular finding with virtually any filter setting desired. Unlike analog filtering, digital filtering does not cause phase shifts. In addition, the same segment of EEG can be easily viewed with a variety of filter settings. For example, if an asymmetry of activity in the alpha frequency range is suspected, then activity outside the 8–13 Hz frequency band can be removed from the record by digital filtering. Reviewing EEGs with montage reformatting and digital filtering is currently somewhat time consuming. It is, however, routinely used for detecting and localizing electrographic seizure activity in epilepsy monitoring units.

7.4.6 *Evoked potentials: Computer averaging.* Sensory stimulation produces electrical responses in the relay stations of the sensory pathways and cortical receiving areas. These responses may be distinguishable in the EEG recorded from the overlying scalp, but they are often small and buried, indistinguishable from the EEG. These responses can be extracted from the EEG, and their details can be enhanced, by administering repetitive stimuli and averaging the EEG recording following each stimulus (Fig. 7.4). By this method, EEG components related to the stimulus are enhanced while components unrelated to the stimulus, also considered 'noise' in this context, are decreased and tend to average to zero.

Routine evoked potential recordings are made with standard EEG disc electrodes. Electrode placement depends on the sensory system under study and may include placements not routinely used in the 10–20 system. In addition, the bandwidth settings of the filters need to be wider than that of routine EEG recordings so that very fast components of the response are not attenuated. Typical filter settings for evoked potentials are 1–300 Hz for visual evoked potentials (VEPs) and 20–3000 Hz for brainstem auditory evoked potentials (BAERs) and SEPs. The output of each amplifier is connected to the input of the ADC in the computer.

A synchronizing pulse between the stimulator and computer triggers the computer to begin recording shortly before or at the beginning of the stimulus. The computer stops recording at the end of each analysis period, or epoch, and begins again with the next stimulus. After a sufficient number of epochs are obtained, they are aligned in time, added together, and then divided by the number of epochs recorded. This yields an average amplitude for the total summed epochs at each point in time. Even though the evoked potential signal is far smaller than the amplitude of the ongoing EEG, it grows in amplitude as successive analysis periods are added because the evoked response always occurs at a fixed time after the stimulus onset, as shown in Fig. 7.5. In contrast, the EEG and non-cerebral activity, which have no fixed relationship in time to the stimulus, will add in a random fashion and be gradually cancelled out. By the same token, only those evoked potentials which occur with the same latency after the stimulus can be averaged in a meaningful fashion. Otherwise they will either cancel each other out. Or, as in the case of flash visual evoked potentials, create a composite waveform with too great a variability to be clinically useful for the analysis of central nervous system conduction times.

The number of analysis periods, or epochs, that must be averaged to obtain an adequate evoked potential recording is best described in terms of the relationship between the signal-to-noise ratio and the number of epochs averaged, where the evoked potential represents the signal and all other activity (i.e., EEG, artifacts, etc.) is considered as noise. Described in this way, the signal-to-noise ratio is proportional to the square root of the number of epochs that are averaged. In one epoch of an imaginary evoked potential the signal-to-noise ratio is $1:1$. As a simple illustration consider that the goal is to increase the ratio to $10:1$. This would mean that the evoked potential has approximately 10 times the amplitude of the noise. To accomplish this would require that 100 analysis periods be averaged (not 10) since the square root of the number of trials is the improvement in the signal-to-noise ratio (i.e., the square root of $100 = 10$). If the signal-to-noise ratio is to be doubled from $10:1$ to $20:1$, then instead of increasing the number of epochs from 100 to

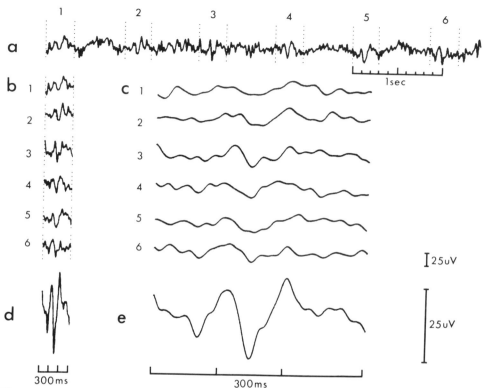

Fig. 7.5. Computer averaging of evoked potentials. The top line a shows cotinuous. EEG recorded between the right occipital and car electrode in a normal subjuct while light flashes were presented at intervals slightly shorter than 1 second (dotted lines at the beginning of periods 1 to 6). The computer sampled the voltage changes during periods of 300 msec after each flash (segments between dotted lines). These segments are arranged vertically in b with the same time scale as in a; they are show in c with an expanded time scale. The samples are added in d and e. The summation enhances features which are common to the individual responses. The sum can be converted into an average by dividing the gain by the number of samples.

148

200, it will be necessary to increase it to 400 ($20^2 = 400$). Therefore, the number of epochs that must be added to improve the signal-to-noise ratio increases exponentially and there is, for example, little to be gained by adding an additional 100 epochs to an average of 2000 epochs to improve noise reduction.

The number of epochs that must be recorded to obtain an adequate evoked potential record are typically in the range of 100–200 for pattern reversal visual evoked potentials and 2000 for BAERs and SEPs. The actual number needed depends largely on the amplitude of the potential, the extent of artifact contamination, and the artifact reduction and filtering methods employed. The amplitudes of most of the components in the evoked potential are usually less than 2 μV for SEPs, less than 0.5 μV for BAERs, and more than 10 μV for VEPs. One of the most effective methods for reducing the number of epochs needed is to visually screen each epoch and select only those with low amplitude noise. Although this is not practical for most routine applications, improved automated methods of artifact rejection are being developed for this purpose.

A critical factor in recording evoked potentials is the demonstration that a set, or ensemble, of averaged epochs is actually reproducible. It is not unusual for random signals to contaminate the average to the extent that the final averaged signal contains a distinctive waveform that is not an evoked potential. This problem is overcome by routinely recording and displaying a second average that confirms the reproducibility of the initial average. *It is not acceptable to draw any conclusions from a single set of averaged epochs without obtaining this confirmation from a second set*. Although certain artifacts may yield a reproducible averaged waveform, these are primarily limited to periodic or rhythmic contaminants such as 50 or 60 cycle interference or rhythmic EEG background activity. (For further details on evoked potential methodology in clinical practice, the reader may consult the American EEG Society Guidelines for Clinical Evoked Potential Studies and the other selected references at the end of the chapter).

149

7.4.7 *Signal comparisons.* Methods that compare signal similarities in frequency, amplitude and phase have been applied to EEG analysis in a number of ways to accomplish such tasks as localizing the mu rhythm, investigating inter- and intrahemispheric cortical relationships, elucidating the role of the thalamus in the generation of the alpha rhythm, and determining the anatomic pathways of spreading electrographic seizure activity. Most of these applications are based on, or derived from, the *cross-correlation* and *coherence functions.*

Cross-correlation evaluates the similarity between signals from two different sources recorded simultaneously. Similarities of both amplitude and shape are measured as the covariance of the signals; similarities of shape regardless of amplitude are expressed by the correlation coefficient which varies between +1, indicating that the signals have identical shape and polarity, and −1, indicating that they have identical shape but opposite polarity. If the two sources generate signals which have similar shape but different timing, the correlation coefficient will vary if the signals are displaced against each other in time; the dependence of the correlation coefficient on the time interval is represented by the correlation function. The correlation coefficient also varies with the frequency of the EEG components; the dependence of the correlation coefficient on the EEG frequency is the coherence function.

7.5 AMBULATORY EEG CASSETTE RECORDING

Ambulatory EEG cassette recording is routinely performed with 8–16 channel systems. Each channel has a preamplifier (made from a solid state amplifier chip) that may be located inside the cassette recording unit worn by the patient or attached near the recording electrode on the patient's head. An additional channel may be used to encode the time as well as to document clinical events each time the patient presses a button. Each cassette tape typically records for 24–36 h. After recording

150

the tapes are scanned on a monitor for the occurrence of electrographic seizure activity. During scanning the EEG signal can also be played through a speaker allowing for the detection of electrographic events by changes in sound pattern. EEG segments with suspected abnormalities are then played out onto an EEG machine for closer inspection and final interpretation.

Ambulatory recording has clearly been shown to be an efficient method for confirming the diagnosis of epilepsy. It is also sometimes helpful for seizure localization. However, monitoring appears to add little to the initial detection of neonatal seizures beyond that gained by performing a routine neonatal EEG recording; neonatal seizures usually occur at frequent intervals. The main disadvantages of ambulatory recording are: (1) the lack of simultaneous visual information, (2) the frequent occurrence of artifacts, and (3) the limited number of recording channels typically availabe. Because of the limited number of channels, and particularly when 2- or 4-channel recorders are used, strategic montage planning is extremely important.

The main clinical indications for ambulatory monitoring are: (1) to determine whether or not abnormal behavioral events are epileptic, (2) to quantify the frequency of epileptic seizures, and (3) to classify the patient's seizure disorder (e.g., partial vs. generalized, absence vs. complex partial).

7.6 EEG RECORDING WITH SIMULTANEOUS VIDEO MONITORING

Prolonged monitoring with closed circuit TV and EEG recording (*CCTV/EEG*) allows the electroencephalographer to combine both EEG and clinical information in the classification of seizure disorders. Indeed, the classification of seizures (see Appendix III) is now based on information obtained from CCTV/EEG monitoring.

CCTV/EEG monitoring is also essential for localizing the anatomical site of seizure onset in patients being evaluated for possible surgical intervention. If

151

behavioral events follow electrographic events, then the site of onset of the ictal activity has localizing value. However, if events precede the electrographic changes, then anatomical localization is less certain.

Current monitoring systems typically consist of the following components: (1) EEG amplifier/encoders, (2) a lightweight, flexible electrode cable to carry the signal from the electrodes to the amplifiers, (3) a decoder, (4) a special effects generator (splitter-inserter), (5) a reformatter, (6) an audio system, (7) a titler/timecode generator, (8) a monitor, and (9) video camera(s).

The encoder combines the signals from all channels into a single signal according to one of a variety of methods of signal multiplexing. The multiplexed signal is reconstructed into the original EEG signal by the decoder. The reformatter transforms the recorded EEG signal into a video display on the monitor and the special effects generator is used to combine the EEG and picture of the patient on the same monitor screen. The titler/timecode generator prints the time on the monitor screen and alphanumerics can be entered onto the picture from a keyboard. Using more than one video camera is helpful, since one camera can be focused on the patient's face (or other area of special interest) while the other provides a wider view of the entire body. The latter view also reduces the likelihood that the patient will move out of the view of the camera entirely.

The storage of the EEG and video signal on videocassette tape obviates the need for an EEG machine during the actual recording. However, to display EEG events for interpretation a printout on an EEG machine or other printing device is currently recommended. The system should allow the user to print out the same recorded segment with montage reformatting so that the same electrographic events can be seen using a variety of montages.

In some systems, instead of a direct lightweight electrode cable connection between the patient and the monitoring equipment (i.e., *cable telemetry*), the EEG electrodes are plugged into a radiotransmitter worn by the patient which transmits the multiplexed EEG signal to a receiver and then to a decoding unit. The potential disadvantages of radiotelemetry are that: (1) the signal may be interrupted if the patient wanders beyond the range of the radiotransmitter and (2) most patients are more likely to remain in view of the camera if a direct cable is used.

Since monitoring typically produces several days worth of data it is important to have an efficient method for reducing the amount of data to be reviewed. This can be accomplished in several ways. First, the patient, or someone with the patient, can press a button which triggers the storage of a time code whenever a seizure occurs. On some systems a list showing the times at which the button was triggered can then be displayed on the monitor screen so that the events can be located on the videotape. Second, electrographic seizure activity can be automatically detected by computer. Although this requires the added expense of a computer and seizure detection software it greatly reduces the likelihood of missing subclinical seizures or seizures that are not noted by the patient. Finally, both methods may be combined.

REFERENCES

Ajmone-Marsan, C. (1986) Depth electrography and electrocorticography. In: M.J. Aminoff (Ed.), Electrodiagnosis in Clinical Neurology, Churchill-Livingstone, New York.
American EEG Society Statement on the Clinical Use of Quantitative EEG (1987) J. clin. Neurophysiol. 4: 75.
Barlow, J.S. (1985) Methods of analysis of nonstationary EEGs, with emphasis on segmentation techniques: A comparative review. J. clin. Neurophysiol. 2: 267–304.
Binnie, C.D., Batchelor, B.G., Bowring, P.A., Darby, C.E., Herbert, L., Lloyd, D.S.L., Smith, D.M., Smith, G.F. and Smith, M. (1978) Computer-assisted interpretation of clinical EEGs. Electroenceph. clin. Neurophysiol. 44: 575–585.
Chiappa, K.H. (1989) Evoked Potentials in Clinical Medicine, Raven, New York.
Cracco, R.Q. and Bodis-Wollner, I. (1986) Evoked Potentials, Liss, New York.
Duffey, F.H., Bartels, P.H. and Burchfiel, J.L. (1981) Significance probability mapping: An aid in the topographic analysis of brain electrical activity. Electroenceph. clin. Neurophysiol. 51: 455–462.

Ebersole, J.S. (1989) Ambulatory Monitoring. Raven, New York.

Fisch, B.J. and Pedley, T.A. (1989) The role of quantitative topographic mapping or 'neurometrics' in the diagnosis of psychiatric and neurological disorders: the cons. Electroenceph. clin. Neurophysiol. 73: 5–9.

Fisch, B.J., Pedley, T.A. and Keller, D.L. (1988) A topographic background symmetry display for comparison with routine EEG. Electroenceph. clin. Neurophysiol. 69: 491–494.

Gasser, T., Bacher, P. and Mocks, J. (1982) Transformations towards the normal distribution of broad band spectral parameters of the EEG. EEG clin. Neurophysiol. 53: 119–124.

Gevins, A.S. and Remond, A. (1987) Methods of Analysis of Brain Electrical and Magnetic Signals. Handbook of Electroencephalography and Clinical Neurophysiology (revised series), Vol. 1, Elsevier, Amsterdam, pp. 31–38.

Gotman, J., Ives, J.R. and Gloor, P. (1985) Long-term monitoring in epilepsy. Electroenceph. clin. Neurophysiol. Suppl. 37: 444.

Gumnit, R.J., Ed. (1987) Intensive Diagnostic Monitoring, Advances in Neurology, Vol. 46, Raven, New York.

Gotman, J. (1985) Practical use of computer-assisted EEG interpretation in Epilepsy. J. clin. Neurophysiol. 2: 251–266.

Kahn, E.M., Weiner, R.D., Brenner, R.P. and Coppola, R. (1988) Topographic maps of brain electrical activity – Pitfalls and precautions. Biol. Psychiatr. 23: 628–636.

Kamp, A. and Lopes da Silva, F.H. (1987) Special techniques of recording and transmission. In: E. Niedermeyer and F.H. Lopes da Silva (Eds.), Electroencephalography: Basic Principles, Clinical Applications and Related Fields, Urban and Schwarzenberg, Baltimore, pp. 619–694.

Lopes da Silva, F.H. (1987) Computerized EEG analysis: A tutorial overview. In: A.M. Halliday, S.R. Butler and R. Paul (Eds.), A Textbook of Clinical Neurophysiology, Wiley, New York, pp. 61–104.

Lopes da Silva, F.H. and Storm van Leeuwen, W.S. (1986) Clinical Applications of Computer Analysis of EEG and Other Neurophysiological Signals. Handbook of Electroencephalography and Clinical Neurophysiology, revised series, Vol. 2, Elsevier, Amsterdam.

Mocks, J. and Gasser, T. (1984) How to select epochs of the EEG at rest for quantitative analysis. Electroenceph. clin. Neurophysiol. 58: 89–92.

Nuwer, M.R. (1988) Quantitative EEG: I. Techniques and problems of frequency analysis and topographic mapping. J. clin. Neurophysiol. 5: 1–44.

Oken, B.S. and Chiappa, K.H. (1986) Statistical issues concerning computerized analysis of brainwave topography. Ann. Neurol. 19: 493–494.

Pfurtscheller, G., Maresch, H. and Schuy, S. (1977) Inter- and intrahemispheric differences in the peak frequency of rhythmic activity within the alpha band. Electroenceph. clin. Neurophysiol. 42: 77–83.

Picton, T.W. (1988) Human Event-Related Potentials. Handbook of EEG (revised series), Vol. 3, Elsevier, Amsterdam.

Porter, R.J. and Sato, S. (1987) Prolonged EEG and video monitoring in the diagnosis of seizure disorders. In: E. Niedermeyer and F.H. Lopes da Silva (Eds.), Electroencephalography: Basic Principles, Clinical Applications and Related Fields, Urban and Schwarzenberg, Baltimore, pp. 634–644.

Roy, O.Z. (1976) Section III. Biotelemetry and telephone transmission. In: Rémond, A. (Ed.), Handbook of Electroenceph. clin. Neurophysiol., Vol. 3A, Elsevier, Amsterdam, pp. 46–66.

Van Hufflen, A.C., Poortvliet, D.C.J. and Van der Wulp, C.J.M. (1984) Quantitative electroencephalography in cerebral ischemia. Detection of abnormalities in 'normal' EEGs. In: G. Pfurscheller, E.J. Jonkman and F.H. Lopes da Silva (Eds.) Brain Ischemia: Quantitative EEG and Imaging Techniques, Elsevier, Amsterdam, pp. 3–28.

Walter, D.O., ed. (1972) Part B. Digital processing of bioelectric phenomena. In: Rémond, A. (Ed.), Handbook of Electroenceph. clin. Neurophysiol., Vol. 4B, Elsevier, Amsterdam.

Yingling, C.D., Galin, D., Fein, G., Peltzman, D. and Davenport, L. (1986) Neurometrics does not detect 'pure' dyslexics. Electroenceph. clin. Neurophysiol. 63: 426–430.

Part B
The normal EEG

Definition of the normal EEG, relation to brain function

8

SUMMARY

(8.1) An EEG is usually called normal not because it contains normal patterns but because it lacks abnormal patterns.

(8.2) A normal EEG does not guarantee the absence of cerebral pathology because not all abnormalities of brain structure and function produce abnormalities of the EEG.

(8.3) An abnormal EEG does not always indicate cerebral abnormality. A few specific mild EEG abnormalities can be seen in some instances in otherwise normal persons.

8.1 DEFINITION OF THE NORMAL EEG

A wide variety of normal EEG patterns can be seen in different persons of the same age, and an even greater variety of normal patterns can occur in different age groups; the waking record generally shows more variability between subjects than the sleep EEG. It is therefore not practical to define the normal EEG by listing all normal patterns and their variations; such a list would be too long. Nor can the normal EEG be defined by requiring that specific normal components be present; in this regard, the EEG differs from other tests such as the electrocardiogram. The problem of defining the normal EEG is therefore better approached in a different way. In contrast to the great variety of normal patterns, there are only a few EEG components, such as spikes and sharp waves, certain slow waves and amplitude changes, which are known to be definitely abnormal in each age group. The normal EEG can therefore be defined more effectively by the absence of abnormal components than by the presence of normal patterns. Conversely, an EEG is considered abnormal if it contains abnormal components regardless of whether or not it also contains normal components. The EEG reader therefore has to know the major features of the normal EEG at different ages and to distinguish from them abnormal components by using a set of precise descriptors (9).

8.1.1 *The normal EEG up to the age of 19 years.* The normal EEG undergoes enormous changes from the early premature period to about the age of 19 years. Characteristic patterns appear at fairly predictable ages and later disappear or change into more mature patterns. The variety of patterns which are accepted as normal is greater during this period than during adulthood. Even abnormalities such as spikes and slow waves have clinical implications which differ from those of similar components in adults. Little is known about the clinical significance of the failure of normal patterns to appear and disappear at expected ages; failure of electrographic maturation is suggestive but not indicative of behavioral retardation.

8.1.2 *The normal EEG of adults.* Between the ages of 20 and 60 years, the normal EEG shows only few changes; these changes have little clinical importance. The limits between normal and abnormal patterns are better defined in this age group than in younger persons and abnormal patterns correspond fairly well with basic types of brain lesions, although not necessarily with specific diseases.

8.1.3 *The normal EEG above the age of 60 years.* The normal EEG at this age is similar to that of younger adults except that a few specific patterns which would be considered abnormal at a younger age become acceptable as normal.

Although acute, severe and large abnormalities of the brain are likely to cause EEG abnormalities, normal EEGs may be seen in some cases of long-standing, mild and small cerebral abnormalities. For instance, a small infarct in the internal capsule far from the recording electrodes may cause a catastrophic hemiplegia but no EEG abnormality. A large infarct near the recording electrodes may cause EEG changes which last for a few weeks or months but then disappear even though the neurological deficit persists. The EEG may remain normal for a long period in slowly progressive, widespread brain diseases, such as senile dementia, which lead to cerebral atrophy and mental changes. An epileptogenic focus may escape detection if it does not fire during the recording or if it is too far from the recording electrodes.

8.3 AN ABNORMAL EEG DOES NOT NECESSARILY MEAN ABNORMAL BRAIN FUNCTION

Most abnormal EEG patterns indicate abnormal brain function. However, abnormal patterns occur occasionally in persons not showing evidence of brain disease. The type and incidence of these patterns is fairly well known in adults. A slight excess of a certain kind of slow waves (21.1.2), and an EEG of unusually low amplitude (24.2.2), occur in about 5–15% of normal persons after the age of 20 years. One might be inclined to call these patterns normal, especially since they occur most commonly in apparently normal persons; however, the same patterns can be seen in patients with mild forms of diseases which, in their more severe stages, are associated with more pronounced expressions of the same EEG patterns. This suggests that in at least some persons, mild manifestations of these patterns indicate mild cerebral abnormalities. In order not to overlook the possibility of such cerebral abnormalities, one should therefore categorize even the mild forms of these patterns as EEG abnormalities. This attitude finds some support in the observation that the incidence of these mild EEG abnormalities decreases in groups of persons who have passed strict examinations, for instance tests used for the selection of flying personnel.

REFERENCES

Goldensohn, E.S. and Koehle, R. (1975) EEG Interpretation: Problem of Overreading. Futura, Mount Kisco, New York.
Hawkes, C.H. and Prescott, R.J. (1973) EEG variation in heatlhy subjects. Electroenceph. clin. Neurophysiol. 34: 197–199.
Hughes, J.R. (1987) Normal limits in the EEG. In: A.M. Halliday, S.R. Butler and R. Paul (Eds.) A Textbook of Clinical Neurophysiology, Wiley, Chichester, pp. 105–154.
Klass, D.W. (1987) Identifying the abnormal EEG. In: A.M. Halliday, S.R. Butler and R. Paul (Eds.) A Textbook of Clinical Neurophysiology, Wiley, Chichester, pp. 189–200.
Kellaway, P. (1979) An orderly approach to visual analysis: The parameters of the normal EEG in adults and children. In: Current Practice of Clinical Neurophysiology, Raven, New York, pp. 69–148.
Maulsby, R.L. (1979) EEG patterns of uncertain diagnostic significance. In: D.W. Klass and D.D. Daly (1979) Current Practice of Clinical EEG, Raven, New York, pp. 411–420.
Maulsby, R.L., Kellaway, P., Graham, M., Forst, J., Proler, M.L., Low, M.D. and North, R.R. (1968) The Normative Electroencephalographic Data Reference Library. Final Report, Contract NAS 9-1200, National Aeronautics and Space Administration, 172 pp.
Van Dis, H., Corner, M., Dapper, R., Hanewald, G. and Hok, H. (1979) Individual differences in the human electroencephalogram during quiet wakefulness. Electroenceph. clin. Neurophysiol. 47: 87–94.
Westmoreland, B.F. (1982) Normal and benign EEG patterns. Am. J. EEG Technol. 22: 3–31.

Descriptors of EEG activity

9

SUMMARY

To analyze the EEG, the reader needs to distinguish: 1. *Wave form*; 2. *repetition*; 3. *frequency*; 4. *amplitude*; 5. *distribution*; 6. *phase relation*; 7. *timing*; 8. *persistence*; and 9. *reactivity*. These features allow the EEG reader to recognize different patterns.

9.1 WAVE FORM

Wave form or *shape* are simple terms used to describe the *configuration* or *morphology* of a wave. Any change in the difference of the electrical potential between two recording electrodes is called a *wave*, regardless of its form. Any wave or sequence of waves is called *activity*. Many waves are *regular*, i.e. they have a fairly uniform appearance due to symmetrical rising and falling phases (Fig. 9.1, Part 1). Some regular waves are similar to sine waves and are called *sinusoidal* (Fig. 9.1, Part 2) while other regular waves may be arch-shaped or saw-toothed. *Irregular waves* have uneven shapes and durations (Fig. 9.1, Part 4).

A *monophasic* wave is a single deflection either up or down from the baseline. A *diphasic* wave has two components on opposite sides of the baseline while a *triphasic* wave has three components alternating about the baseline. A *polyphasic* wave has two or more components of different direction. These terms do not indicate whether a wave has positive or negative electrical polarity (3.4.1) nor whether it was recorded with bipolar or referential electrode montages (4.1).

A *transient* is an event which clearly stands out against the background. It consists of either a single wave or a *complex*, i.e. a sequence of two or more waves which have a characteristic form or recur with a fairly consistent shape (Fig. 9.1, Part 5).

A *sharp transient* is a wave of any duration which has a pointed peak at conventional EEG recording speed. Sharply contoured waveforms which are not abnormal epileptiform waveforms are often referred to sharp transients. *Epileptiform* is a term used to describe EEG patterns that are identical to those that have been specifically associated with seizures or epilepsy. Epileptiform patterns usually consist of apiculate waveforms referred to as *spikes* or *sharp waves*. A *spike* is a sharply contoured waveform with a duration of 20–70 msec (Fig. 9.1, Part 7). A *sharp wave* has a duration of 70–200 msec and may not be as sharply contoured as a spike (Fig. 9.1, Part 6). Sharply contoured waveforms that: (1) appear as part of the background rhythm (e.g., the mu rhythm); (2) appear at different times either in isolation or as part of the background rhythm (e.g., wicket spikes; 19.4.5); (3) demonstrate a varying morphology; or (4) only occur once in the entire record are often referred to as sharp transients because they have less significance in the diagnosis of seizure disorders than do stereotyped spikes or sharp waves (see also 17.1.1).

A spike may be followed by a slow wave and form a *spike-and-wave complex* (Fig. 9.1, Part 8) which may repeat at regular intervals. Spike-and-wave complexes recurring at rates below 3 Hz are called *slow-spike-and-wave complexes*. A sharp wave may be followed by a slow wave and form a *sharp-and-slow-wave complex;* complexes of this kind usually last longer than a third of a second and therefore do not repeat at rates over 3 Hz. In some cases, two or more spikes occur in sequence, forming *multiple spike complexes*, also called *polyspike complexes* (Fig. 9.1, Part 9). These complexes may be followed by a slow wave and thus form part of a *multiple spike-and-slow-wave complex* or *polyspike-and-slow-wave complex* (Fig. 9.1, Part 10). Spikes recorded in the EEG should not be confused with action potentials of single nerve cells which are recorded through microelectrodes inserted

164

into the brain and which last only about 1 msec (1.1.3); they too are often called spikes but are never observed in the surface EEG. *< 3 sec*

Single spikes and sharp waves, and complexes which contain spikes and sharp waves and last for less than a few seconds are called *interictal epileptiform activity*; longer lasting activity of this type and of some other types is referred to as a *seizure pattern* or *ictal pattern* (17.1). Although seizure patterns are often associated with clinical seizure manifestations, they may occur without such correlates and are then called *subclinical seizure patterns*. Both interictal and ictal patterns are here called *epileptiform* in contrast to the definition in the glossary of the International Federa-

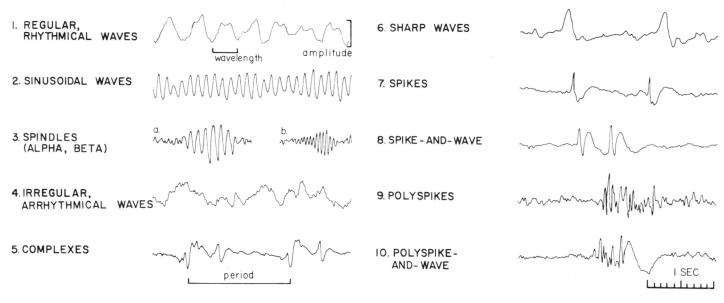

Fig. 9.1. Characteristic wave forms.

165

tion of Societies for Electroencephalography and Clinical Neurophysiology which uses the term 'epileptiform' only for interictal patterns.

A *paroxysm* or a *paroxysmal discharge* consists of one or more waves which begin abruptly, reach maximum amplitude rapidly, and disappear suddenly. These waves clearly stand out against the background, are usually abnormal, and are often seen in epileptiform patterns. Paroxysms often consist of complexes (Fig. 9.1, Part 5), but not all complexes begin and end abruptly, and not all paroxysms recur with a similar shape.

It is important to note that although the terms spike(s), sharp wave(s), paroxysm, and paroxysmal discharges are often used to describe epileptiform patterns, they are not synonymous with epileptiform activity. Thus, if epileptiform activity is considered to be present, then the term epileptiform must be added to any other descriptive terms used. For example, if the activity seen is considered to be epileptiform then in the interpretation of the EEG it would be incorrect to simply state: The EEG is abnormal due to the presence of spikes localized to the left anterior temporal lobe. Instead it should be rephrased as: The EEG is abnormal due to the presence of epileptiform spikes localized to the left temporal lobe.

9.2   REPETITION

Repetition of waves may be rhythmical or arrhythmical. *Rhythmical* repetitive waves have similar intervals between individual waves; they are usually regular and often sinusoidal in shape (Fig. 9.1, Parts 1–3). *Spindles* are groups of rhythmical repetitive waves which gradually increase and then decrease in amplitude (Fig. 9.1, Part 3). Rhythmical repetitive waves were formerly called 'monorhythmic' or 'monomorphic'. *Arrhythmical* repetitive waves are characterized by variable, irregular intervals between individual waves (Fig. 9.1, Part 4). They can be considered to be a sequence of waves of different frequency. They often have irregular

166

shape. Arrhythmical irregular waves were formerly called 'polyrhythmic' or 'poly-morphic'.

Frequency refers to the number of times a repetitive wave recurs in one second. A wave completing three cycles in one second is called a wave of 3 Hertz (Hz) or of 3 per sec. The frequency of single or repetitive waves can be determined by measuring the duration of an individual wave, the *wavelength* (Fig. 9.1, Part 1), and calculating the reciprocal. For instance, a wave lasting 250 msec or 1/4 second is said to have a frequency of 4 Hz, regardless of whether or not it repeats. Single waves and complexes may repeat at intervals longer than the wavelength and are then called 'periodic', the *period* being the time interval between them (Fig. 9.1, Part 5).

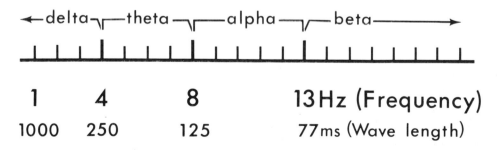

Fig. 9.2. Frequency bands. Delta, theta, alpha and beta frequency bands, defined by wave frequency and length.

The frequency of EEG waves is often divided into four groups or *frequency bands*, namely:

- delta frequency band: under 4 Hz
- theta frequency band: from 4 to under 8 Hz
- alpha frequency band: from 8 to 13 Hz
- beta frequency band: over 13 Hz (Fig. 9.2).

These divisions are somewhat arbitrary; many EEGs contain waves of frequencies extending across the boundaries of the bands, for instance waves of 3–5 Hz. Nonetheless, the frequency bands help to set apart the most important normal and abnormal waves in the EEG, and frequency is one of the most important criteria for assessing abnormality in clinical EEG. Although waves under 8 Hz are commonly called *slow waves* and waves over 13 Hz are commonly called *fast waves*, it is more accurate and therefore preferable to either state the frequency of the activity (e.g., 3–5 Hz) or describe it according to the frequency band(s) it occupies (e.g., delta and theta activity). Activity that is less than 1/2 Hz or more than 20 Hz is of limited clinical utility in routine scalp recordings because it is often unclear if such activity is of cerebral origin (6.1–3).

9.4 AMPLITUDE

Amplitude of EEG waves is measured in microvolts (μV). It is determined by measuring and comparing the total vertical distance of a wave (Fig. 9.1, Part 1) to the height of a calibration signal recorded at the same gain and filter settings (3.3.1). Thus, if the height of an EEG wave measures 14 mm and a calibration signal of 50 μV measures 7 mm, the amplitude of the wave is 100 μV. If the sensitivity of an amplifier is known to be 7 μV/mm (3.4.2), a wave of 7 mm can be inferred to have an amplitude of 50 μV without direct comparison with a calibration pulse.

Amplitude should not be expressed in terms of the height of the pen deflection because this varies with the amplifier settings.

In clinical EEG, amplitude is often not reported in terms of microvolts but described loosely as *low* (under 20 μV), *medium or moderate* (20–50 μV), or *high* (over 50 μV). However, these terms often are used to describe amplitude of certain waves relative to that of other waves in the same record. For instance, a wave of 60 μV cannot be said to be of high amplitude if it occurs on a background of 40–50 μV.

An important abnormality is *asymmetry* of amplitude of the activity that is recorded simultaneously from corresponding parts of the two sides of the head. Even slight differences of amplitude may be of clinical importance (23.2) if they persist; this is true especially of the adult EEG, with the exception of the alpha rhythm (11.1).

Differences of amplitude are sometimes caused by factors outside the brain, especially by unequal spacing and impedance of the recording electrodes; the technician should therefore verify correct electrode placements (2.3) and impedances (2.2) before accepting that abnormal amplitude is genuine.

9.5 DISTRIBUTION

Distribution refers to the occurrence of electrical activity recorded by electrodes positioned over different parts of the head. EEG patterns may appear over large areas on both sides of the head, over one side only, or in a restricted, small area.

9.5.1 *Widespread, diffuse or generalized* distribution refers to activity which occurs at the same time over most or all of the head. Generalized activity may have a clear maximum within its field of distribution, recognized by the highest amplitude in referential recordings and by phase reversal in bipolar recordings from that area (4.1).

169

9.5.2 *Lateralized* distribution refers to activity which appears only or mostly on one side of the head. Lateralized activity is abnormal and suggests a cerebral abnormality either on the side where abnormal activity is present or on the side where normal activity is absent. Some normal patterns may appear on one side of the head at one time and then occur on the other side a few seconds or minutes later (9.7).

9.5.3 *Focal* activity is that which is restricted to one or a few electrodes over an area of the head. Some of the neighboring electrodes may pick up the same activity with lower amplitude. This restricted distribution must be distinguished from a wide or generalized distribution which may have a maximum in one area. This distinction is important especially with regard to abnormal slow waves and to sharp waves. Criteria which sometimes help in this distinction are that *focal slow waves* often have a lower frequency at the area of maximum amplitude whereas generalized slow waves do not. *Focal sharp waves* with a tendency to spread can often be distinguished from generalized sharp waves with a local maximum of amplitude by their greater persistence at the focus.

Activity arising from a single unilateral focus is always abnormal. Activity from a midline focus or from two foci located symmetrically in the two hemispheres may be part of a normal pattern.

9.6 PHASE RELATION

Phase refers to the timing and polarity of components of waves in one or more channels. Waves of different frequency may occur in different channels so that the troughs and peaks occur at the same time; these waves are said to be *in phase*. If they do not coincide in this manner, they are said to be *out of phase*. The phase difference may be expressed in terms of phase angle. For instance, peaks pointing in opposite directions are said to be 180° out of phase. Such a *'phase reversal'* is the major indicator of the origin of EEG potentials in bipolar recordings (4.1.1). In a single channel, phase refers to the time relationship between different components of a rhythm; for instance, the peak of a sine wave is said to 'lead' the preceding crossing of the zero line by 90° and to 'lag' behind the next following peak by 360°.

9.7 TIMING

Timing of waves in different areas of the head may be similar or different. The terms *'simultaneous'* and *'synchronous'* are used to indicate that two events occurred at the same time. These terms are usually used with the same meaning, but 'synchronous' is sometimes used to denote precise coincidence while 'simultaneous' may be used more broadly to indicate the coincidence that is recognizable only imprecisely within the limits of the relatively slow recording speed of the EEG. The eye can hardly distinguish a horizontal difference of less than 1 mm between corresponding points on two waves even in neighboring channels. A horizontal distance of only 1 mm corresponds to a time difference of 33 msec at the conventional EEG recording speed. The resolution of time relations deteriorates if more distant channels are compared and if the writing units are not perfectly aligned; because of the curvilinear movement of the pens, synchronous excursions of different amplitude seem to have occurred at different times (3.6.1).

Waves which occur at the same time on both sides of the head are called *'bilaterally synchronous'* or *'bisynchronous'*. These terms consider mainly the relationship between the two sides but not necessarily that on the same side; thus, bilaterally synchronous waves may be out of phase in the same hemisphere. In some instances, waves are delayed against each other by the same amount in successive channels which record activity from electrodes placed from the front to the back of the head, giving the impression that these waves spread from front to back. For instance, this type of delay can be seen in triphasic waves of metabolic encephalopathies (19.2.6).

Waves which occur in different channels without constant time relation to each other are called *'asynchronous'*. This usually implies that the waves are present in different areas at the same time even though they do not fall in phase with each or do not have the same frequency. If waves occur in one area at one time and in other areas at another time, they are usually said to be *'independent'*; for instance, spikes in both temporal lobes may occur bisynchronously or independently; each case has different implications regarding a possible triggering mechanism.

9.8 PERSISTENCE

Persistence describes how often a wave or pattern occurs during a recording. Some waves occur only occasionally or intermittently, either in the form of a single wave or trains of waves; other waves are present through most or all of the recording. The persistence of waves can be estimated by measuring the proportion of time during which these waves appear. This is called the *index*. For instance, a delta index of 20% means that delta activity was present during one-fifth of a recording. Because the clinical importance of EEG patterns often depends not only on their persistence but also on their amplitude, the persistence and amplitude are often described together in terms of their *quantity, amount or prominence*. The term 'abundance', previously used to describe this combination of persistence and amplitude, is now obsolete.

Single waves and complexes may occur with a high, moderate or low persistence or incidence; the persistence of these events is best expressed as their average number in one second or one minute. They may occur periodically or at irregular intervals. Irregular and infrequent occurrence is sometimes called *'sporadic'*. The terms 'random' and 'diffuse' should not be used to describe persistence of EEG patterns.

9.9 REACTIVITY

Reactivity refers to changes which can be produced in some normal and abnormal patterns by various maneuvers. Some patterns are induced or increased, diminished or blocked by opening or closing the eyes, hyperventilation, photic or sensory stimuli, changes in levels of alertness, movements or other maneuvers. Abnormal slow waves in toxic and metabolic encephalopathies are often diminished by alerting and enhanced by hyperventilation and drowsiness whereas abnormal slow waves seen in cases of structural lesions usually show a less attentuation or blocking during alerting maneuvers.

Thus, a recording should not be considered complete unless at least simple alerting maneuvers have been performed to demonstrate the effects of arousal on the EEG. These maneuvers include eye opening and closing (this may be passively performed for infants or other individuals who cannot respond to verbal commands) and questions testing memory and simple calculations. If the patient is unable to respond to verbal commands then vigorous auditory and tactile stimulation should be applied. These maneuvers will also help clarify if background slowing is actually present or if the patient was merely excessively drowsy during the recording.

REFERENCES

Binnie, C.D. (1987) Electroencephalography and epilepsy. In: A. Hopkins (Ed.) Epilepsy, Demos, New York, pp. 169–200.

Blume, W.T. and Lemieux, J.F. (1988) Morphology of spikes in spike-and-wave complexes. Electroenceph. clin. Neurophysiol. 69: 508–515.

Chatrian, G.E., Bergamini, L., Dondey, M., Klass, D.W., Lennox-Buchthal, M. and Petersén, I. (1974) A glossary of terms most commonly used by clinical electroencephalographers. Electroenceph. clin. Neurophysiol. 37: 538–548.

Gastaut, H. (1975) Section I. The significance of the EEG and of ictal and interictal discharges with respect to epilepsy. In: Rémond, A. (Ed.), Handbook of Electroenceph. clin. Neurophysiol., Vol. 13A, pp. 3–6.

Niedermeyer, E. (1987) Abnormal EEG patterns. In: E. Niedermeyer and F. Lopes da Silva (Eds.), Electroencephalography: Basic Principles, Clinical Applications and Related Fields, Urban and Schwarzenberg, Baltimore, pp. 183–208.

Pedley, T.A. (1980) Interictal epileptiform discharges: Discriminating characteristics and clinical correlations. Am. J. EEG Technol. 20: 101–109.

The normal EEG from premature age to the age of 19 years

10

SUMMARY

The development of the normal EEG parallels the maturation of the brain. Milestones are summarized in Table 10.1 and 10.2. The most abrupt changes occur between the early premature age and the first three months of life. The EEG of the premature baby depends on the conceptual age, i.e. the gestational age plus the time since birth. The premature baby develops new EEG patterns and modifies the acquired ones within fairly narrow ranges of conceptional age. One may distinguish patterns characterizing the periods of the conceptional ages.

(10.1.1)   *Less than 29 weeks*

(10.1.2)   *29 to 31 weeks*

(10.1.3)   *32 to 34 weeks*

(10.1.4)   *34 to 37 weeks*

(10.1.5)   *At the conceptual age of 38 weeks* the premature infant has developed EEG patterns similar to those of the full-term (40 weeks conceptual age) newborn.

(10.2)   *After 46 weeks conceptual age*, the neonatal patterns are replaced by patterns which show different rhythms in different areas. This differentiation, and the frequency of the rhythms, increases rapidly during the first year of life.

(10.3)   *During the first 3 months of life* there is a gradual loss of the neonatal patterns and a posterior dominant amplitude gradient develops during wakefulness and quiet sleep. Between 3 and 4 months of age approximately three-fourths of normal infants demonstrate a 3–4 Hz occipital rhythm during wakefulness that is activated by passive eye closure and attenuated by passive eye opening or alerting.

(10.4)   *During childhood and late adolescence*, several age-specific patterns appear transiently, but background activity during wakefulness continues to shift towards the alpha and beta frequency range.

(10.5)   *EEG abnormalities* are less sharply defined below the age of 20 years. Patterns that are abnormal in adults may be normal at younger ages; synchrony, distribution and relation to sleep stages must be taken into consideration when deciding whether a particular activity is normal or abnormal.

10.1   NEONATAL EEG

Neonatal EEG recording places special demands on both the electroencephalographer and the technologist because: (1) there are a number of age-specific normal electrographic features that are prominent for only several weeks at a time; (2) many of the patterns occurring in the neonatal period have different implications than when seen at later ages (such as multifocal sharp transients or discontinuous patterns); and (3) special recording techniques are used (5.2).

With few exceptions, the EEG of the neonate is a function of the actual age of the brain. The actual age of the neonate from the time of conception is referred to as the *conceptual age*. Knowledge of the conceptual age is critical for accurate EEG interpretation and should always be noted on the record by the technologist. It is determined by adding the estimated *gestational age* (the number of weeks and days of intrauterine life since the last menstrual period) to the *legal age* (the number of days and weeks since the time of birth). Thus, the EEG of a normal 4-week-old neonate who was born at 30 weeks gestation will show the same kinds of EEG patterns as a 1-week-old born at 33 weeks of gestation since they both have the same conceptual age (34 weeks). Under abnormal circumstances a pattern that is appropriate at one conceptual age may appear at a later age. This persistence or reappearance of patterns with immature features is referred to as *dysmaturity* or *anachronism*. Dysmaturity may be transient and associated with reversible cerebral disorders (such as electrolyte disturbances or mild anoxia due to pulmonary disease), or may be present on repeated recordings and associated with more enduring disorders of cerebral function (e.g., ischemic-hypoxic encephalopathy or intraventricular hemorrhage). When a much more mature EEG pattern than expected is seen it is usually because the conceptual age has been underestimated.

The EEG and other physiological findings that define the behavioral state of the neonate develop together in an organized and predictable fashion. Behavioral states can be assessed from the EEG and from electrographic recordings of body movements, eye movements, respiratory pattern and EMG. In addition, frequent notations by the technologist verify the accuracy of the electrographic monitors and provide essential information regarding body, eye, and respiratory movements, artifacts, and the presence of other individuals in the recording environment. Body movements in the neonate can usually be characterized as phasic (rapid) or tonic (slow and sustained muscle contractions). Respiration can be described as regular (appearing as monorhythmic fluctuations in recordings from nasal thermistor or thoracic strain gauge monitors) or irregular (in repetition rate and amplitude).

Each neonatal recording should ideally include the following monitors (as described in Chapter 4): (1) eye movement monitors (2 channels); (2) a submental EMG activity monitor; (3) an electrocardiogram monitor recorded in one channel using electrodes placed on either arm (this channel can also be useful for detecting body movements); and (4) two respiratory monitors: a thoracic strain gauge (or a motion transducer) to detect chest wall movements in one channel and a nasal or oral thermistor to detect airflow in the other channel. Chest wall movements can also be recorded using electrodes placed on the left and right sides of the chest that measure skin impedance (impedance pneumogram). As in adults, *central apnea* (an absence of breathing due to a complete interruption of both diaphragmatic and chest wall movement) will appear as the cessation of activity in both monitors, whereas *obstructive apnea* (a block in air flow due to intermittent upper airway obstruction) will appear as continuing chest wall movement without evidence of airflow (activity in the chest wall movement monitor without activity in the thermistor).

Neonatal EEG recordings may be performed with electrodes placed either at all the standard 10–20 positions or with a reduced array. A reduced number of electrode positions is preferred (see Table 4.4 and Section 5.2) because: (1) the relatively small head size of the neonate allows for an adequate sampling of EEG activity with fewer electrodes; (2) the crowding together of a full set of electrodes increases the likelihood of inadvertently connecting adjacent electrodes with salt bridges; and (3) the use of fewer electrodes simplifies the recording procedure which is often performed in fragile patients and under difficult circumstances.

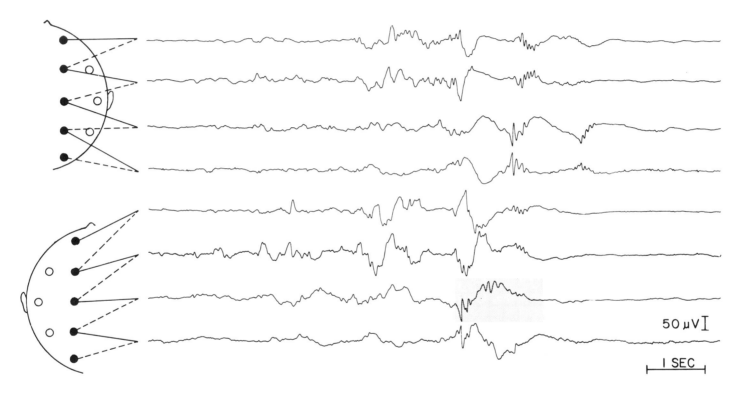

Fig. 10.1. Pattern of discontinuous activity of quiet sleep in a normal premature baby of a conceptional age of 34 weeks, recorded 5 days after birth. Delta brush is marked by shading.

Although premature and full-term neonatal EEG recordings are often run at routine paper recording speeds of 3 cm per second, it is helpful to perform part or all of the recording at a slower speed of 1.5 cm per second. Slower recording speeds make it easier to appreciate discontinuous background changes, transitions between continuous and discontinuous backgrounds, and the symmetry and rhythmicity of slower waveforms. The duration of the routine neonatal record should be approximately 45–60 min. This usually allows for the recording of the neonate's typical behavioral states. In the full-term infant sleep cycles usually last 45–60 min and consist of about 25 min of active sleep and 20 min of quiet sleep.

10.1.1 *Premature infants of less than 29 weeks conceptual age.* At approximately 28 weeks of life the major sulci of the brain are just beginning to appear. At this time there is relatively little variation in behavior except for occasional fluctuations in body motility. Eye movements are rare and respiration is continuously irregular. When body movements do occur they are mostly tonic. Single or repetitive jaw jerks may also be seen.

EEG background activity this early in life is always discontinuous (a finding which is universal among mammalian species) and consists of bursts of moderate to high amplitude waveforms that are usually maximal over the posterior head regions and interrupt an otherwise nearly flat background. The intervals between the bursts have an average duration of 6 sec but may last up to 25–30 sec. This pattern is commonly referred to as *tracé discontinue*. The duration of the relative flattening becomes shorter during periods of increased motor activity and with increasing age. Under abnormal circumstances, such as cerebral hypoxia, the interburst interval becomes longer in duration. With increasing age the tracé discontinu pattern gradually gives way to a discontinuous pattern with shorter duration and higher amplitude interburst periods commonly referred to as *tracé alternant*. The tracé alternant pattern first appears between 34 and 36 weeks conceptual age (10.1.4) and

179

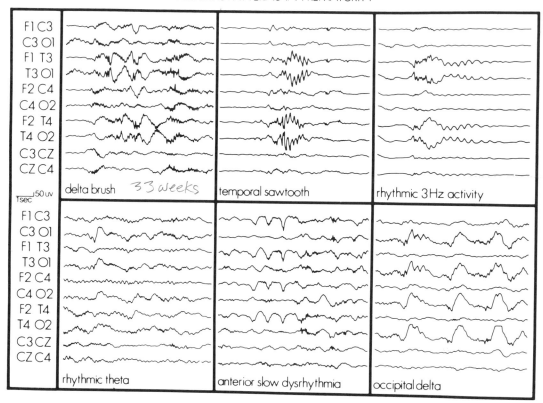

Fig. 10.2. These normal patterns seen in premature infants are sometimes mistaken for abnormalities. They were recorded at (from left to right, above to below): 33 weeks, 30 weeks, 28 weeks, 29 weeks, 35 weeks and 28 weeks conceptual age. (Courtesy S.S. Werner, J.E. Stockard and R.G. Bickford, Atlas of Neonatal EEG, Raven, New York, 1977).

may be seen as late as 46 weeks conceptual age. *Interhemispheric synchrony* (i.e., the time of onset of EEG activity in one hemisphere compared to the other) is well developed at this age and approximately 90–100% of bursts begin within 1.5 sec of each other. Indeed, interhemispheric synchrony is often better developed than intrahemispheric synchrony at this age.

The characteristic EEG feature seen at this age is the *delta brush pattern*. It consists of moderate to high voltage (25–200 μV) 0.3–1.5 Hz delta waves with superimposed 10–150 μV rhythmic fast activity. The 'brush', or fast activity, is typically in the 8–22 Hz range, although somewhat slower, 4–6 Hz activity, may be also seen, particularly at this age. *Delta brushes* are located predominantly over the central and occipital head regions, but as the neonate becomes older they become more prominent over the temporal head regions. Delta brushes are most abundant between 32 and 35 weeks conceptual age (Figs. 10.1 and 10.2), occur infrequently at term, and are not seen in normal neonates beyond 42–43 weeks conceptual age.

10.1.2 *Premature infants of 29 to 31 weeks of age.* Behavior at this age is characterized by more prominent variations between quiescence and body motility, rare periods of regular respiration, and irregular rapid eye movements (REM).

Active sleep, characterized by the appearance of continuous EEG activity in association with REM, irregular respiration and increased body motility occurs rarely. *Quiet sleep*, characterized by discontinuous EEG activity, reduced eye and body movements and regular respiration is also infrequent. Thus, in the majority of routine recordings quiet and active sleep still cannot be clearly differentiated. *Delta brushes* are now more abundant, appear over the central, occipital and temporal head regions, and occur most often during periods of REM. In contrast, after 33–34 weeks conceptual age they occur most frequently during non-REM periods. Interhemispheric synchrony is lowest between 31 and 32 weeks of conceptual age with approximately 50–70% of the onset bursts occurring within 1.5 sec of each other.

181

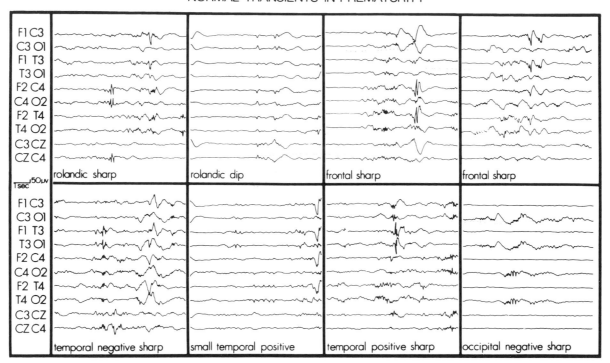

Fig. 10.3. These records illustrate the variability in location, amplitude, and duration of transients recorded in normal prematures at (from left to right, above to below): 33 weeks, 30 weeks, 28 weeks, 28 weeks, 33 weeks, 30 weeks, 33 weeks and 30 weeks. (Courtesy S.S. Werner, J.E. Stockard and R.G. Bickford, Atlas of Neonatal EEG, Raven, New York, 1977)

Theta bursts with amplitudes up to 200 μVs occur frequently ove the temporal head regions and occasionally resemble delta brushes (Fig. 10.2). They may appear in a unilateral or bisynchronous fashion. They are also seen, although far less often, prior to 29 weeks and as late as 35 weeks conceptual age.

10.1.3 *Premature infants of 32 to 34 weeks of age.* Motor activity is now more often phasic than tonic. Eye movements tend to occur in clusters and periods of regular respiration are more frequent.

Although activity consistent with active and quiet sleep (as described in 10.1.2) is more likely to be seen than previously, much of the recording still contains *transitional or indeterminate sleep* (sleep states which are not identifiable as either quiet or active sleep). Continuous activity is seen more frequently and is associated with REM, active sleep and wakefulness. *Tracé discontinu* contains shorter duration periods of relative inactivity. However, by 32 weeks CA these periods should not exceed 10 sec. Intermittent amplitude gradients appear with greater amplitude activity in the delta frequency range over the posterior head regions. Delta brushes are present predominantly over the central and occipital head regions.

Two other distinctive changes also occur at this age. The first is an increase in the number of *multifocal sharp transients* (Fig. 10.3) in all states. The second is the appearance of EEG reactivity: stimulation of the neonate now produces clear changes in the EEG.

10.1.4 *Premature infants of 34 to 37 weeks of age.* EEG reactivity is now present in all states and appears as either a widespread attenuation of activity or, less often, as an augmentation of activity. Active sleep is further defined by: (1) the appearance of more active eye movements during REM periods (including more vertical eye movements than seen previously) and (2) a decrease in EMG activity (revealed by an attenuation of activity in the submental EMG monitor). Quiet sleep is seen more often in association with longer periods of regular respiration.

183

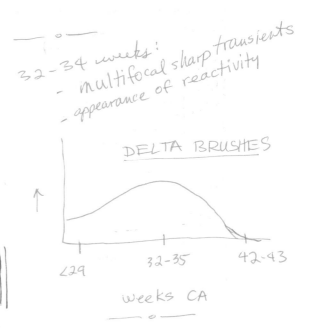

During periods of continuous EEG activity a spatial amplitude gradient is maintained with predominantly lower amplitude faster activity appearing maximally over the anterior head regions and predominantly higher amplitude delta activity appearing maximally over the posterior head regions. *Delta brushes* are now more frequent during quiet sleep than during active sleep. It is also during this stage of life that

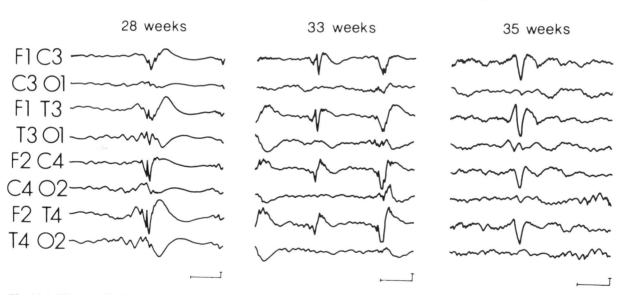

Fig. 10.4. High-amplitude 'spikey' or polyphasic transients are seen in frontal regions before 36 weeks conceptual age. Calibration is 50 μV and 1 sec. (Courtesy S.S. Werner, J.E. Stockard and R.G. Bickford, Atlas of Neonatal EEG, Raven, New York, 1977)

the overall abundance of delta brushes begins to decline and this trend continues until they disappear at approx. 42–43 weeks conceptual age. The *tracé alternant* pattern (10.1.1) gradually replaces the *tracé discontinu* pattern. The onset of 60–80% of all bursts between hemispheres (interhemisphere synchrony) differs by no more than 1.5 sec during tracé discontinu and tracé alternant at 33–34 weeks of age. This degree of interhemispheric synchrony increases to 70–85% at 35–36 weeks of age.

Multifocal sharp transients are less abundant, but well developed *frontal sharp waves* (also referred to as *encoches frontales*) are first seen at this age (Fig. 10.4). Frontal sharp waves are biphasic, sharply contoured waveforms that may be unilateral, asymmetric, or bilateral and synchronous. They are maximal in amplitude over the frontal and mid-frontal head regions. They occur most often during sleep and are rarely seen up to 48 weeks conceptual age.

Monorhythmic frontal slowing (also referred to as *anterior slow dysrhythmia*) occurs frequently at this age and persists into the perinatal period. It consists of short runs of bilateral, monomorphic or rhythmic, 2–4 Hz, 50–150 μV activity (Fig. 10.2). It should not be confused with abnormal patterns, particularly neonatal epileptiform patterns.

Prior to this age wakefulness is difficult to record because it occurs infrequently and is often associated with movement related artifacts. At this age quiet wakefulness appears more often and consists of activity similar to that seen during active sleep. It is relatively low in amplitude with little evidence of an anterior–posterior amplitude gradient; a pattern sometimes referred to as *activité moyenne* (Fig. 10.5).

10.1.5 *Infants of 38 to 42 weeks of age.* Wakefulness and active and quiet sleep are now clearly differentiated. Four main EEG patterns are seen. The first consists of continuous widespread 25–50 μV theta activity with intermixed lower amplitude delta activity and is present during quiet wakefulness and active sleep. This pattern

185

[handwritten margin notes]

34 – 37 weeks:
- tracé alternant *
- encoches frontales (up to 48 weeks)
- monorhythmic frontal slowing (FIRDA-like)
- activité moyenne △

* during NREM sleep
△ " wakefulness

—o—

38 – 42 weeks

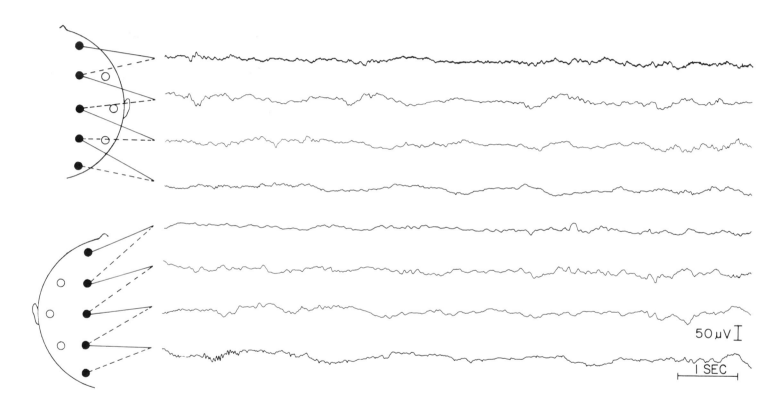

Fig. 10.5. Pattern of low voltage irregular theta and delta waves ('activité moyenne') in a wakeful normal full-term infant, 10 days old.

186

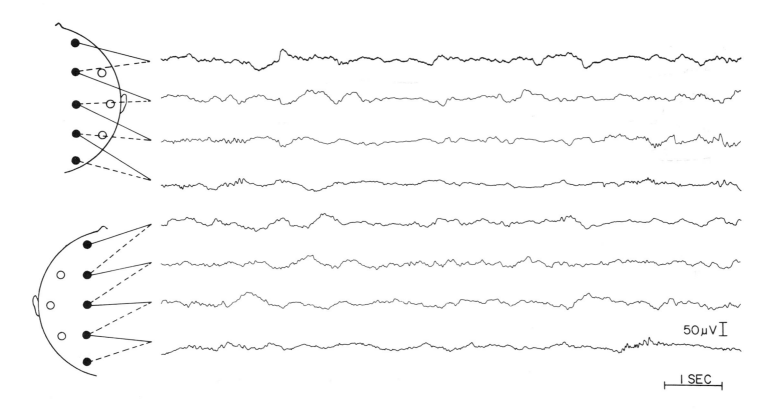

Fig. 10.6. Pattern of low voltage irregular slow waves, including larger delta waves, during active sleep in a normal full-term infant, 10 days old.

"mixed pattern"

also seen in wakefulness

187

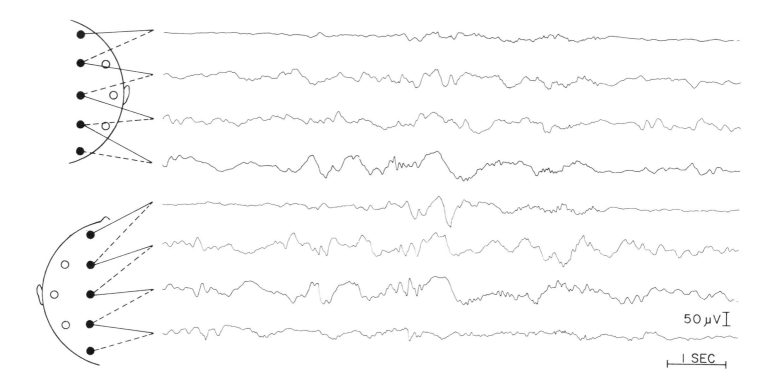

50 µV

1 SEC

Fig. 10.7. Pattern of continuous high amplitude slow waves of quiet sleep in a normal full-term infant, 4 days old.

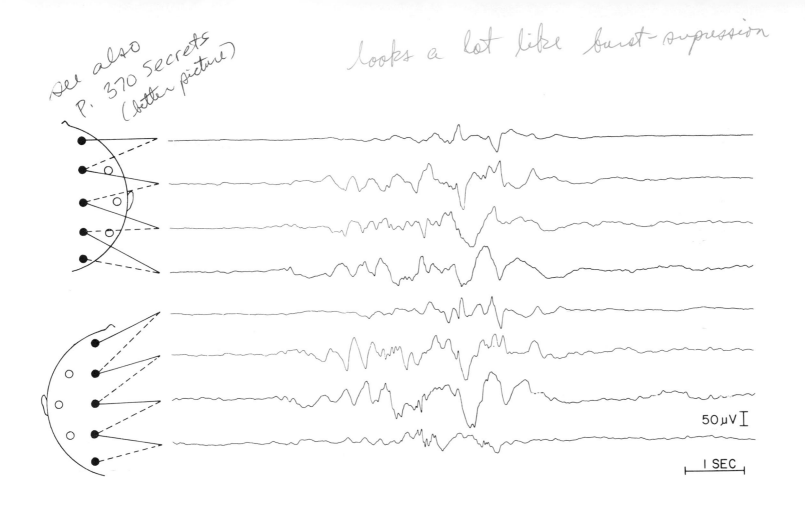

See also
P. 370 Secrets
(better picture)

looks a lot like burst-supression

50 μV

1 SEC

Fig. 10.8. Pattern of quiet sleep ('tracé alternant') in a normal full-term infant, 4 days old.

189

is referred to as the *low voltage irregular pattern*, or activité moyenne (Fig. 10.5), although the voltage is low only in relation to other activity present at this age. The second type of pattern contains similar features but also has intermixed intermittent higher amplitude 2–4 Hz delta waveforms. Because it combines low and high amplitude components it has been referred to as the *mixed pattern* (Fig. 10.6). It is also seen during wakefulness and active sleep. The other two patterns occur during quiet sleep. In one there is continuous 25–150 μV slow delta activity, referred to as either the *high voltage slow pattern* or *continuous slow wave pattern* (Fig. 10.7). However, at term nearly all quiet sleep is dominated by the fourth pattern: *tracé alternant* (Fig. 10.8). Nearly 100% of the bursts of activity occurring in the tracé alternant pattern are synchronous by 40 weeks conceptual age. Brushes are very infrequent and, if present, occur almost exclusively during quiet sleep.

Frontal sharp waves (*encoches frontales*) and *monorhythmic frontal delta* (*slow anterior dysrhythmia*) occur frequently, particularly during indeterminate (transitional) sleep. Sharp transients are regularly seen over the central and temporal head regions. Because multifocal sharp transients in the neonate are sometimes misinterpreted as being suggestive of a seizure disorder, the following points warrant emphasis. Sporadic multifocal sharp transients in either wakefulness or sleep in a 28–42 week CA infant are a normal finding. Moreover, although they decrease in occurrence after 40 weeks CA, rare (2–3/h) multifocal spikes in any state are considered normal up to 44 weeks CA. In addition to frontal sharp waves, sharp transients commonly occur as part of the burst phase of the tracé alternant pattern and may occur sporadically over the rolandic head regions during quiet sleep. An abnormal increase in the abundance of multifocal sharp transients represents a nonspecific response to any encephalopathic process and does not specifically suggest the presence of a seizure disorder. If it is the only abnormal finding, then the EEG is interpreted as mildly abnormal. Frequent sharp transients occurring in any location during wakefulness or active sleep after 42 weeks CA are abnormal (see also 19.1).

190

(see also 19.1).

Between term and the end of the first 3 months of life precursors of adult patterns appear and neonatal patterns gradually disappear. The tracé alternant pattern occurs less and less frequently until it disappears at 46 weeks CA. At term, and thereafter, interhemispheric synchrony during tracé alternant is present nearly 100% of the time. As noted in 10.1.5, frontal sharp transients (encoches frontales) and monorhythmic frontal delta (slow anterior dysrhythmia) are associated with sleep, particularly transitions between active and quiet sleep, and are commonly seen up to 41 weeks CA. However, it has not been determined beyond what CA their presence constitutes a significant abnormality and frontal sharp transients may occur very rarely up to 48 weeks CA. Multifocal sharp transients, which are most commonly seen in all states between 32 and 34 weeks CA, decline in frequency and retreat into quiet sleep, becoming rare by 42 weeks CA and finally disappearing at 44 weeks CA.

Drowsiness between full term and 5 months of life is usually characterized by gradual generalized background slowing which increases in amplitude and progresses smoothly into sleep. This often occurs when the infant appears to be awake and resting with the eyes partially or fully open. Because of the frequent lack of obvious EEG and behavioral changes during drowsiness, the reliable detection of the onset of drowsiness by clinical observation is difficult in the first 5 months of life.

At term approximately 80% of episodes of sleep onset consist of active sleep. But by 46 weeks CA the majority of sleep onset episodes begin with quiet sleep. This shift in sleep state at sleep onset is roughly paralleled by a shift in the relative time occupied by active and quiet sleep; from 40 to 48 weeks CA active sleep decreases from approximately 50% to 40% of total sleep time. Background activity during quiet sleep shifts from the tracé alternant pattern (which occupies nearly 100% of quiet sleep at term) to the high voltage slow (continuous slow wave) pattern which

191

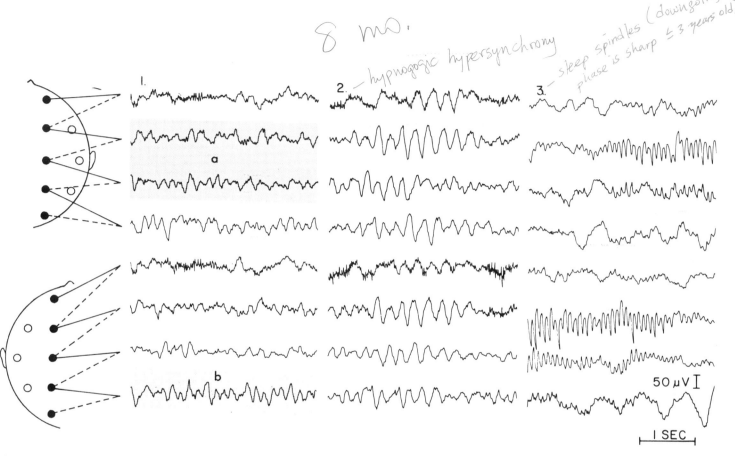

Handwritten annotations:

8 mo.
2. - hypnogogic hypersynchrony
- sleep spindles (downgoing phase is sharp ≤ 3 years old)

Fig. 10.9. Patterns of wakefulness (1), drowsiness (2) and sleep (3) in a normal 8 month old infant. 1. During wakefulness, rhythmical theta waves of 4–5 Hz in the central regions (a) can be distinguished from a rhythm of 6 Hz in the occipital areas (b); 2. Drowsiness is associated with high amplitude bisynchronous waves of 3–4 Hz; 3. During sleep, prominent spindles appear in the central regions, slightly asynchronous on the two sides; they are superimposed on generalized slow waves of under 2 Hz.

predominates by 45–46 weeks CA. As the name implies, the high voltage slow pattern consists of predominantly theta and delta waveforms. At 40 weeks CA this activity is often maximal over the posterior head regions and by 3 months of age an amplitude gradient with greater amplitude activity over the posterior than the anterior head regions is well established and persists until approximately 10 years of age.

Sleep spindles may be present in rudimentary form at 40 weeks CA, but they are not consistently seen until 2–3 months of age. They appear as 12–14 Hz runs of low to moderate amplitude rhythmic activity with maximal amplitude over the central and parasagittal head regions that usually last 3–5 sec. In the first 3 years of life sleep spindles often have a characteristic rectified morphology (the negative, or downgoing phase, is sharply contoured) that differentiates them from the more sinusoidal appearing sleep spindles in older individuals (Fig. 10.9, Part 3). Until approximately 8 months of life they are frequently asynchronous over the 2 hemispheres and appear to shift from one side to the other. After this time asynchronous sleep spindles occur less and less often and after 2 years of age asynchronous sleep spindles are considered abnormal. In addition to asynchrony, sleep spindles also frequently demonstrate a shifting asymmetry or occur more often on one side compared to the other. Sleep spindles should be considered abnormal only if they appear unilaterally or demonstrate a consistent amplitude asymmetry of more than 50%.

Tactile or auditory stimulation during sleep can produce one of several nonspecific reactions in the EEG: (a) a negative vertex spike up to 100 μV; (b) generalized flattening; (c) bursts of generalized slow waves; (d) bursts followed by flattening; and (e) change in sleep stage, especially from tracé alternant to diffusely slow or low voltage pattern. In addition, more specific responses may be elicited during wakefulness and sleep in the form of visual evoked potentials in response to single flashes (5.2; 7.6.1; 14.3.1) in approximately 60% of newborns. This response

193

is typically a high amplitude (75 to 200 μVs), sharply contoured triphasic waveform that has a much longer latency of onset following the flash (up to 200 msec) than that seen in adults. It fatigues rapidly and occurs only with single flashes or at slow rates of stimulation (1 per second or less). It may be elicited at the onset or cessation of more rapid rates of stimulation (sometimes referred to as the on and off response). Rarely, lambda waves (occipital waveforms evoked by looking at complex patterns; 11.4) appear when the infant is looking around the room. When present (as in childhood and adulthood) lambda waves are usually associated with a prominent flash evoked response.

10.3 INFANTS FROM 3 MONTHS TO 12 MONTHS OF AGE

10.3.1 *Wakefulness* is characterized by patterns which begin to show regional differences and to react to stimulation.

Background activity consists of rhythmical and arrhythmical slow waves in the delta and theta frequency range. These waves are generalized, and often more prominent over the occipital areas. They may appear synchronously over wide areas of both hemispheres. Delta waves become more rhythmical and diminish considerably during the first year. Before the age of 5 months, rhythmical occipital activity develops from the diffuse theta activity which is most prominent over the central and posterior regions (Fig. 10.9, Part 1). The absence of rhythmical theta activity after 5 months of age is considered abnormal.

Occipital rhythms which can be clearly distinguished from the background first appear at the age of about 3 months.* These rhythms have frequencies of 3–4 Hz and are reduced in amplitude by eye opening. They become more regular and increase in frequency to about 5 Hz at 5 months of age and to 6–8 Hz at the end of the first year of life (Fig. 10.9, Part 1). The amplitude decreases from 50–100 μV to 50–75 μV at

* tabla Rubén

194

12 months. The trend of alpha frequency in relation to age in a group of normal individuals is shown in Fig. 10.10.

10.3.2 *Drowsiness* up to the age of 6–8 months is associated with a smooth transition from patterns of wakefulness to those of sleep; the EEG shows a generalized and progressive increase of amplitude and a decrease of frequency to 2–3 Hz. At 3 months of age approximately 30% of infants show a specific pattern of drowsiness referred to as *hypnogogic hypersynchrony* which consists of rhythmical and bisynchronous 3–5 Hz waves of high amplitude (75–200 μV; Fig. 10.9, Part 2). These waves begin rather abruptly and are widely distributed. They sometimes have an anterior, temporal or posterior predominance, and occur intermittently or continuously for up to several minutes at the beginning and at the end of sleep. Nearly 100% of normal infants between 6 and 8 months of age show this pattern and it is present in the majority of infants and children between 4 months and 2 years of age. Hypnogogic hypersynchrony vanishes gradually and is rarely seen by 12 years of age. The rhythmical slow waves lose amplitude and become asynchronous and are thus transformed into the adult pattern of drowsiness. A few infants do not show this pattern of drowsiness but instead show occipital or widespread rhythmical and asynchronous 4–5 Hz waves of low to medium amplitude; this pattern more closely resembles the adult patterns of drowsiness.

10.3.3 *Sleep* activity shows several major changes during the first year of life: Active sleep develops into a sleep stage characterized by rapid eye movements (REM); the two infantile EEG patterns previously seen during active sleep are transformed into electrical patterns which gradually come to resemble the low amplitude patterns of the adult REM stage of sleep (12.2.6). REM sleep, at first occupying about one-half of the total sleep time, decreases to about 40% of total sleep time at the age of 3–5 months, and to about 30% in the second half of the first year. The tracé

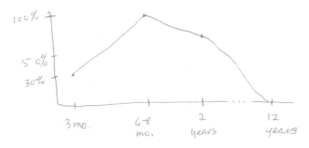

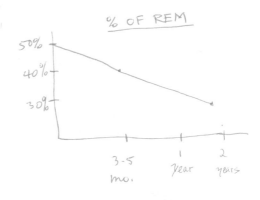

195

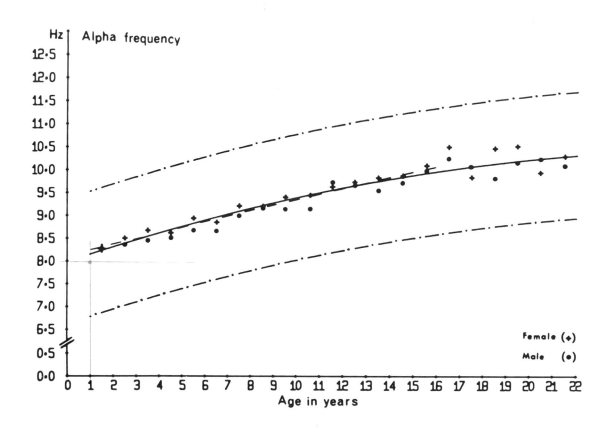

Fig. 10.10. Alpha frequency in relation to age in highly selected normals (continuous line). The diagram is based on a second degree polynomial (parabolic function). The dot–dash lines indicate 95% confidence limits. (Courtesy P. Kelleway, Current Practice of Clinical EEG, Raven, New York, 1979)

196

fig 10.7

alternant and high voltage slow patterns of quiet sleep disappear 4–6 weeks after
term and are replaced by sleep patterns which contain elements resembling those of
adults. At the age of about 6 months, the EEG begins to show features similar to
those which distinguish the adult non-REM sleep stages I–IV (12.2). After the age
of 3 months, sleep no longer begins with the active phase: infants now fall directly
into non-REM sleep and go into REM sleep 40–50 minutes later. During non-REM
sleep there is generalized, posterior dominant, delta activity with occasional intermixed moderate to high amplitude bi- or tri-phasic delta waveforms that appear
over the occipital head regions. These intermixed occipital waveforms have a prominent negative phase and are referred to as *cone waves*, or 'O' waves. They are most
prominent during stages 2 and 3 sleep and are commonly observed up to 5 years of
age.

Sleep stages in this age group are characterized by the following combinations of
EEG patterns and behavioral characteristics.

REM sleep can generally be distinguished from non-REM sleep by EEG patterns,
by the occurrence of eye and limb movements, and by irregular breathing. However,
in infants and young children the behavioral manifestations of REM sleep are not
very tightly correlated with the EEG pattern of REM sleep. For example, irregular
breathing, characteristic of REM sleep in adults, occurs also in non-REM sleep in
infants. Furthermore, the EEG patterns of REM sleep in infants consist of delta and
theta waves which gradually change towards the pattern of low amplitude diffuse
asynchronous slow waves characteristic of the adult EEG during REM sleep. In
contrast to adults, normal infants may have sharp waves in the occipital regions
during REM sleep.

Non-REM sleep is usually associated with regular breathing, absence of movements and presence of tonic neck muscle activity. Non-REM sleep can be divided
into four stages characterized by EEG patterns similar to those of adults (12.2).
These patterns begin to become distinguishable in the second half of the first year
after the elements of these patterns are established.

197

The most important elements of sleep activity acquired during the first year of life are sleep spindles, vertex sharp transients and K complexes.

Sleep spindles continue to increase in distribution and abundance up to 3–6 months of age to the point where they typically occur in prolonged runs lasting 8 sec or longer separated by intervals of less than 10 sec. After that time, the duration of spindle bursts decreases. An absence of sleep spindles between the ages of 5 and 12 months may be considered abnormal, but only if the duration of uninterrupted recorded sleep exceeds approximately 30 min (i.e., a reasonable sample of non-REM sleep states is obtained). Spindles are commonly asynchronous over the two hemispheres until the age of 8 months in normal infants; continuously asynchronous spindles after 2 years of age are abnormal. Spindle bursts are fairly asymmetrical in normal infants, but a marked and persistent reduction on one side raises the suspicion of a unilateral depression of activity.

Vertex sharp transients (V waves) and K complexes can be distinguished in rudimentary form in some infants during the neonatal period. They appear in well developed form for the first time at the age of 5 to 6 months. *V waves* have negative polarity, an amplitude of up to 250 μV, a wide distribution about the vertex, and a duration of usually less than 200 msec. V waves in the neonatal period tend to be smaller, longer lasting and more asymmetrical than later. In infants and young children, vertex waves often appear in short bursts (Fig. 10.11, Part 3a) or repetitive runs and tend to have a sharper configuration compared to those seen in adolescents and adults. K complexes consist of a sharp, negative, high amplitude wave (often over 200 μVs in ear reference recordings) followed by a moderate to high amplitude longer duration positive wave. Their topography is similar to that of vertex waves, but they are readily distinguished by their longer duration (greater than 0.5 sec). They occur spontaneously during non-REM sleep and can be elicited during sleep by sensory stimulation (particularly auditory). The positive component usually occurs approximately 0.75 sec after the stimulus. They may or may not be followed by a 1–2 sec run of sleep spindles.

198

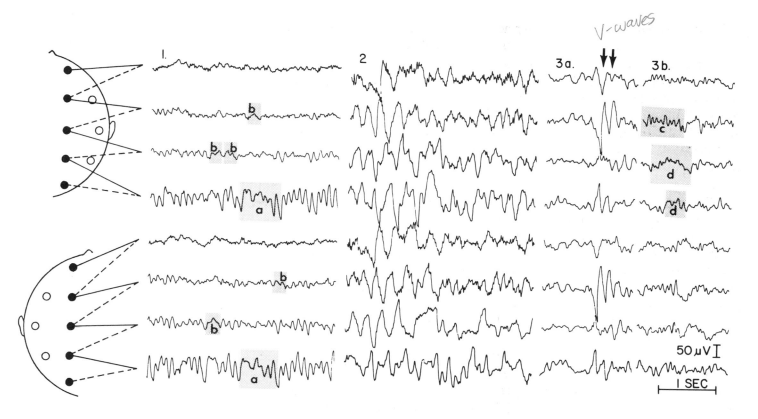

Fig. 10.11. Patterns of wakefulness (1), drowsiness (2) and sleep (3) in a normal boy of 12 years. 1. Wakefulness is associated with well developed occipital alpha rhythm of 9–10 Hz superimposed on bilaterally synchronous intermittent slow waves of 1–2 Hz (a), and with central theta waves (b); 2. Drowsiness is characterized by generalized bilaterally synchronous slow waves of 2–4 Hz of high amplitude; 3. Sleep is associated with repetitive V waves (arrows) in 3a, and with sleep spindles (c) and slow waves (d) in 3b.

The EEG during resting wakefulness can now be recorded more reliably and at greater length and shows differentiation of patterns towards those seen in adults. The waking record becomes the major indicator of structural lesions and metabolic abnormalities of the brain; the sleep EEG becomes useful for the activation of epileptiform activity. Hyperventilation and photic stimulation during wakefulness can be used as test conditions which may add information to that of the spontaneous EEG.

Resting wakefulness is often associated with a mixture of an alpha rhythm and slow waves of theta frequency. POSY

The alpha rhythm develops from the rhythmical background activity in the occipital regions (Fig. 10.11, Part 1). It consists of sinusoidal waves of 8–13 Hz which are greatest in amplitude over the posterior head regions and may extend forward to the central regions and beyond. The alpha rhythm appears during relaxed wakefulness, usually while the eyes are closed. It is blocked or clearly attenuated by eye opening, attention, and by mental effort. The alpha rhythm slows in frequency and then disappears in drowsiness. The frequency of the alpha rhythm increases gradually with age (Fig. 10.10) and reaches 8 Hz in over 80% of children by 3 years of age. Between childhood and adolescence it reaches the 9–11 Hz range.

The amplitude of the alpha rhythm also increases up to the age of 10 years and averages 50–60 μVs (measured in T5-O1) between the ages of 3 and 15. In some children (particularly those between 6 and 9 years of age) the amplitude may exceed 100 μVs. Children rarely show low amplitude (less than 20 μVs in T5-O1) alpha rhythms and, in contrast to adults, either absent or very low amplitude alpha rhythms (less than 15 μVs in T5-O1) are abnormal between 3 and 12 years of age. The alpha rhythm is frequently asymmetric, usually with greater amplitude on the

200

right. However, the hemisphere with greater alpha amplitude should not exceed the amplitude of the opposite hemisphere by more than 1.5 times.

Slow waves decrease in prominence with age. Theta waves are more prominent than alpha waves up to the age to 4 years. Between 5 and 6 years, the amounts of alpha and theta activity are about equal. After this age, alpha waves are normally more prominent than theta waves. Rhythmical theta waves during wakefulness in the teenage years are usually most prominent over the temporal and posterior head regions (Fig. 10.11, Part 1). They also appear over the frontocentral head regions in approximately 15–20% of normal individuals between 8 and 16 years of age. Frontocentral theta may even occur in early adulthood. Therefore, the presence of 5–7 Hz frontal or frontocentral theta in runs lasting several seconds are a normal finding in young individuals. Anterior theta activity should only be considered abnormal if it occurs during wakefulness with amplitudes of 100 μVs or greater in bipolar montages or when the amplitude clearly exceeds that of the alpha rhythm. Random frontal delta activity diminishes rapidly after 5 years of age and is rarely seen after 9 years of age.

Intermixed random theta and delta waveforms are commonly seen over the posterior head regions during childhood and adolescence. They occur less often thereafter but may still be seen in over 5% of normal individuals up to 30 years of age. These waveforms, like frontocentral theta, are commonly misinterpreted as an abnormal finding. Rhythmic, 1–3 sec runs of 2.5–4.5 Hz activity of less than 100 μVs make up less than 2% of the waking record in up to 25% of children between the ages 1 and 15 years. This activity is most likely to be seen between 5 and 7 years of age. It is occasionally accentuated by hyperventilation.

Between the ages of 6 months and 2 years moderate to high amplitude, diphasic, approximately 0.75-sec duration, waveforms appear over the occipital head regions immediately following the onset of eye blinks. They may have a sharp component

201

but should not be mistaken for abnormal background slowing or abnormal epilep-tiform waves. They have been referred to as *shut eye waves*.

After 8 years of age prominent occipital slow waves normally occurring during wakefulness often fall into the categories of either the *slow alpha variant* (Fig. 11.1, Part 4) or *posterior slow waves of youth* (Fig. 10.11, Part 1a). The *slow alpha variant* occurs rarely and consists of a series of waves with approximately half the frequency of the surrounding alpha rhythm. Because of its morphology, distribution, and frequency, and because it demonstrates the same reactivity as the alpha rhythm, it is considered to be a subharmonic of the alpha rhythm.

Posterior slow waves of youth are also considered to be formed by the alpha rhythm and therefore share the same distribution and reactivity to eye opening. They are most likely to be seen between the ages of 8 and 14 years, but occur commonly between 2 and 21 years of age. Although they occur infrequently after 21 years of age, if clearly identifiable, they should be considered a normal variant at any age. Each waveform has the duration of 4–6 combined waveforms from the surrounding alpha rhythm. They may occur in rapid succession or be separated from each other by one to several seconds. They often have a characteristic fused alpha wave morphology in which individual alpha waves appear with increasing definition during the second half of the waveform.

The precise point at which posterior slowing becomes abnormal, particularly in children, is poorly defined. As noted above, a substantial portion of normal slow waves that occur over the posterior head regions do not fall into the categories of either posterior slow waves of youth or the alpha variant. The correct interpretation of posterior slow waves in individuals less than 9 years of age is also made difficult by the fact that posterior dominant slowing frequently occurs as a nonspecific response to a variety of diffuse cerebral dysfunctions such as head injury, CNS infection and toxic or metabolic encephalopathies. After 9 years of age, anterior dominant or generalized slowing predominates. There are, however, several useful guidelines for identifying normal posterior slowing during wakefulness that include the following: (1) in children over 1 year of age a monorhythmic occipital rhythm that attenuates with eye opening (performed passively by the technologist when necessary) that has a normal frequency for the age of the child should be present; (2) slower waveforms should rarely exceed the amplitude of the alpha rhythm by more than 1.5 times; (3) asymmetries of slower waveforms should conform to a similar asymmetry in the ongoing alpha rhythm; (4) the slow waves should also have approximately the same topographic distribution as the alpha rhythm; and (5) the slow waves should attenuate with the alpha rhythm during alerting. As in adults, rhythmical, bisynchronous, occipital slow waves of about half the frequency of alpha rhythm may alternate or mix with alpha rhythm to form slow alpha variants (11.1.7). Unlike adults, some normal teenagers show intermittent or briefly repetitive posterior slow waves of medium or high amplitude which transiently replace alpha rhythm.

Beta activity occurs only rarely in children and adolescents during wakefulness. At any age beyond the neonatal period the voltage of beta activity recorded during wakefulness between adjacent electrodes (e.g., F3-C3) should not exceed 25 μVs. Excessive beta activity, particularly in the 18–25 Hz band, is almost always seen as a medication effect. It is reliably produced in most individuals by benzodiazepenes and barbiturates, even at nonsedating levels. For this reason, chloral hydrate, which rarely produces excessive beta activity at the minimal doses required for sedation, is commonly used for sedation in the EEG laboratory. However, higher doses of chloral hydrate will also produce beta activity. Aside from drug induced beta activity, the clinical significance of excessive beta activity during wakefulness is uncertain. A more important clinical finding is an asymmetry of beta activity. In general, the difference in amplitude between homologous hemispheric head regions should be less than approximately 35% of the amplitude of the side with the greater amplitude. If an abnormal asymmetry is present, then in contrast to activity that

203

is below the beta range, it is almost always the case that the abnormal side is the side with lower amplitude. A notable exception is the situation in which a skull defect (with or without an associated underlying lesion) may result in an ipsilateral increase in beta amplitude.

Mu rhythm may begin in childhood or adolescence and is similar to that in the adult (11.3).

Drowsiness may be associated with the following patterns:

(1) Between the ages of 6 months and 2 years the majority of children demonstrate *hypnogogic hypersynchrony*; it is rarely seen after 12 years of age. This pattern may at times appear abruptly on an otherwise quiescent background with intermixed low amplitude spike-like waves. Because of its paroxysmal appearance and occasional accompanying sharply contoured waveforms it is frequently misinterpreted as an abnormal epileptiform pattern (Figs. 19.17 and 19.18).

(2) Between 6 months and 2 years an increase in beta activity in the predominantly 20–25 Hz range often appears maximally over the central and posterior head regions during drowsiness and stages 1 and 2 sleep. In older children and adults beta activity may also be activated by drowsiness, but it appears more anteriorly; over the frontocentral head regions.

(3) At approximately 10 years of age adult patterns of drowsiness become more common. The earliest sign of drowsiness, when present, is often the appearance of *slow lateral eye movements*. These movements produce waveforms of 1 Hz or less that have maximal amplitude and opposite polarity at the F7 and F8 electrodes. They frequently occur at a time when the alpha rhythm is still present. With continued drowsiness the alpha rhythm may slow by 1–2 Hz. *Therefore, it is extremely important that the frequency of the alpha rhythm be determined during wakefulness, and that wakefulness is clearly established by performing specific alerting maneuvers* (e.g., ask the patient to respond to verbal commands or answer questions about orientation to place, time, or person, or to perform mental calcula-

204

tions). These maneuvers should be followed or preceded by eye opening and closing on command.

(4) Between 10 and 20 years of age prominent frontal rhythmic theta activity occurs commonly during drowsiness.

Sleep activity shows maturation of stages and the development of new patterns.

The sleep stages I–IV of non-REM sleep and the *stage of REM sleep* become more similar to those of adults (12.2) and can be distinguished more easily from each other. Sleep cycles also mature. The proportion of time spent in REM sleep gradually drops from about 30% of the total sleep time at 1–2 years to the adult fraction of about 25%.

see p. 195

Positive occipital sharp transients of sleep (POSTs) similar to those of adults (12.1.2) begin to appear in light sleep during childhood.

Fourteen and 6 Hz positive bursts are frequently seen during drowsiness and sleep in children and adolescents and are more common at these ages than in adults. They are most likely a normal phenomenon (19.4.2).

Vertex waves in children, particularly between the ages of 3 and 5, often have a very sharply contoured morphology and may occur in repetitive runs. Because of these features they are sometimes misinterpreted as abnormal central epileptiform spikes.

Cone waves (10.3) are often present during non-REM sleep from infancy until 5 years of age.

10.5 MAJOR ABNORMALITIES DURING THE NEONATAL PERIOD AND INFANCY

Because normal and abnormal patterns in the first year of life differ greatly from those seen later in life, the major EEG abnormalities during infancy are also presented in this chapter.

Mild or moderate deviations from normal neonatal EEG patterns occur frequently as a nonspecific response to many disorders (e.g., sepsis or abnormalities of pulmonary function, cerebral blood flow, nutrition, hydration, and electrolyte balance). Indeed, because birth itself is a stressful event, if the EEG is obtained within the first 3 days after delivery, a number of transient abnormalities may be seen. In contrast, major neonatal EEG abnormalities are always associated with a severe degree of cerebral dysfunction in which the prognosis for normal development or survival is poor. Such records are also frequently associated with cerebral structural abnormalities. As a general rule, in the neonatal period definitive clinical correlations are best made by obtaining repeated recordings. Mild or moderate abnormalities such as dysmaturity, which may have little prognostic significance on a single recording, gain significance if they persist on repeated recordings. Similarly, a moderate to severe EEG abnormality which persists over a period of weeks is far more suggestive of a severe and enduring disorder than one which is seen on a single recording.

Major abnormalities associated with a poor outcome after 36 weeks CA can be grouped into the following 5 main categories from most to least severe:

(1) *The isoelectric pattern* or pattern of electrocerebral inactivity (ECI) is characterized by the absence of obvious activity of cerebral origin. Recording techniques used to determine electrocerebral inactivity in adults are applied (i.e., long interelectrode distances, sensitivity of at least 2 μV/mm, over 30 min of recording, etc.). In the typical neonatal ICU setting random activity will be less than 5 μVs. The prognosis with ECI is very poor except in some cases complicated by hypothermia, hypotension, sedative medications, or severe blood gas abnormalities. The majority of patients die and those who survive have severe neurological deficits. Among the survivors, the isoelectric pattern is often gradually replaced by a pattern of poorly reactive, generalized, excessive slowing. Because of the serious implications of ECI it is recommended that a second record be obtained to help rule out the presence of transient complicating disorders.

206

[handwritten margin note:]
poor prognosis patterns
(after 36 weeks CA)! *
1 - ECS
2 - burst-supression
3 - low voltage patterns (<30µV)
4 - diffuse delta pattern
5 - asynchronous pattern

* all are unreactive

[handwritten bottom note:] * not required in adults

(2) The *paroxysmal* or *suppression-burst pattern* is characterized by synchronous or asynchronous bursts of activity usually lasting 0.5–10 sec separated by a generalized isoelectric pattern that often lasts more than 10 sec. The morphology of the bursts of activity vary in complexity and amplitude from one individual to another. Unlike tracé discontinu, it is the only pattern present throughout the recording and it shows little or no alteration to external stimuli. If it only occurs in the first 24 h of life it may be associated with normal development.

When the suppression-burst pattern occurs with complete asynchrony, or the tracé alternant or early infantile patterns occur with excessive asynchrony, the diagnosis of agenesis of the corpus callosum should be considered. If the suppression-burst pattern occurs in a female patient and is either unilateral or is bilateral with complete asynchrony, then a diagnosis of *Aicardi's syndrome* should be considered. Aicardi's syndrome occurs in females and includes three essential features: (1) partial or total agenesis of the corpus callosum, (2) infantile spasms, and (3) choroidal or chorioretinal lacunae. All three features are necessary for the diagnosis, although the retinal lesions are thought to be virtually pathognomonic. Other intracranial malformations, such as porencephalic cysts, and extracranial malformations, particularly costovertebral anomalies, occur frequently. Infantile spasms are present within the first 3 months of life.

(3) *Low voltage patterns* are characterized by background activity less than 30 μVs in all states (usually between 5 and 25 μVs). They suggest a very poor prognosis when there is no evidence of reactivity. Low voltage patterns with intermixed runs of focal or multifocal low amplitude theta activity frequently evolve into an isoelectric pattern. Caution is indicated when interpreting low voltage records in neonates younger than 42 weeks CA, particularly if reactivity is present. Although such records are abnormal, they are not uncommon in full term newborns in the first week of life at which time they have little prognostic significance. However, if persistent beyond 43 weeks CA, they correlate with a poor outcome.

(4) *The diffuse delta pattern* consists of irregular, <u>continuous</u> delta waveforms over all head regions that <u>do not react</u> to external stimuli. Activity in other frequency ranges is conspicuously absent. This <u>invariant</u> pattern is not often encountered but must be distinguished from other normal delta patterns such as the *high voltage slow (continuous slow wave) pattern* of quiet sleep and *monorhythmic frontal slowing (anterior slow dysrhythmia).*

(5) The *asynchronous pattern* is identified in records with predominantly discontinuous or paroxysmal patterns. The asynchrony should clearly and continuously exceed normal limits (10.1). As noted above, asynchronous suppression-burst patterns are more often associated with congenital malformations, particularly those which include agenesis of the corpus callosum.

Premature newborns demonstrate major abnormalities similar to those seen in full term neonates, but the significance of those abnormalities depends even more on establishing their persistence with repeated recordings. In addition, careful allowance must be given for normal conceptual age related features that would be grossly abnormal at other ages.

Structural abnormalities that may or may not be associated with normal development have been associated with *positive sharp waves* and with a *persistent interhemispheric asymmetry greater than 50%.* <u>P</u>ositive sharp waves that appear over the <u>central</u> head regions and clearly stand out in amplitude and morphology from other sharply contoured waveforms were first reported in association with <u>intraventricular hemorrhage</u>. Although epileptiform in appearance, they are <u>not correlated with seizures</u>. Moreover, they may be a <u>normal finding up to 32 weeks</u> CA. After that time they probably occur in less than 20% of clinically normal newborns. They are seen in approximately <u>60–80%</u> of <u>newborns with intracranial hemorrhages</u> of various etiologies and have also been noted in the settings of hydrocephalus and anoxia. Regardless of the etiology, in newborns <u>beyond 32 weeks</u> CA they are currently thought to be an electrographic correlate of periventricular <u>leukomalacia</u>.

208

A persistent interhemispheric asymmetry greater than 50% is usually associated with an underlying structural abnormality of the hemisphere with lower amplitude. When assessing hemispheric asymmetries it is important to rule out the presence of the following technical problems: (1) asymmetrical electrode placement; (2) uneven spacing between electrodes; (3) salt bridges produced by connecting adjacent electrodes with conductive jel or intravenous fluid from scalp IV sites; or (4) scalp edema produced by intravenous fluid infiltration. Subdural hematomas may also produce asymmetries, but they are rare at this age. It is also important to recognize that transient asymmetries and asymmetries of less than 50% are a common and normal finding in the neonatal and early infantile periods of life.

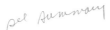

REFERENCES

Andersen, C.M. and Torres, F. (1985) The EEG of the early premature. Electroenceph. clin. Neurophysiol. 60: 95–105.

Aso, K., Scher, M.S. and Barmada, M.A. (1989) Neonatal electroencephalography and neuropathology. J. clin. Neurophysiol. 6: 103–124.

Blume, W.T. (1982) Atlas of Pediatric EEG. Raven, New York.

Blume, W.T. and Dreyfus-Brisac, C. (1982) Positive rolandic sharp waves in neonatal EEG: Types and significance. Electroenceph. clin. Neurophysiol. 53: 277–282.

Clancy, R.R. and Tharp, B.R. (1984) Positive rolandic sharp waves in the electroencephalograms of premature neonates with intraventricular hemorrhage. Electroenceph. clin. Neurophysiol. 57: 395–404.

Clancy, R.R. and Tharp, B.R. (1984) EEG in premature infants with intraventricular hemorrhage. Neurology 34: 583–590.

Dreyfus-Brisac, C. and Curzi-Dascalova, L. (1975) Section II. The EEG during the first year of life. In: Rémond, A. (Ed.), Handbook of Electroenceph. clin. Neurophysiol., Vol. 6B, Elsevier, Amsterdam, pp. 24–30.

Dreyfus-Brisac, C. and Monod, N. (1975) Section I. The electroencephalogram of full-term newborns and premature infants. In: Rémond, A. (Ed.), Handbook of Electroenceph. clin. Neurophysiol., Vol. 6B, Elsevier, Amsterdam, pp. 6–23.

Eeg-Olofsson, O. (1971) The development of the electroencephalogram in normal adolescents from the age of 16 through 21 years. Neuropaediatrie 3: 11–45.

Ellingson, R.J. (1979) The EEGs of premature and full-term newborns. In: D.W. Klass and D.D. Daly (Eds.), Current Practice of Clinical Electroencephalography, Raven, New York, pp. 149–169.

Ellingson, R.J. and Peters, J.F. (1980) Development of EEG and daytime sleep patterns in normal full-term infants during the first 3 months of life: Longitudinal observations. Electroenceph. clin. Neurophysiol. 49: 112–124.

Hanley, J.W. (1981) A step-by-step approach to neonatal EEG. Am. J. EEG Technol. 21: 1–13.

Hahn, J.S., Monyer, H. and Tharp, B.R. (1989) Interburst interval measurements in the EEGs of premature infants with normal neurological outcome. Electroenceph. clin. Neurophysiol. 73: 410–418.

Holmes, G.L. (1986) Morphological and physiological maturation of the brain in the neonate and young child. J. clin. Neurophysiol. 3: 209–238.

Holmes, G., Rowe, J., Hafford, J., Schmidt, R., Testa, M. and Zimmerman, A. (1982) Prognostic value of the electroencephalogram in neonatal asphyxia. Electroenceph. clin. Neurophysiol. 53: 60–72.

Hughes, J.R. (1987) Normal limits in the EEG. In: A.M. Halliday, S.R. Butler and R. Paul (Eds.), A Textbook of Clinical Neurophysiology, Wiley, Chichester, pp. 105–154.

Jankel, W.R. and Niedermeyer, E. (1985) Sleep spindles. J. clin. Neurophysiol. 2: 1–36.

Kellaway, P. (1979) An orderly approach to visual analysis: parameters of the normal EEG in adults and children. In: D.W. Klass and D.D. Daly (Eds.), Current Practice of Clinical Electroencephalography, Raven, New York, pp. 69–147.

Lacey, D.J., Topper, W.H., Buckwald, S., Zorn, W.A. and Berger, P.E. (1986) Preterm very-low-birth-weight neonates: Relationship of EEG to intracranial hemorrhage, perinatal complications, and developmental outcome. Neurology 36: 1084–1087.

Laget, P. (1987) The abnormal EEG in childhood. In: A.M. Halliday, S.R. Butler and R. Paul (Eds.), A Textbook of Clinical Neurophysiology, Wiley, Chichester, pp. 201–230.

Lombroso, C.T. (1979) Quantified electrographic scales on 10 pre-term healthy newborns followed up to 40–43 weeks of conceptional age by serial polygraphic recordings. Electroenceph. clin. Neurophysiol. 46: 460–474.

Lombroso, C.T. (1987) Neonatal Electroencephalography. In: E. Niedermeyer and F. Lopes da Silva (Eds.), Electroencephalography: Basic Principles, Clinical Applications and Related Fields, Urban and Schwarzenberg, Baltimore, pp. 725–762.

Mizrahi, E.M. (1986) Neonatal Electroencephalography: Clinical features of the newborn, techniques of recording, and characteristics of the normal EEG. Am. J. EEG Technol. 26: 81–103.

Monod, N., Pajot, N. and Guidasci, S. (1972) The neonatal EEG: Statistical studies and prognostic value in full-term and pre-term babies. Electroenceph. clin. Neurophysiol. 32: 529–544.

Niedermeyer, E. (1987) Maturation of the EEG: Development of waking and sleep patterns. In: E. Niedermeyer and F. Lopes da Silva (Eds.), Electroencephalography: Basic Principles, Clinical Applications and Related Fields, Urban and Schwarzenberg, Baltimore, pp. 133–158.

Novotny, E.J., Tharp, B.R., Coen, R.W., Bejar, R., Enzmann, D. and Vaucher, Y.E. (1987) Positive rolandic sharp waves in the EEG of the premature infant. Ann. Neurol. 37: 1481–1486.

Pampiglione, G. (1977) Development of rhythmic EEG activities in infancy. (Waking state). Rev. electroencephalogr. Neurophysiol. 7: 327–333.

Petersén, I., Eeg-Olofsson, O. and Selldén, U. (1968) Paroxysmal activity of normal children. In: Kellaway, P. and Petersén, I. (Eds.), Clinical Electroencephalography of Children. Almqvist and Wiksell, Stockholm, pp. 167–187.

Petersén, I. and Eeg-Olofsson, O. (1970) The development of the electroencephalogram in normal children from the age of 1 through 15 years. Nonparoxysmal activity. Neuropadiatrie 2: 247–304.

Petersén, I. and Eeg-Olofsson, O. (1971) The development of the electroencephalogram in normal children from the age of 1 through 15 years – non-paroxysmal activity. Neuropaediatrie 2: 247–304.

Petersén, I., Selldén, U. and Eeg-Olofsson, O. (1975) Section III. The evolution of the EEG in normal children and adolescents from 1 to 21 years. In: Rémond, A. (Ed.), Handbook of Electroenceph. clin. Neurophysiol., Vol. 6B, Elsevier, Amsterdam, pp. 31–68.

Rowe, J.C., Holmes, G.L., Hafford, J., Baboval, D., Robinson, S., Philipps, A., Rosenkrantz, T. and Raye, J. (1985) Prognostic value of the electroencephalogram in term and preterm infants following neonatal seizures. Electroenceph. clin. Neurophysiol. 60: 183–196.

Slater, G.E. and Torres, F. (1979) Frequency-amplitude gradient. A new parameter for interpreting pediatric sleep EEGs. Arch. Neurol. 36: 465–470.

Tharp, B.R. (1986) Neonatal and pediatric electroencephalography. In: M.J. Aminoff (Ed.), Electrodiagnosis in Clinical Neurology, Churchill Livingstone, New York, pp. 77–124.

Tharp, B.R. (1987) The electroencephalographic aspects of ischemic hypoxic encephalopathy and intraventricular hemorrhage. In: H. Yabuuchi, K. Watanabe and S. Okada (Eds.), Neonatal Brain and Behavior, University of Nagoya Press, pp. 86–100.

Tharp, B.R., (1990) Electrophysiological brain maturation in premature infants: An historical perspective. J. clin. Neurophysiol. 7: 302–314.

Tharp, B.R., Cukier, F. and Monod, N. (1981) The prognostic value of the electroencephalogram in premature infants. Electroenceph. clin. Neurophysiol. 51: 219–236.

Werner, S.S., Stockard, J.E. and Bickford, R.G. (1977) Atlas of Neonatal EEG. Raven, New York.

Westmoreland, B.F. and Sharbrough, F.W. (1975) Posterior slow wave transients associated with eye blinks in children. Am. J. EEG Technol. 15: 14–19.

The normal EEG of wakeful resting adults of 20–60 years of age

SUMMARY

The normal EEG of the wakeful adult at rest may show various types of activity alone or in combination:

(11.1)   *The alpha rhythm* is most common and consists of sinusoidal 8–13 Hz waves maximal over the posterior head region which are blocked by eye opening and various alerting maneuvers and disappear in drowsiness and sleep.

(11.2)   *Beta rhythms* are less common and consist of waves over 13 Hz which appear either in a wide distribution, or limited to the frontal or posterior head regions.

(11.3)   *Mu rhythm*,

(11.4)   *Lambda waves*,

(11.5)   *Vertex sharp transients*,

(11.6)   *Kappa rhythm*,

(11.7)   *Intermittent posterior theta rhythms* are rarer than alpha and beta rhythms.

(11.8)   *Low voltage activity* may be the only pattern of the EEG in some normal adults.

(11.9)   *Abnormalities* include epileptiform spikes and sharp waves, more than a minimum of slow waves, asymmetrical or very low amplitude activity, or specific deviations from normal patterns.

11.1   THE ALPHA RHYTHM

The alpha rhythm is defined by its frequency, its distribution and its reactivity (Fig. 11.1, Parts 1–5). Thus, the terms *alpha rhythm* and *alpha frequency* or *activity* are not synonymous.

11.1.1   The *wave form* is regular and often, but not always, sinusoidal. Alpha waves may have sharp points at the top or bottom. Single alpha waves with sharp peaks may be distinguished from abnormal sharp waves by the similarity to other, repetitive alpha waves in the same recording.

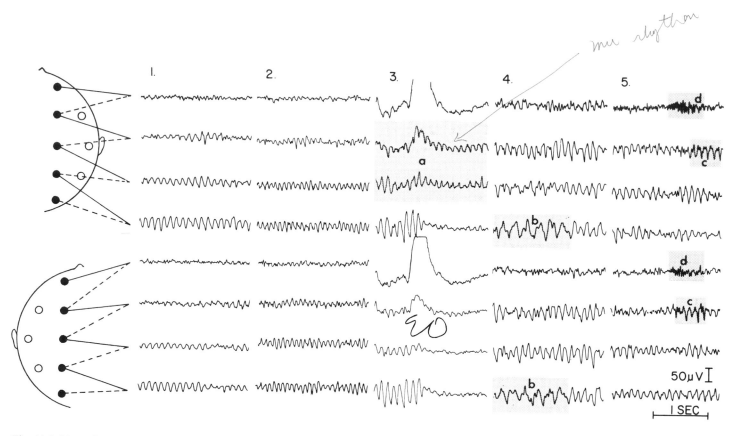

mu rhythm

Fig. 11.1. Normal patterns of wakefulness in adults. 1. An alpha rhythm of 9 Hz in the posterior head regions and minimal beta activity in the frontal regions; 2. An alpha rhythm of 12–13 Hz extending from the posterior to the central regions; 3. An alpha rhythm of 9–10 Hz in the posterior head regions is present at the beginning and is then blocked by eye opening (E/O); a central mu rhythm on the right side persists after eye opening (a); 4. Slow alpha variant of 4–5 Hz, maximal in the occipital regions (b), alternates with an alpha rhythm of about 9 Hz in a wider posterior distribution; a beta rhythm is present in the frontal regions; 5. An alpha rhythm of 8–9 Hz posteriorly, mu rhythm of similar frequency fronto-centrally (c), and beta rhythm frontally (d).

11.1.2   The *frequency* ranges from 8 to 13 Hz in different subjects. It is fairly constant in a given subject but may decrease by 1 Hz or more with drowsiness and increase momentarily after eye closure. This brief increase in frequency immediately following eye closure is sometimes referred to as the *squeak phenomenon*. Because of this constancy, the alpha rhythm within the normal frequency range may be found to be abnormally slow or fast when compared with other recordings in the same subject.

   The frequency of the alpha rhythm in the two hemispheres should be the same at any moment; even a slight difference is suspicious of abnormality if it persists, and a difference of over 1 Hz at any time is definitely abnormal. The hemisphere with the lower frequency is abnormal.

11.1.3   The *phase relation* of the alpha rhythm over different parts of the brain may vary. Individual alpha waves are often not in phase in different areas in normal EEGs, even though the alpha rhythm normally appears and disappears simultaneously in the two hemispheres.

11.1.4   The *distribution* of the alpha rhythm is posterior: The alpha rhythm has the greatest amplitude and is most persistent in the occipital and parietal areas. It often extends into the temporal areas and sometimes into the central areas, especially in young subjects. The alpha rhythm may appear in recordings from a frontal electrode referred to an electrode on the ear, the mastoid or other posterior placements because these reference electrodes pick up the alpha rhythm in posterior locations (4.1.2; Fig. 11.2). Rhythms of alpha frequency which appear only or mainly in the frontal regions in an adult are abnormal (25.3.1). During the early stages of drowsiness, activity in the alpha frequency range may become more prominent over the frontocentral head regions when recorded using a neck/chest, average, or ear reference. This shift in the topography of alpha activity during drowsiness occurs more often in older individuals. It may not be apparent if longitudinal bipolar montages are used.

11.1.5 The *amplitude* of the alpha rhythm often waxes and wanes. While the amplitude may differ on the two sides at different times, an estimate of the average amplitude of the alpha rhythm during a recording may show it to be symmetrical on the two sides. However, even persistent asymmetries of the alpha rhythm are not necessarily abnormal. A higher amplitude of the alpha rhythm on the right side is fairly common, but the amplitude on the left side should be no less than 50% that on the right side (Fig. 11.1). Some normal subjects have an alpha rhythm of slightly higher amplitude on the left side. The normal asymmetry of the alpha rhythm is probably due to an asymmetry of occipital bone thickness. It does not seem to depend on whether a subject is right-handed or left-handed. Abnormal asymmetries can be seen in many conditions (23.7.1).

The amplitude and persistence of the alpha rhythm decreases with age from its maximum in childhood (10.7.1). Because of the wide variation of the alpha rhythm between normal adults, low amplitude, rare occurrence, or even complete absence of the alpha rhythm in adults (11.8) is not abnormal.* Therefore, no clinical significance can be attached to distinctions which have been made between dominant and rare alpha rhythms, or between 'plus' or persistent ('P-type'), reactive ('R-type') and 'minus' or minimal ('M-type') alpha rhythms. Only if the alpha rhythm changes significantly between sequential recordings from the same subject (24.1.2; 24.1.4) can one suspect the development of an abnormality (24.7).

11.1.6 The *reactivity* of the alpha rhythm can be tested with various maneuvers. The alpha rhythm is blocked by eye opening (Fig. 11.1, Part 3), sudden alerting, attention to visual and other stimuli, and mental concentration. The degree of reactivity varies in different subjects and in the same subject at different times. The

216

*it is abnormal in children

alpha rhythm may be blocked completely for many seconds or its amplitude may be attenuated only briefly. However, the complete absence of any reduction suggests an abnormality (25.2.2). Unilateral blocking of the alpha rhythm always indicates the presence of an abnormality of the non-reactive hemisphere.

The alpha rhythm also attenuates when alertness decreases to the level of drowsiness (12.2.2). This attenuation may be associated with a decrease of frequency and is often gradual and intermittent. Drowsiness can also produce a normal variation of alpha blocking, namely a *paradoxical alpha rhythm* which appears on eye opening as the result of partial alerting. This alpha rhythm will disappear with eye closure if drowsiness returns (Fig. 11.2, Top). A normal alpha rhythm can also be demonstrated in most individuals who have a paradoxical alpha rhythm (Fig. 11.2, Bottom).

The effect of eye opening should be studied in every routine clinical EEG recording to: (a) study the reactivity and symmetry of alpha blocking; (b) demonstrate the artifacts produced by eye opening, eye closing and eye movements and to distinguish them from frontal slow waves; (c) bring out rhythms hidden by the alpha rhythm; (d) test the reactivity of other EEG activity; and (e) precipitate abnormal reactions to eye opening and eye closing, for instance paroxysmal discharges.

11.1.7 *Alpha variants* are normal rhythms which resemble the alpha rhythm in distribution and reactivity but differ from it by having slower or faster frequency.

Slow alpha variants are rhythms of 3.5–6.5 Hz; half the frequency of the alpha rhythm that appears elsewhere in the same record (Fig. 11.1, Part 4). It appears over the posterior head, usually alternates with the alpha rhythm of the usual frequency, and blocks like the alpha rhythm. Slow alpha variants are rare but normal and should not be confused with the intermittent occipital slow waves seen in children (10.4) and adults (11.7.2).

Fast alpha variants are described with beta rhythms (11.2).

217

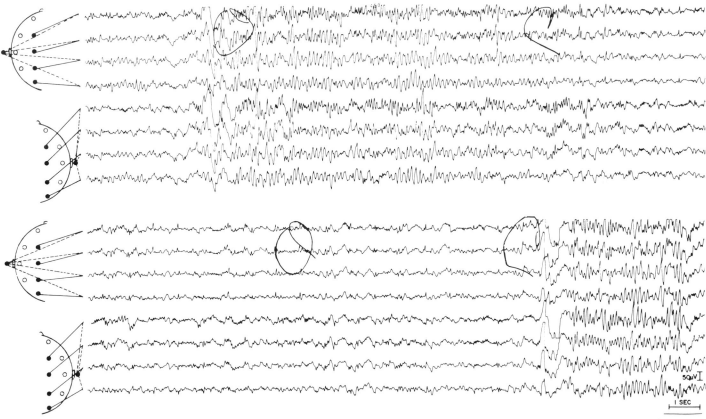

Fig. 11.2. Paradoxical alpha rhythm (top) and normal return of the alpha rhythm (bottom) in a normal drowsy teenager. *Top*: The alpha rhythm appears on eye opening (O) and disappears soon after eye closure (C); activity characteristic of drowsiness is present before and after the period of eye opening; *Bottom*: The alpha rhythm appears after eye closure (C); activity before eye opening (O) and until shortly before eye closing is characteristic of drowsiness; the bottom section was recorded about 1 minute after the top section.

11.1.8 The *physiological significance* of the alpha rhythm remains unknown. The posterior distribution, blocking with eye opening, and other characteristics of the alpha rhythm indicate that it is integrated with visual system function and possibly represents activity which appears in the absence of specific input to that system. Like other rhythmic cortical activities it is modulated by thalamic and cortical interactions.

11.2 BETA RHYTHMS

Unlike the alpha rhythm, beta rhythms are defined only by frequency, although they can be further subdivided according to distribution and reactivity.

11.2.1 The *frequency* of beta rhythms is over 13 Hz. Although any rhythmical activity above that frequency is called beta rhythm, beta rhythms of over 30 Hz have usually very low amplitude and are difficult to record with conventional EEG techniques (3.5.2).

11.2.2 The *distribution* and reactivity of beta rhythms varies. Three types can be distinguished. All of them disappear in drowsiness and sleep, but the first two usually persist longer during drowsiness than does the alpha rhythm.

Frontal beta rhythm is the most common type. It often extends into the central regions (Fig. 11.1, Part 5). In some instances, this type of beta rhythm is blocked by movement, the intention to move, and tactile stimulation. The blocking effect is greater in the hemisphere contralateral to the moved or stimulated side.

Widespread beta rhythm can be recorded over most areas of the head, usually at the same time (Fig. 11.3, Part 1). It is not blocked by any stimulus.

Posterior beta rhythm or *fast alpha variant* has a frequency of about twice that of the alpha rhythm (usually 16–20 Hz) and either intermixes or alternates with the

219

similar to mu rhythm

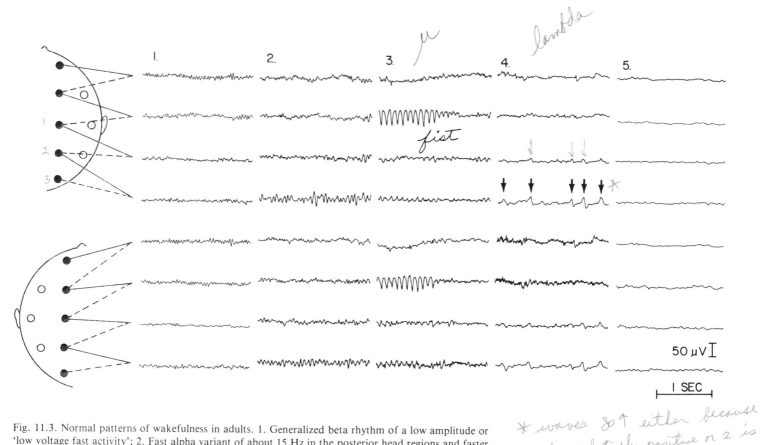

Fig. 11.3. Normal patterns of wakefulness in adults. 1. Generalized beta rhythm of a low amplitude or 'low voltage fast activity'; 2. Fast alpha variant of about 15 Hz in the posterior head regions and faster beta rhythm elsewhere; 3. Fronto-central mu rhythm, blocked by making a fist; posterior alpha rhythm is blocked by eye opening during this recording; 4. Lambda waves (arrows) in the occipital areas, triggered by visual scanning of a picture; 5. Low voltage pattern; subject was alert and had eyes closed during the recording.

220

Handwritten annotations:

μ

lambda

fist

if 3 was negative, the waves in this last channel should go ↓ (G2 neg.)

* waves go ↑ either because 3 is relatively positive or 2 is relatively negative. If 2 was negative, then the waves in the adjacent channel should go ↓ (G2 negative). But since they go ↑, 3 must be positive.

also if 2 was negative, there should be a phase reversal at 2.

alpha rhythm or replaces it (Fig. 11.3, Part 2). This beta rhythm is blocked by maneuvers which block the alpha rhytm.

11.2.3 The *amplitude* of beta activity is usually lower than that of alpha activity in the same record, but amplitude and persistence of beta rhythm may be abnormally high (24.8). Amplitude and distribution of all normal beta rhythms is symmetrical; amplitude in homologous head regions should not differ by more than 35%.* A significant (>35%) asymmetry or unilateral or focal appearance of beta rhythm is abnormal (19.3.6; 23.7.2).

11.2.4 The *persistence* of beta rhythms in the EEG of individuals and the incidence of beta rhythms in the general population increase with age. Since alpha activity tends to decrease during adult life (11.1.5), the ratio of beta to alpha activity increases with age (13.2). However, these age-dependent changes do not have definite clinical implications for a single subject. Only in a general manner does the presence of beta activity in an older person signal better cerebral function than does its absence.

Excessive prominent beta activity is usually the result of a medication effect, most reliably produced by benzodiazepenes or barbiturates. Otherwise excessive generalized beta activity is of little diagnostic significance.

11.2.5 The *physiological significance* of beta rhythms is not clear. The blocking mechanism of frontal beta rhythm suggests a relationship between this type of beta rhythm and sensorimotor functions of the underlying cortex; a similar relationship may be postulated for mu rhythm (11.3). Posterior beta rhythm probably has the same significance as the alpha rhythm (11.1.8); it is of no clinical importance.

* alpha can differ by 50%

11.3 MU RHYTHM

Older names for this rhythm which should no longer be used are 'wicket', 'comb' or 'arceau' rhythm. Mu rhythm, seen in less than 10% of EEGs and most commonly in younger adults, consists of arch-shaped waves at 7–11 Hz which appear in trains of usually up to a few seconds over the central or centro-parietal regions (Fig. 11.3, Part 3). These trains often appear at different times on the two sides of the head. They are better seen in bipolar than in referential recordings. Mu waves intermix or alternate with beta activity (Fig. 11.1, Part 5) and then often have half the frequency of the beta waves. Because the mu rhythm has a frequency similar to that of the alpha rhythm, it usually is best recognized when the alpha rhythm is blocked by eye opening (Fig. 11.1, Part 3). The appearance of the mu rhythm is said to be facilitated while a subject scans visual images.

Like the frontal beta rhythm, the mu rhythm is often blocked by voluntary, reflex or passive movement, by the intention to move, or by tactile stimuli (Fig. 11.3, Part 3). The effect is greatest over the hemisphere opposite the side of the movement or stimulation. If the alpha rhythm is present while the mu reactivity is tested, the alpha rhythm may be blocked along with the mu rhythm if the test alerts the subject. A paradoxical mu rhythm is a mu rhythm which is induced by contralateral movement or touch after mu rhythm has dropped out in drowsy subjects. The same events which induce a paradoxical mu rhythm may also alert the subject, and a paradoxical alpha rhythm may be induced at the same time.

Because mu rhythm is normally intermittent and asynchronous, an EEG is not abnormal if it shows only a few trains of mu rhythm on one side, or only a moderate difference in the incidence of mu rhythm on the two sides. However, frequent trains of mu rhythm appearing only on one side, or a consistent asymmetry of amplitude or frequency of mu rhythm suggests an abnormality on the side of the lower amplitude or frequency.

222

The physiological significance of mu rhythm may be related to somatosensory processes associated with movement. This is suggested by the distribution of mu rhythm, by the blocking effect of sensory stimuli and of passive movement, and by the onset of the mu blocking before actual and intended movement. Mu rhythm, like the alpha rhythm, may represent the idling of a sensory system not processing specific input from thalamic nuclei.

11.4   LAMBDA WAVES

Sharp transients of sawtooth shape and of positive polarity occur in the occipital regions of some subjects when they look at images containing visual detail (Fig. 11.3, Part 4). Lambda waves are therefore rarely encountered in routine clinical EEGs. Neither the presence nor the absence of lambda waves is abnormal, but a marked asymmetry suggests an abnormality on the side of lower amplitude. Lambda waves resemble visual evoked potentials elicited by intermittent flash stimuli in many regards including distribution, wave form and latent period between the change of visual input and the wave peak. Each lambda wave is preceded by a scanning eye movement, sometimes recognizable as an eye movement artifact in frontal derivations. It is therefore likely that lambda waves partly represent visual evoked potentials. However, they persist to some extent after eye movements in the dark and probably also reflect other events, perhaps processes related to eye movement or to the blocking of visual input during changes of gaze.

they look similar to POSTS

11.5   VERTEX SHARP TRANSIENTS (V WAVES)

Sharp transients of negative polarity at the vertex are a common element of normal sleep activity (12.1.3). They occur very rarely in wakeful adults following a sudden loud noise or other unexpected stimuli, but are more easily evoked in children, for example by percussing the hands or feet. The amplitude of V waves during wakefulness is usually much lower than that of V waves occurring during sleep. V waves may form part of a generalized response to startling stimuli; such a response may also include eye blinks and scalp movements.

V waves probably represent a late component of evoked potentials which is non-specific insofar as it does not depend on the modality of the sensory stimulus and appears in a larger region of the cortex than the relatively small specific sensory area. Because of its wider distribution, evoked vertex waves are more likely to be recorded in the EEG than the earlier parts of sensory responses which are restricted to the specific sensory pathways and cortical receiving areas and usually need enhancement by computer averaging to be seen clearly (7.6).

11.6   KAPPA RHYTHM

This rhythm consists of bursts of very low amplitude waves of alpha or theta frequency which have been recorded in a few instances in the temporal regions of subjects engaged in mental activity and are rarely seen in routine clinical recordings. It is not clear whether these waves represent electrocerebral activity in the temporal lobes generated by mental effort or whether they are due to fine rhythmical eye movements associated with eyelid flutter.

11.7   NORMAL POSTERIOR THETA RHYTHMS

Two very rare patterns of rhythmical theta activity can be distinguished in some normal EEGs. Their distribution and reactivity resembles that of alpha rhythms. They are the only exceptions to the rule that synchronous and repetitive theta waves in the EEG of wakeful resting adults are abnormal (11.9.2).

11.7.1 *Slow alpha variant* has been described (11.1.7).

11.7.2 *Rhythmical slow waves of about 4–5 Hz* appear intermittently in the occipital and temporal areas in probably less than one percent of normal adults. Even though the distribution of these rhythms differs slightly from that of alpha waves, they are blocked by eye opening and alerting and disappear in drowsiness and sleep. The incidence of this pattern decreases during adult life.

11.8 THE LOW VOLTAGE EEG

Some EEGs show no activity over 20 μV in recordings from any part of the head (Fig. 11.3, Part 5). At a high gain, a wide range of frequencies can be distinguished, including beta, theta and some delta waves, and sometimes posterior alpha waves (Fig. 11.4). The term 'low voltage fast EEG', which has sometimes been used to describe this pattern, is therefore not appropriate. Waves of higher amplitude can sometimes be induced by hyperventilation, photic stimulation and sleep.

Low voltage EEGs are not seen in normal children, but they become more common with advancing age. They are sometimes seen in tense subjects who show normal amplitude when relaxed. However, low voltage EEGs may be abnormal reflecting bilateral reduction of amplitude which can be recognized only if a prior record from the same subject shows normal amplitude. Very low voltage, i.e. no activity over 10 μV, is more likely to be abnormal (24.2.2).

Low voltage EEGs must be clearly distinguished from recordings showing electro-cerebral inactivity, i.e. absence of cerebral activity of over 2 μV (5.4).

11.9 MAJOR ABNORMALITIES

11.9.1 *Spikes and sharp waves* are abnormal except for (a) vertex sharp transients (11.5); (b) lambda waves which can easily be recognized by their shape and distri-

225

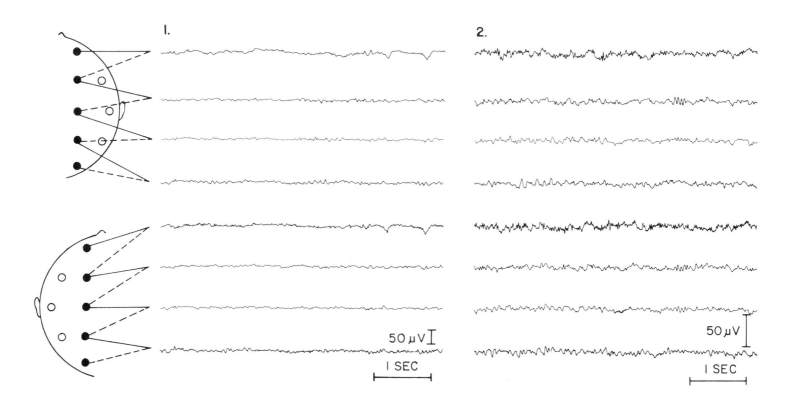

Fig. 11.4. Low voltage pattern in a normal adult. 1. Recording at the usual sensitivity shows an EEG without distinctive features; 2. Continuation at a higher sensitivity shows a mixture of a wide range of frequencies.

bution and by the specific precipitating mechanisms (11.4); (c) most 6 Hz spike-and-slow-wave complexes (19.5.1); and other normal variants described in 19.5.

11.9.2 *Slow waves* of less than 8 Hz should be absent or very rare. They can be accepted as normal only if they are single, of theta frequency, without focal, regional or lateral predominance, asynchronous and not much higher in amplitude than the background. Slow waves are abnormal if they are repetitive or frequent, of delta frequency, of focal, regional or lateral distribution, bilaterally synchronous or of clearly higher amplitude than the background. A rare exception are the bilaterally synchronous theta rhythms in the posterior head regions of a few adults (11.7).

11.9.3 *Low amplitude* generally can best be diagnosed as being abnormal if the amplitude can be shown to be decreased in comparison with a preceding or subsequent record from the same subject. Moderately low amplitude observed in a single recording, although strictly an abnormal EEG feature, is often not associated with clinical abnormalities (24.2.2). However, a single recording of very low amplitude often indicates an abnormality.

11.9.4 *Deviations from normal patterns* such as changes of the frequency or reactivity of alpha rhythm and the occurrence of alpha frequency patterns in coma and seizures may indicate important abnormalities (25).

REFERENCES

Adrian, E.D. and Matthews, B.H.C. (1934) The Berger rhythm: Potential changes from the occipital lobes in man. Brain 57: 355–385.

Barlow, J.S. and Ciganek, L. (1969) Lambda responses in relation to visual evoked responses in man. Electroenceph. clin. Neurophysiol. 26: 183–192.

Chapman, R.M., Armington, J.C. and Bragdon, H.R. (1962) A quantitative survey of kappa and alpha EEG activity. Electroenceph. clin. Neurophysiol. 14: 858–868.

Chatrian, G.E. and Lairy, G.C. (eds.) (1976) Part A. The EEG of the waking adult. In: Rémond, A. (Ed.), Handbook of Electroenceph. clin. Neurophysiol., Vol. 6A, Elsevier, Amsterdam.

Fourment, A., Calvet, J. and Bancaud, J. (1976) Electrocorticography of waves associated with eye movements in man during wakefulness. Electroenceph. clin. Neurophysiol. 40: 457–469.

Gibbs, F.A. and Gibbs, E.L. (1951) Atlas of electroencephalography, Vol. 1: Methodology and Controls, 2nd Ed., Addison-Wesley Publishing Co., Reading.

Gloor, P. (1969) Hans Berger on the electroencephalogram of man. The fourteen original reports on the human electroencephalogram. Electroenceph. clin. Neurophysiol., Suppl. 28.

Hoovey, Z.B., Heinemann, U. and Creutzfeldt, O.D. (1972) Inter-hemispheric 'synchrony' of alpha waves. Electroenceph. clin. Neurophysiol. 32: 337–347.

Hughes, J.R. and Cayaffa, J.J. (1977) The EEG in patients at different ages without organic cerebral disease. Electroenceph. clin. Neurophysiol. 42: 776–784.

Hughes, J.R. (1987) Normal limits in the EEG. In: Halliday, A.M., Butler, S.R. and Paul, R. (Eds.), A Textbook of Clinical Neurophysiology, Wiley, Chichester, pp. 105–154.

Kellaway, P. (1979) An orderly approach to visual analysis: The parameters of the normal EEG in adults and children. In: Klass, D.W. and Daly, D.D. (Eds.), Current Practice of Clinical Electroencephalography, Raven Press, New York, pp. 69–148.

Kozelka, J.W. and Pedley, T.A. (1990) Beta and mu rhythms. J. clin. Neurophysiol. 7: 191–208.

Kuhlman, W.N. (1978) Functional topography of the human mu rhythm. Electroenceph. clin. Neurophysiol. 44: 83–93.

Lehmann, D. (1971) Multichannel topography of human alpha EEG fields. Electroenceph. clin. Neurophysiol. 31: 439–449.

Leissner, P., Lindholm, L.-E. and Petersén, I. (1970) Alpha amplitude dependence on skull thickness as measured by ultrasound technique. Electroenceph. clin. Neurophysiol. 29: 392–399.

Liske, E., Hughes, H.M. and Stowe, D.E. (1967) Cross-correlation of human alpha activity: Normative data. Electroenceph. clin. Neurophysiol. 22: 429–436.

Markand, O. (1990) Alpha rhythms. J. clin. Neurophysiol. 7: 163–190.

Niedermeyer, E. (1987) The normal EEG of the waking adult. In: Niedermeyer, E. and Lopes da Silva, F. (Eds.), Electroencephalography: Basic Principles, Clinical Applications and Related Fields, Urban and Schwarzenberg, Baltimore, pp. 97–118.

Perez-Borja, C., Chatrian, G.E., Tyce, F.A. and Rivers, M.H. (1962) Electrographic patterns of the occipital lobe in man: A topographic study based on use of implanted electrodes. Electroenceph. clin. Neurophysiol. 14: 171–182.

Pfurtscheller, G., Maresch, H. and Schuy, S. (1977) Inter- and intrahemispheric differences in the peak frequency of rhythmic activity within the alpha band. Electroenceph. clin. Neurophysiol. 42: 77–83.

Schoppenhorst, M., Brauer, F., Freund, G. and Kubicki, S. (1980) The significance of coherence estimates in determining central alpha and mu activities. Electroenceph. clin. Neurophysiol. 48: 25–33.

Westmoreland, B.F. (1982) Normal and benign EEG patterns. Am. J. EEG Technol. 22: 3–31.

SUMMARY

The sleep EEG of adults shows less variation of patterns between individuals than does the waking EEG.

(12.1)   The *elements* of the sleep EEG differ from those of the waking EEG and consist of slow waves, sleep spindles, positive occipital sharp transients of sleep (POSTs), vertex sharp waves, K complexes and sawtooth waves. Eye movements and muscle activity may be picked up incidentally from routine electrode placements but are often recorded intentionally with special electrode placements.

(12.2)   *Sleep stages* are distinguished by EEG patterns consisting of different combinations of electrographic elements. These patterns serve to distinguish *stages I–IV of slow wave sleep*, representing progressively deeper levels of dreamless sleep, and the *stage of rapid eye movement (REM) sleep*, which has characteristics of both very light and very deep sleep and is associated with dreaming.

(12.3)   *Sleep cycles* are characteristic sequences of sleep stages. Cycles are best studied in all-night sleep recordings. Heart beat, respiration and other parameters are included in such recordings.

(12.4)   *Abnormalities* which can be found in sleep recordings include spikes and sharp waves, REM periods at the onset of sleep ('sleep onset REM periods'), and sleep disorders characterized by disturbances of sleep cycles and of respiration. The multiple sleep latency test (12.4.5) is used to detect REM onset sleep in patients with suspected narcolepsy.

12.1   ELEMENTS OF NORMAL SLEEP ACTIVITY

12.1.1   *Slow waves* occur in a wide distribution and are often more prominent posteriorly than anteriorly. In lighter stages of non-REM sleep they are generally less persistent, more asynchronous, of lower amplitude and faster frequency (Fig. 12.1, Parts 2 and 3) than in deeper stages (Fig. 12.2, Parts 1 and 2).

12.1.2   *Positive occipital sharp transients* of sleep (POSTs) are monophasic, triangular waves in the occipital regions (Fig. 12.1, Parts 2 and 3; Fig. 12.2, Part 1). Because they have positive electrical polarity, they produce upgoing pen deflections in channels connected to the occipital electrodes through input 2 (3.4.1). POSTs occur intermittently and apparently spontaneously, either simultaneously or independently, on the two sides of the head. They usually recur irregularly at intervals of over 1 second, but they may repeat up to 4–6 times a second. Their amplitude is moderate in most cases, but may be high. Intermittent independent POSTs of high amplitude may resemble focal epileptiform discharges but should not be confused with them.

POSTs have also been called 'lambdoid waves' because they resemble lambda waves in shape and distribution (11.4); like lambda waves, they depend on normal central visual acuity. However, because the mechanisms responsible for generating the two types of waves are not known, the term 'lambdoid' should not be used.

Individuals with prominent lambda waves are more likely to demonstrate both POSTs and prominent photic driving. Awareness of this relationship is sometimes helpful in distinguishing high amplitude asymmetric POSTs from epileptiform activity.

12.1.3 *Vertex sharp transients (V waves)* are bilaterally synchronous waves which have a maximum of amplitude at the vertex and often extend into frontal, temporal and parietal areas (Fig. 12.1, Part 3). V waves have negative electrical polarity and therefore cause upgoing pen deflections in channels connected to an electrode closer to the vertex through input 1 and to a more distant electrode through input 2, whereas they cause a downgoing pen deflection in channels connected to electrodes near the vertex through input 2 and to more distant electrodes through input 1 (3.4.1; 4.1). V waves are symmetrical on average even though their amplitude on either side may fluctuate transiently. They are single and often recur at irregular intervals, rarely more often than two times a second. They sometimes appear in response to a sensory stimulus (11.5).

230

12.1.4 *Sleep spindles* have a frequency of 11–15 Hz, usually 12–14 Hz, a duration of > 0.5 sec, and may last up to a few seconds (Fig. 12.1, Part 3, Fig. 12.2, Part 1). They have a wide distribution, with a maximum over the central regions. They appear simultaneously and are approximately symmetric. *– unlike mu*

12.1.5 *K complexes* resemble V waves in distribution, reaction to sensory stimuli and polarity of the major component, but they are typically longer in duration and less sharply contoured (Fig. 12.2, Part 1). A more detailed description is given in 10.3.

12.2   SLEEP STAGES

12.2.1 *Stage W* or wakefulness at the transition to drowsiness may show some slowing and greater prominence of alpha rhythm (Fig. 12.2, Part 1). Beta rhythms may be present and continue into stage I of sleep; they are especially prominent when sleep is induced by sedatives. Movement and muscle artifacts may obscure the EEG at the transition to sleep.

Slow lateral eye movements (SEMs), typically less than 0.5 Hz, are often the first obvious electrographic sign of drowsiness and often occur at a time when the alpha rhythm is still present. Earlier stages of drowsiness can be detected using a sensitive movement transducer taped over the outer aspect of the upper eyelid. By this technique wakefulness during eye closure is characterized by the presence of *mini-blinks* (rapid eye deflections; predominantly vertical) that occur 5–10 times per 10 sec, each with a duration of less than 400 msec. They correspond to low amplitude deflections in the eye lead monitors. The earliest stage of drowsiness occurs when mini-blinks disappear. In approximately one third of normal individuals with further drowsiness the mini-blinks are replaced by *small fast irregular eye movements*. The latter have a faster repetition rate (5–30/sec) and are lower in amplitude than

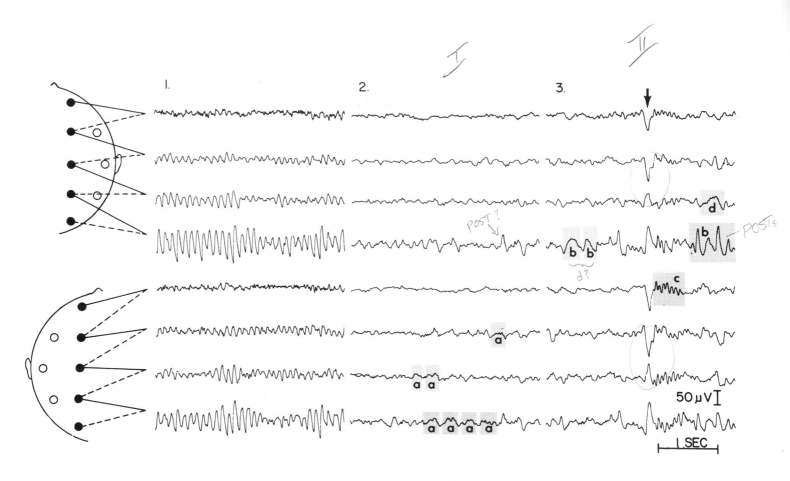

Fig. 12.1. Normal patterns of wakefulness and light sleep in an adult. 1. Stage W (wakefulness) with alpha rhythm and frontal beta rhythm; 2. Stage I (drowsiness) with irregular slow waves at 3–7 Hz (a); 3. Stage II (light sleep) with a V wave (arrow), POSTs (b), sleep spindles (c), and slow waves of 2–7 Hz (d).

232

mini-blinks. Finally, SEMs appear. In approximately one-third of normal individuals SEMs are accompanied by *small fast rhythmic* (3–8 Hz) eye movements.

12.2.2 *Sleep stage I* begins with the disappearance of the alpha rhythm and the appearance of slow waves of 2–7 Hz (Fig. 12.1, Part 2). At the early part of this stage, most persons show low amplitude activity of mixed frequencies, but some have medium amplitude slow wave bursts immediately after the disappearance of the alpha rhythm. Alpha waves may recur briefly; this is the time when paradoxical alpha rhythm appears on slight alerting (11.1.6). Muscle activity diminishes. Slow eye movements may occur and last for several seconds.

Slow waves and paroxysmal slowing during drowsiness and stage I sleep may at times be difficult to distinguish from pathological slowing, particularly since many abnormal changes appear predominantly during eye closure at rest or early drowsiness. Normal slowing during drowsiness is most likely to occur in patients who have either been sedated in order to obtain a sleep recording or who spontaneously achieve stages 1 and 2 sleep during the recording. Other findings consistent with drowsiness are the presence of SEM and a reduction in muscle artifact. Finally, alerting maneuvers should be performed at some point in *every* recording to produce a state of clear wakefulness. It is best to assess the frequency of the alpha rhythm during alerting maneuvers since during drowsiness it may slow by 1–2 Hz. Alerting maneuvers should *always* include more than the simple commands to open and close the eyes (e.g., mental calculation, orientation to time, or other questions appropriate to age and clinical condition), otherwise sustained wakefulness may not occur.

In deeper parts of stage I, slow waves are of medium amplitude and may form irregularly spaced bursts. V waves may occur in response to alerting stimuli or apparently spontaneously in this stage and in stage II. At the end of stage I, POSTs appear in many subjects.

233

12.2.3 *Stage II* is characterized by the presence of sleep spindles of at least half a second in duration, K complexes or both (Fig. 12.1, Part 3). Slow waves of 2–7 Hz continue to be seen and are often bilaterally synchronous; slow waves of less than 2 Hz are absent or not prominent. POSTs often persist in stage II.

12.2.4 *Stage III* is characterized by the presence of a moderate amount of very slow waves of high amplitude: 20–50% of the recording time is occupied by waves of 2 Hz or less of over 75 μV (Fig. 12.2, Part 1). K complexes are often present. Sleep spindles may be present or absent. POSTs can usually be distinguished.

12.2.5 *Stage IV* is characterized by more slow wave activity than is present in stage III. Over 50% of the recording time is occupied by waves of 2 Hz or less over 75 μV. K complexes blend with slow waves. Spindles and POSTs may be seen but are rare (Fig. 12.2, Part 2).

12.2.6 *Stage REM* is characterized by low voltage EEG patterns, rapid eye movements, and generally reduced muscle activity; it is associated with dreaming. Although the EEG and some behavioral changes suggest that sleep is lighter during this stage, the threshold for arousal by auditory stimuli is increased, suggesting a deeper stage of sleep. These conflicting findings have prompted the use of the term '*paradoxical* sleep'.

The EEG during REM sleep shows asynchronous low voltage waves of mixed frequency (Fig. 12.2, Part 3). It may resemble the pattern of stage I sleep except that it contains no V waves but may contain waves of sawtooth shape at the central and frontal regions. Alpha waves of 1–2 Hz less than the frequency of the alpha rhythm during wakefulness may be present.

Rapid eye movements are often picked up with routine prefrontal electrode placements but are more reliably monitored with recording electrodes placed near the

234

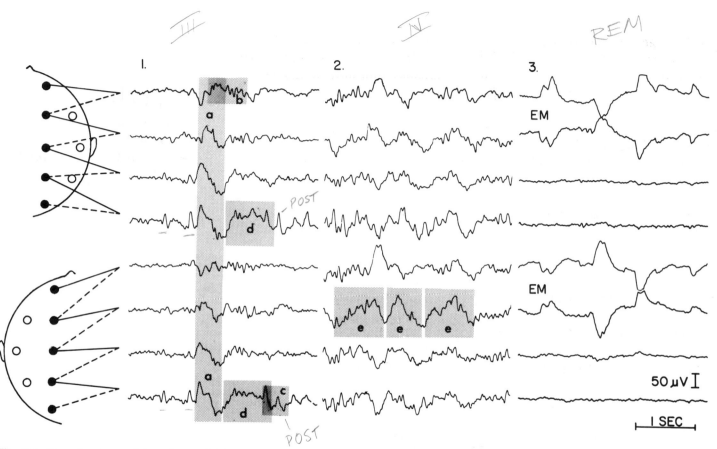

Fig. 12.2. Normal patterns of deep sleep and REM sleep in an adult. 1. Stage III (deep sleep) with a K complex (a), sleep spindle (b), POSTs (c), and slow waves of less than 2 Hz (d); 2. Stage IV (very deep sleep) with slow waves of less than 2 Hz and over 75 μV during over 50% of the recording (e); 3. Stage REM (rapid eye movement sleep) with eye movements indicated by eye movement monitors (EM) used during this part of the recording.

eyes (4.3.1). Such recordings show irregular deflections with extremely fast initial components due to rapid lateral changes of eye position (Fig. 12.2, Part 3).

Changes of muscle tone and other activity are sometimes monitored. Muscle tone can be recorded with EEG electrodes placed on neck muscles below the chin (4.3.4) and reaches its lowest level during the REM stage of sleep. However, paroxysms of muscle activity may appear in such recordings and often are associated with vigorous bursts of REM and brief twitches of face and limb muscles. Blood pressure and heart rate increase, breathing becomes faster and irregular, and gastrointestinal movement ceases; males have erections during almost every REM period.

REM sleep is rarely encountered during routine adolescent and adult recordings because the latency of REM sleep exceeds routine recording times. Therefore, the appearance of REM sleep in a routine recording raises the question of a sleep disorder.

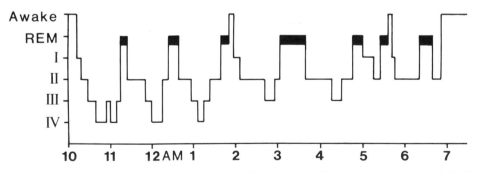

Fig. 12.3. Diagram of sleep cycles during an all-night sleep recording in a normal young adult. Sleep stages are plotted against time of the night.

236

Normal nightly sleep is organized in characteristic sequences of sleep stages (Fig. 12.3). The first cycle begins with stage I and proceeds through increasingly deeper stages of non-REM sleep to REM sleep. This resets the depth of sleep to a much lighter level and is followed by another cycle of gradual descent through non-REM sleep to REM sleep. Normally, people go through about 5–7 such cycles during a night. The first cycle is the shortest, but later cycles do not vary much in length and last about 80–120 minutes. REM sleep normally occurs only at the end of each cycle and thus first appears 70–90 minutes after the onset of sleep.

Several features of sleep vary with age. Although total sleep time is fairly constant through adulthood, the number and duration of the individual sleep stages changes. A normal young adult spends about 30–50% of sleep time in stage II, 20–40% in stages III and IV, and 5–10% in stage I. The percentage of stages III and IV decreases with age so that greater amounts of sleep time are spent in lighter stages. The proportion of REM sleep decreases slightly from about 25% in young adults to about 20% in the fifth decade.

To chart sleep stages, an all-night sleep recording is scored during successive periods of usually 20 or 30 seconds. The sleep stage prevailing during these periods is plotted as a function of time from the onset of sleep. To identify the sleep stages accurately, eye movements and muscle activity are recorded in addition to the EEG (5.3). A thorough study of sleep cycles requires that recordings be made during more than one night to overcome the distorting 'first night effect' which is due to the subject's unfamiliarity with the environment of the sleep laboratory and the recording procedures.

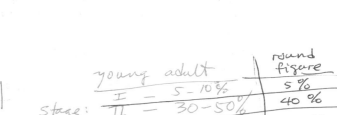

Epileptiform activity, short latency to sleep onset, REM periods at sleep onset and other sleep disorders are often looked for in sleep recordings made as part of a routine EEG during the day. Such recordings are satisfactory for the detection of short sleep latency and may activate epileptiform activity, but all-night sleep recordings are more reliable for the study of sleep disorders.

12.4.1 *Spikes and sharp waves* appear during sleep in many patients with convulsive disorders. Therefore sleep is often used as an activation procedure in the diagnosis of epilepsy (14.2.1). Spikes and sharp waves must be carefully distinguished from positive occipital sharp transients (12.1.2) and vertex sharp transients (12.1.3).

12.4.2 *Short latency to sleep onset* of an average of less than 5 minutes can be found in patients with narcolepsy and other disorders (25.4.3) when they are given the opportunity to fall asleep during the day ('multiple sleep latency test').

12.4.3 *Sleep onset REM periods* are characteristically seen in patients with narcolepsy and may occur in patients with sleep apnea (25.4.3). Daytime naps are not reliable indicators of this disorganization of the first sleep cycle because naps occasionally begin with REM sleep in persons without sleep disorders, and may begin without REM periods in some patients with narcolepsy and in many patients with sleep apnea.

12.4.4 *Disorders of sleep cycles* such as abnormal length, number and distribution of sleep stages occur in various conditions (25.4.5). To diagnose these conditions, it is often necessary to record extracerebral physiological activity in addition to the EEG (4.3). For example, respiratory body movement and air flow must be monitored to study sleep apnea, characterized by frequent and long periods without breathing which can be the cause of undiagnosed daytime symptoms.

12.4.5   The multiple sleep latency test (MSLT) is used to detect: (1) the presence of REM onset sleep in patients with suspected narcolepsy and, (2) to evaluate complaints of excessive daytime drowsiness. Since REM onset sleep and excessive drowsiness may both be caused by sleep deprivation, the MSLT is most revealing when performed in a controlled inpatient setting that allows for the observation of the patient's sleep pattern prior to testing. However, the MSLT is useful as an outpatient screening test to confirm the diagnosis of narcolepsy or to select patients for further testing.

The MSLT is performed by giving the patient 5 opportunities to fall asleep during the day. The first nap should begin at approximately 10:00 AM and the remaining are performed at 2-hour intervals. For each nap the patient is given 20 min to fall asleep. *Sleep onset* is defined as either (1) three consecutive 30-sec epochs of stage 1 sleep, or (2) any single epoch of stage 2, 3, or REM sleep. Each nap is terminated if the patient is not asleep at 20 min after the onset of testing or the patient sleeps for 15 consecutive min. The nap is also terminated if the patient awakens at any time beyond 20 min from the onset of the test. Wakefulness is defined as 2 consecutive 30-sec epochs of wakefulness.

The *mean sleep latency* (i.e., the time between the beginning of the nap period and the beginning of *sleep onset*) is calculated for each of the 5 naps. A mean sleep latency of less than 5 min is considered abnormal and suggests the presence of excessive drowsiness. The number of nap periods with REM sleep is also calculated. If 2 or more nap periods contain REM sleep, then a diagnosis of narcolepsy is highly likely. However, it is important to be aware that MSLT results are extremely difficult to interpret in individuals who are either sleep deprived or taking medications that may alter sleep (e.g., amphetamines or antidepressant medications).

239

REFERENCES

Association of Sleep Disorders Centers and the Association for the Psychophysiological Study of Sleep. (1979) Glossary of terms used in the sleep disorders classification. Sleep 2: 123–129.

Broughton, R. (1987) Polysomnography: Principles and applications in sleep and arousal disorders. In: Niedermeyer, E. and Lopes da Silva, F. (Eds.), Electroencephalography: Basic Principles, Clinical Applications and Related Fields, Urban and Schwarzenberg, Baltimore, pp. 687–724.

Browman, C.P., Krishnareddy, S.G., Yolles, S.F. and Mitler, M. (1986) Forty-eight hour polysomnographic evaluation of narcolepsy. Sleep 9: 183–188.

Daly, D.D. and Yoss, R.E. (1957) Electroencephalogram in narcolepsy. Electroenceph. clin. Neurophysiol. 9: 109–120.

Decoster, R. and Foret, J. (1979) Sleep onset and first cycle of sleep in human subjects: Change with time of day. Electroenceph. clin. Neurophysiol. 46: 531–537.

Dement, W. and Kleitman, N. (1957) Cyclic variations in EEG during sleep and their relation to eye movements, body mobility, and dreaming. Electroenceph. clin. Neurophysiol. 9: 673–690.

Dement, W.C. (1976) Daytime sleepiness and sleep 'attacks'. In: Guilleminault, D., Dement, W.C. and Passouant, P. (Eds.), Narcolepsy, Spectrum, New York, pp. 17–42.

Dement, W.C. (1990) A personal history of sleep disorders medicine. J. clin. Neurophysiol. 7: 17–47.

Erwin, C.W., Somerville, E.R. and Radtke, R.A. (1984) A review of electroencephalographic features of normal sleep. J. clin. Neurophysiol. 1: 253–274.

Guilleminault, C. and Baker, T.L. (1984) Sleep and electroencephalography: Points of interest and points of controversy. J. clin. Neurophysiol. 1: 275–291.

Hughes, J.R. (1985) Sleep spindles revisited. J. clin. Neurophysiol. 2: 37–44.

Jankel, W.R. and Niedermeyer, E. (1985) Sleep spindles. J. clin. Neurophysiol. 2: 1–36.

Kales, A. and Kales, J.D. (1974) Sleep disorders. Recent findings in the diagnosis and treatment of disturbed sleep. New Engl. J. Med. 290: 487–499.

Lavie, P., Gadoth, N., Gordon, C.R., Goldhammer, G. and Bechar, M. (1979) Sleep patterns in Kleine-Levin syndrome. Electroenceph. clin. Neurophysiol. 47: 369–371.

Mitler, M.M., van den Hoed, J., Carskadon, M.A., Richardson, G., Park, R., Guilleminault, C. and Dement, W.C. (1979) REM sleep episodes during the multiple sleep latency test in narcoleptic patients. Electroenceph. clin. Neurophysiol. 46: 479–481.

Mitler, M. (1984) The multiple sleep latency test as an evaluation for excessive somnolence. In: Guilleminault, C. (Ed.), Sleeping and Waking Disorders, Indications and Techniques, Addison-Wesley, Reading, pp. 145–153.

Niedermeyer, E. (1987) Sleep and EEG. In: Niedermeyer, E. and Lopes da Silva, F. (Eds.), Electroencephalography: Basic Principles, Clinical Applications and Related Fields, Urban and Schwarzenberg, Baltimore, pp. 119–132.

Oswald, I. (1987) The normal record of sleep. In: Halliday, A.M., Butler, S.R. and Paul, R. (Eds.), A Textbook of Clinical Neurophysiology, Wiley, Chichester, pp. 173–185.

Parkes, J.D. (1985) Sleep and Its Disorders, Saunders, Philadelphia.

Passouant, P. (1975) EEG and sleep. In: Killam, E.K. and Killam, K. (Eds.), Handbook of EEG and Clinical Neurophysiology, Elsevier, Amsterdam, Vol. 7A, pp. 5–25.

Rechtschaffen, A. and Kales, A. (1968) A Manual of Standardized Terminology, Techniques and Scoring System for Sleep Stages of Human Subjects. PHS, U.S. Government Printing Office, Washington, D.C.

Richardson, G.S., Carskadon, M.A., Flagg, W., van den Hoed, J., Dement, W.C. and Mitler, M.M. (1978) Excessive daytime sleepiness in man: Multiple sleep latency measurement in narcoleptic and control subjects. Electroenceph. clin. Neurophysiol. 45: 621–627.

Roth, M., Shaw, J. and Green, J. (1956) The form, voltage distribution and physiological significance of the K-complex. Electroenceph. clin. Neurophysiol. 8: 385–402.

Santamaria, J. and Chiappa, K.H. (1987) The EEG of Drowsiness, Demos, New York.

Vignaendra, V., Matthews, R.L. and Chatrian, G.E. (1974) Positive occipital sharp transients of sleep: Relationships to nocturnal sleep cycle in man. Electroenceph. clin. Neurophysiol. 37: 239–246.

Williams, R.L., Karacan, I. and Hursch, C.J. (1974) Electroencephalography (EEG) of Human Sleep. Wiley, New York.

241

The normal EEG of adults over 60 years of age

13

SUMMARY
The normal EEG of adults over 60 years of age is similar to that of younger adults with a few exceptions.
   (13.1)   The alpha rhythm may be slower, less persistent and less reactive.
   (13.2)   *Beta activity* is often more prominent.
   (13.3)   *Sporadic generalized slow waves* may be slightly more common than in younger adults.
   (13.4)   *Intermittent temporal slow waves* appear in some apparently normal subjects, especially on the left side.
   (13.5)   *Sleep* is less deep and more often interrupted by wakefulness.
   (13.6)   *Major abnormalities* at this age is similar to those of younger adults except that a wider range of slow waves is acceptable as normal in old age.

13.1   ALPHA RHYTHM

Alpha rhythm decreases in frequency, prominence and reactivity.

13.1.1   The *frequency* of alpha rhythm drops from mean values of about 10–11 Hz in groups of young adults to means of about 9 Hz in persons over 60 years and of 8–9 Hz in centenarians. This progression to slower rates can be seen in recordings from the same individual made at different ages.

   The frequency of the alpha rhythm may fall below 8 Hz in adults; although such rhythms are abnormal and outside the alpha frequency range, they are commonly, however imprecisely, called 'alpha rhythm' as long as they retain the distribution and reactivity of the alpha rhythm. It was previously thought that a frequency as

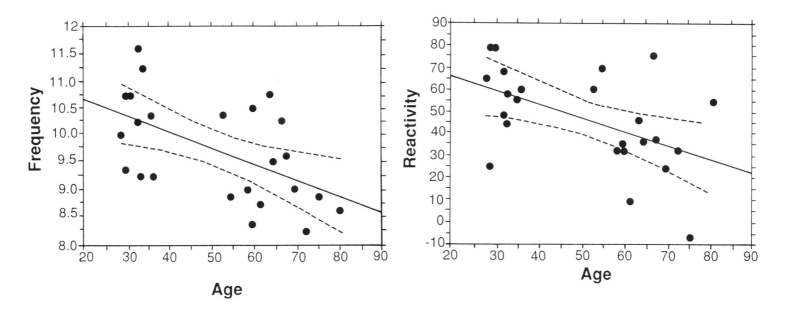

Fig. 13.1. Age vs. absolute peak frequency in the 8–13 Hz range in a group of carefully screened (medication-free) normal individuals. The spectral peak frequency of activity recorded in O1-A1A2 derivation was determined by computer analysis. The amplitude spectra analyzed was obtained from an average of 4 eight second epochs (yielding a frequency resolution of 0.125 Hz).

Fig. 13.2. Age vs. alpha reactivity recorded in T5-O1 in a group of carefully selected (medication-free) normal individuals. Alpha reactivity was calculated by subtracting the 8–13 Hz amplitude spectral band value during eye opening from the 8–13 Hz band value during eye closure and then dividing the difference by the 8–13 Hz band value during eye closure. The final value multiplied by 100 yields the percentage of change in the eyes closed 8–13 Hz band caused by eye opening. The spectra used for these calculations were obtained by averaging four 8-sec epochs in each condition (eyes opened and eyes closed). During the recording the subjects were instructed to hold their eyes open or closed every 10 sec.

low as 7.0 Hz was not abnormal in persons between 60 and 70 years of age and that frequencies of 6–7 Hz could be normal in some persons over 70 years. But an alpha rhythm of 8.0 Hz or less is now generally considered abnormal, even in elderly persons (Fig. 13.1). The frequency of the alpha rhythm becomes a more sensitive indicator of cerebral dysfunction if a previous baseline recording is available for comparison. For example, provided that the alpha rhythm is assessed during definite wakefulness (e.g., with alerting maneuvers), even a well sustained alpha rhythm of 9.0 Hz is an abnormal finding if the individual's baseline alpha rhythm is 11.0 Hz.

13.1.2 The *voltage and persistence* of alpha rhythm decrease with age. Low voltage patterns (11.8) become more common after age 60.

13.1.3 The *reactivity* of the alpha rhythm is decreased. The percentage of attenuation of the alpha rhythm in response to eye opening decreases with age. This has recently been demonstrated by computerized quantitative EEG analysis (as shown in Fig. 13.2). It is also thought that the onset of attenuation following eye closure is delayed and the degree of sustained attenuation is of shorter duration.

13.1.4 The *topography* of activity in the alpha frequency range when recorded with non-cephalic, common average, or ear reference montages is often shifted from a posterior to a more frontocentral dominant location during eye closure at rest. This occurs more often in elderly individuals than in young adults, particularly during drowsiness.

13.2 BETA RHYTHM

The incidence and amplitude of beta rhythms increase during middle life (11.2.4). Beta activity is found in at least half of the elderly, more commonly in women than in men. Fast activity tends to disappear in very old age. Its disappearance is probably not a normal phenomenon but generally correlates with the development of cerebral atrophy.

13.3   SPORADIC GENERALIZED SLOW WAVES

Sporadic generalized slow waves are not much more prominent between 60 and 75 years than in younger adults. After age 75, a slight increase of slow waves mainly in the theta range may represent normal, age-dependent EEG changes, but more continuous theta activity or the appearance of generalized delta waves represents an EEG abnormality. Abnormal generalized slow waves correlate more strongly than other age-related EEG changes with dementia of Alzheimer's type. However, senile dementia may progress to considerable severity before the EEG shows any deviation from the normal range.

13.4   INTERMITTENT TEMPORAL SLOW WAVES

Intermittent temporal slow waves of elderly persons have several characteristic features. They appear in the form of either single waves or of brief bursts of theta or delta activity (Fig. 13.4). Although these bursts have medium or high amplitude, they occur infrequently and remain separated from each other by normal background activity. Approximately two-thirds arise from the left temporal area. Similar slow waves of lower amplitude sometimes appear simultaneously or independently in the right temporal regions. Since such slow waves usually are distributed either evenly over the left and right temporal areas or more frequently on the left, the finding of a right-sided predominance should raise the question of an underlying right temporal abnormality.

Although these slow waves are probably not the result of normal aging but of degenerative and perhaps vascular cerebral changes, they are often found in apparently normal elderly individuals. They are best seen in bipolar or Cz reference montages and least well seen in ipsilateral ear reference montages. They can usually be distinguished from an abnormal slow wave focus by their clearly intermittent occurrence between long periods of normal background activity and by their restricted distribution. *'Normal' temporal slowing in the delta frequency range should occupy less than 1% of the waking record. 'Normal' temporal slowing in the theta frequency range should occupy less than 10% of the waking record.* In contrast, abnormal focal slow waves of comparable amplitude occur more frequently, may extend in to neighboring areas, especially the frontal regions, and are often associated with generalized slow waves. Sharp transients that may infrequently occur with some temporal slow wave bursts occasionally resemble focal epileptiform sharp waves (17.1.2), but their configuration usually shows greater variability.

see Nidermeyer

Fig 13.3 (arrows)

13.5 SLEEP

13.5.1 *Sleep onset* may be associated with fairly prominent slow waves beginning abruptly as soon as alpha activity has dropped out. Some normal old persons show trains of bilaterally synchronous delta waves in drowsiness.

13.5.2 *Sleep depth* is reduced. The proportion of time spent in stages III and IV decreases through adult life and reached a minimum of less than 10% in old age. The time spent awake between periods of sleep increases with age.

see p. 237

13.5.3 *REM sleep* decreases to less than 20% of total sleep time at the ages of 70–80 years.

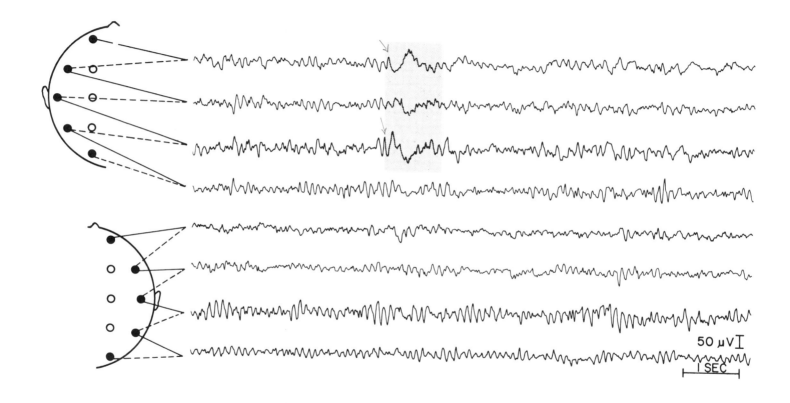

Fig. 13.3. Sporadic left temporal slow waves with sharp contours in 61-year-old subject without clinical abnormalities (shaded).

248

13.6 MAJOR ABNORMALITIES

13.6.1 *Slow waves* in excess of those acceptable as normal at this age (13.3) indicate abnormality. Abnormal slow wave patterns at this age, in contrast to those of younger adults, consist more often of bilaterally synchronous trains of rhythmical delta waves and less often of focal slow waves.

13.6.2 *Extremely low amplitude* and *asymmetry of amplitude* are abnormal; the standards are the same as for younger adults (11.9.3).

13.6.3 *Spikes and sharp waves* are abnormal with the same exceptions as for younger adults during wakefulness (11.9.1) and sleep (12.4.1).

REFERENCES

Arenas, A.M., Brenner, R.P. and Reynolds, C.F. (1986) Temporal slowing in the elderly revisited. Am. J. EEG Technol. 26: 105–114.

Bennet, D.R. (1981) Electroencephalographic and evoked potential changes with aging. Sem. Neurol. 1: 47–51.

Celesia, G. (1986) EEG and event related potentials in aging and dementia. J. clin. Neurophysiol. 3: 99–112.

Erwin, C.W., Somerville, E.R. and Radtke, R.A. (1984) A review of electroencephalographic features of normal sleep. J. clin. Neurophysiol. 1: 253–274.

Hubbard, O., Sunde, D. and Goldensohn, E.S. (1976) The EEG in centenarians. Electroenceph. clin. Neurophysiol. 40: 407–417.

Ingvar, D.H., Sjölund, B. and Ardö, A. (1976) Correlation between dominant EEG frequency, cerebral oxygen uptake and blood flow. Electroenceph. clin. Neurophysiol. 41: 268–276.

Katz, R.I. and Horowitz, G.R. (1982) Electroencephalogram in the septuagenarian: Studies in a normal geriatric population. J. Amer. geriat. Soc. 30: 273–275.

Kellaway, P. (1979) An orderly approach to visual analysis: The parameters of the normal EEG in adults and children. In: Klass, D.W. and Daly, D.D. (Eds.), Current Practice of Clinical Electroencephalography, Raven, New York, pp. 69–148.

Marsh, G.R. and Thompson, L.V. (1977) Psychophysiology of aging. In: Handbook of the Psychology of Aging. In: Birren, J.E. and Schaie, K.W. (Eds.), Reinhold van Nostrand, New York, pp. 219–248.

Mundy-Castle, A.C., Hurst, L.A., Beerstecher, D.M. and Prinsloo, T. (1954) The electroencephalogram in the senile psychoses. Electroenceph. clin. Neurophysiol. 6: 245–252.

Niedermeyer, E. (1987) EEG and old age. In: Niedermeyer, E. and Lopes da Silva, F. (Eds.), Electroencephalography: Basic Principles, Clinical Applications and Related Fields, Urban and Schwarzenberg, Baltimore, pp. 301–308.

Obrist, W.D., Sokoloff, L., Lassen, N.A., Lane, M.H., Butler, R.N. and Feinberg, I. (1963) Relation of EEG to cerebral blood flow and metabolism in old age. Electroenceph. clin. Neurophysiol. 15: 610–619.

Obrist, W.D. (1976) Section V. Problems of aging. In: Rémond, A. (Ed.), Handbook of Electroenceph. clin. Neurophysiol., Vol. 6A, Elsevier, Amsterdam, pp. 275–292.

Otomo, E. and Tsubaki, T. (1966) Electroencephalography in subjects sixty years and over. Electroenceph. clin. Neurophysiol. 20: 77–82.

Pedley, T.A. and Miller, J.A. (1983) Clinical neurophysiology of aging and dementia. In: Mayeux, R. and Rosen, W.G. (Eds.), The Dementias, Raven, New York, pp. 31–49.

Prinz, P.N., Peskind, E.R., Vitaliano, P.P., Raskind, M.A., Eisdorfer, C., Zemcuznikov, N. and Gerber, C.V. (1982) Changes in the sleep and waking EEGs of nondemented and demented elderly subjects. J. Amer. geriat. Soc. 30: 86–93.

Soininen, H., Partanen, V.J., Helkala, E.-L. and Riekkinen, P.J. (1982) EEG findings in senile dementia and normal aging. Acta neurol. Scand. 65: 59–70.

Torres, F., Faoro, A., Loewenson, R. and Johnson, E. (1983) The electroencephalogram of elderly subjects revisited. Electroenceph. clin. Neurophysiol. 56: 391–398.

Visser, S.L., Hooijer, C., Jonker, C., Van Tilburg, W. and De Rijke, W. (1987) Anterior temporal focal abnormalities in EEG in normal aged subjects; correlations with psychopathological and CT brain scan findings. Electroenceph. clin. Neurophysiol. 66: 1–7.

Activation procedures

14

SUMMARY

Activation procedures are used to induce, enhance or better define abnormal EEG patterns. These procedures also may induce normal patterns which are not seen in the spontaneous EEG.

(14.1) *Hyperventilation* is used routinely in most laboratories. The normal response consists of a buildup of generalized slow waves; this response is seen especially in persons who are young or in those who are hypoglycemic. Abnormal responses include spike-and-wave discharges, spikes, sharp waves, focal slow waves or enhancement of abnormal slow waves and of asymmetries.

(14.2) *Sleep* recordings are made after routine daytime waking records in many laboratories and are indicated especially in patients who are suspected of having epilepsy but show no epileptiform activity in the waking record; all-night sleep recordings are occasionally used for that purpose. Recordings after a period of *sleep deprivation* should be used in patients who give a history of having seizures after insufficient sleep.

(14.3) *Photic stimulation* with stroboscopic flashes of diffuse light is used in some laboratories. Normal responses are visual evoked potentials to intermittent flashes and photic driving to repetitive flashes. Photomyoclonic responses are unusual; photoconvulsive responses are abnormal.

(14.4) *Other stimuli* such as patterned light, startling noise, or musical sounds should be used during EEG recordings in those patients who are known to react to these stimuli with behavior suspected of representing seizure activity.

(14.5) *Pentylene tetrazol* and other convulsant drugs are used only rarely and for very narrowly defined reasons.

14.1 HYPERVENTILATION

Hyperventilation should be performed for 3–5 minutes in all routine recordings with the few exceptions described in 5.1.

14.1.1 *Normal responses* consist of generalized slow waves which may begin soon

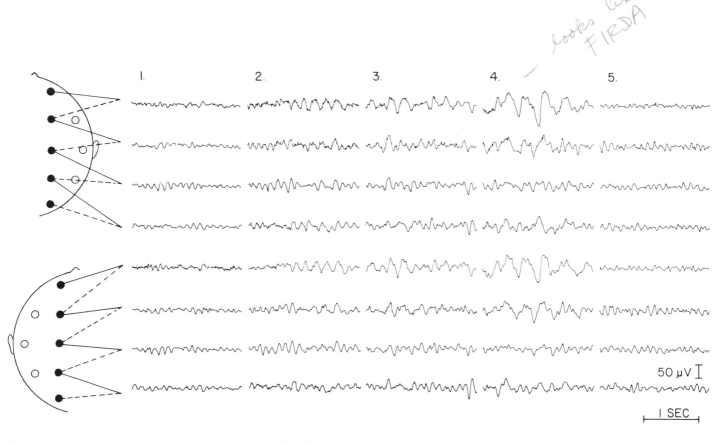

looks like FIRDA

50 μV

1 SEC

Fig. 14.1. Normal hyperventilation response in 45-year-old subject, 4–5 hours after the last meal. 1. Before hyperventilation: Normal EEG; 2. After 1 minute of hyperventilation: Rhythmical theta waves with frontal maximum; 3. After 2 minutes of hyperventilation: Theta and delta waves with frontal maximum; 4. After 3 minutes of hyperventilation: Fairly rhythmical delta waves, maximal frontally; 5. 1 minute after the end of hyperventilation: Return to initial EEG pattern.

252

after the onset of hyperventilation (Fig. 14.1). Initially, the slow waves are often intermittent and may appear in the form of bilaterally synchronous bursts containing waves with sharp contours. The slow waves sometimes start as, or often develop into, long trains of rhythmical, bisynchronous, generalized delta waves of high amplitude which may become continuous. Normal slow waves of hyperventilation are not focal or lateralized in distribution even though they may have a maximum in the frontal or occipital regions. In children the response to hyperventilation usually begins or remains maximal over the posterior head regions. In contrast, in teenagers and adults the response is almost always maximal over the anterior head regions. The normal response ends within one minute after the patient stops hyperventilating. The hyperventilation response may also be induced by sobbing or crying.

14.1.2 *The incidence and intensity* of the hyperventilation response in normal individuals depends on age, blood sugar level and cerebral responsiveness to hypocarbia. Hyperventilation responses are most common and most pronounced in children and teenagers. They diminish in young adults and are rare in old persons, presumably because of reduced respiratory effort, reduced gas exchange across alveolar membranes, and reduced reactivity of neuronal structures to blood gas changes. Hyperventilation responses are more prominent in persons with low serum glucose or cerebral ischemia at the time of hyperventilation. The EEG changes produced by hyperventilation are generally thought to arise from constriction of cerebral blood vessels which leads to reduced cerebral blood flow and decreased delivery of oxygen and glucose to the brain. However, this mechanism of action has not been established conclusively, and other explanations, such as a brainstem-mediated response to hypocarbia, have also been proposed.

14.1.3 *Abnormal responses* to hyperventilation can occur at any age. Subjective symptoms in a patient's history such as dizziness, numbness, tingling, transient blurring of vision, episodic changes of consciousness or awareness, or ringing in the ears often raise the clinician's suspicion of a convulsive disorder and prompt an EEG examination. The specific symptoms of the patient may be reproduced during hyperventilation. If the EEG at that time shows no epileptiform abnormalities, it is very unlikely that the symptoms are due to a seizure disorder. This is one of the most common and useful pieces of information which can be obtained from hyperventilation. The technician should therefore document whether hyperventilation reproduced any of the patient's symptoms (5.1), and the EEG reader should report the reproduction and state whether or not it was associated with EEG abnormalities (26.1.3).

An extremely intense or abnormally prolonged hyperventilation response, especially if occurring in a person after adolescence, raises the suspicion of low blood sugar or cerebral anoxia. However, it is also difficult to tell by bedside observation at what point an individual actually stops hyperventilating, even after being instructed to breathe normally. For this reason in routine recordings the point at which a response can be considered abnormally prolonged is uncertain. (>2 min (?))

A prominent asymmetric response, or *a response which reappears* after hyperventilation has stopped and the background has returned to baseline, suggests the presence of cerebrovascular insufficiency. In children and young adults these findings should always raise the question of Moyamoya disease.

Epileptiform discharges may be induced or enhanced by hyperventilation in some cases. Spike-and-wave discharges of 3 Hz are particularly sensitive to hyperventilation and in many cases appear only during this procedure.

Slow waves in a wide distribution, if present in the spontaneous recording, may be enhanced during hyperventilation, but they may merge with the generalized slow waves of a normal hyperventilation response and are then difficult to recognize as abnormal. Hyperventilation is more likely to enhance rhythmical and generalized slow waves than arrhythmical and focal slow waves.

Asymmetries of background activity may be enhanced and become clearly significant during hyperventilation, or they may become less prominent and reduce the suspicion of an abnormality. Persistent asymmetries of the hyperventilation response itself are abnormal. It may be difficult to determine whether the underlying abnormality is on the side of higher or lower amplitude.

14.2 SLEEP

14.2.1 *Sleep recordings* can help in the diagnosis of epilepsy (12.4.1). Although most epileptiform abnormalities can be found in waking records, recordings which contain a period of sleep can help to (1) detect these abnormalities in some patients who do not show them during wakefulness and (2) discover or delimit an epileptogenic focus in patients showing epileptiform activity without clear focal origin during wakefulness. Foci in the temporal lobes are especially likely to fire in sleep. An attempt should therefore be made to obtain a sleep recording, either spontaneous or drug-induced (5.1), (a) in all patients who are suspected of having a convulsive disorder and who do not show epileptiform discharges in the waking EEG, and (b) in patients whose clinical findings or waking EEG suggest a focal epileptiform abnormality but whose waking EEG does not clearly indicate a focus. Epileptiform activity may occur in any non-REM stage of sleep and is less likely to appear during REM sleep.

14.2.2 *Sleep deprivation* has been used in the past as a method for inducing epileptiform activity in susceptible individuals. Currently, its use is considered limited because: (1) it has been difficult to clearly establish that sleep deprivation offers significant advantages over the activating effect of spontaneous or drug-induced sleep in most individuals with epilepsy; (2) paroxysmal and perhaps epileptiform ab-

255

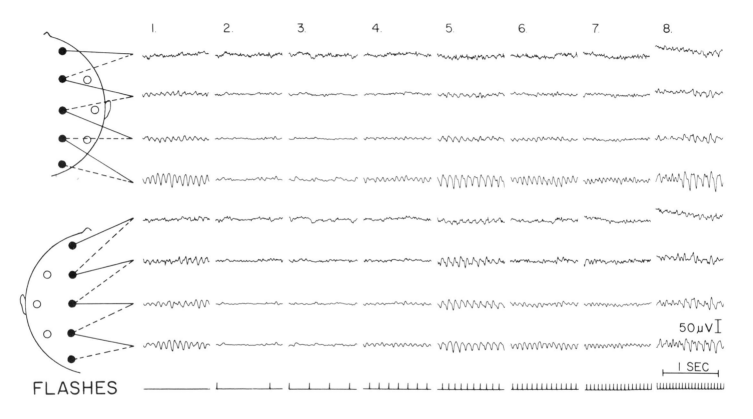

FLASHES

Fig. 14.2. Normal responses to photic stimulation in a 58-year-old subject with closed eyes. Flashes are indicated on the bottom line. 1. Before stimulation: Normal EEG with posterior alpha rhythm; 2. to 8. During photic stimulation at rates of 1, 3, 6, 9, 12, 15 and 18 Hz. Note that the posterior responses have the highest amplitude at a rate near that of the alpha rhythm (Part 5) and at twice that rate (Part 8).

normalities may also be produced by sleep deprivation in persons without convulsive disorders; and (3) in practice it is difficult to keep most individuals awake for more than 20 h. However, sleep deprivation should still be considered as a method of activation in patients who have a history of seizures after insufficient sleep and who do not show epileptiform activity in routine waking and sleep recording.

14.3 PHOTIC STIMULATION

14.3.1 *Normal cerebral responses* to stimulation with flashes of diffuse light (5.1) consist of visual evoked potentials produced by intermittent flashes, and of photic driving in response to repetitive flashes. These responses appear mainly in the occipital areas but may extend into the parietal, posterior temporal and even more anterior areas.

Visual evoked potentials recorded in the EEG usually consist of a monophasic wave of positive polarity with a peak appearing 50 to 150 msec after the flash. When extracted from the ongoing EEG by computer averaging techniques, the potential often shows additional smaller components (7.6.1).

Photic driving usually occurs at flash rates over 3 Hz (Fig. 14.2). At these rates, individual components of the visual evoked potential merge into rhythms which consist of some components having the frequency of the stimulus and of other components often having harmonic or subharmonic frequencies. The response may develop gradually and change in amplitude and configuration as the repetitive stimulation continues. The response on one side may differ from that on the other, both in wave form and in amplitude; these differences may vary with the stimulus rate. The largest responses are often obtained with stimulus frequencies at or near the frequency of the subject's alpha rhythm.

While the amplitude of photic driving, like that of alpha rhythm, is often higher

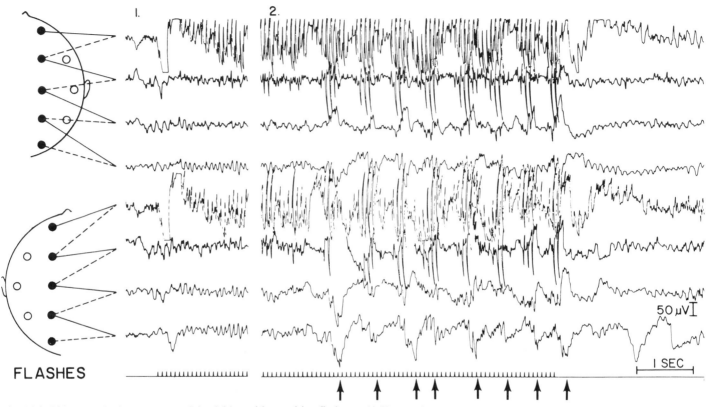

FLASHES

Fig. 14.3. Photomyoclonic response. 1. Stimulaltion with repetitive flashes at 13 Hz, monitored at the bottom, causes muscle artifact in the frontal regions at the rate of the flashes. The posterior head regions show the beginning of photic driving. 2. Five seconds after part 1, the muscle artifact is spreading to the posterior head regions and repetitive movement artifacts at 1–2 Hz (arros) develop, corresponding with jerking of the head and neck. Muscle and movement artifacts end promptly at the end of the flash stimuli. This 37-year-old woman has a history of syncope, headaches and high blood pressure; the neurological examination was normal.

258

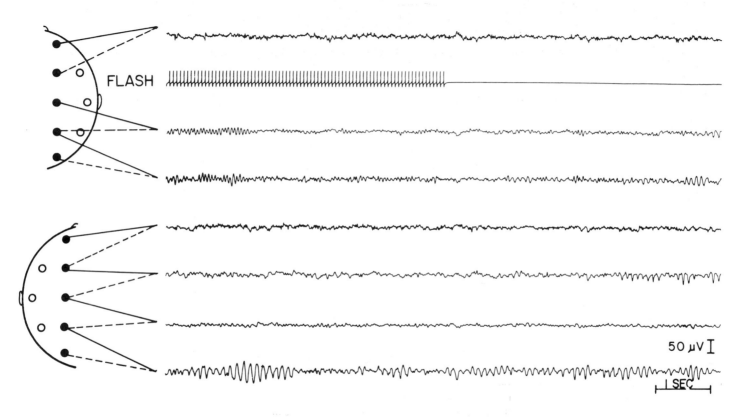

Fig. 14.4. Significant asymmetry of photic driving. Stimulation with repetitive flashes, monitored in channel 2, elicits moderate driving in the right parietal and occipital areas; there is no response on the left where alpha waves continue. This is a part of a recording also used in Fig. 25.1 to illustrate unilateral failure of alpha blocking on eye opening.

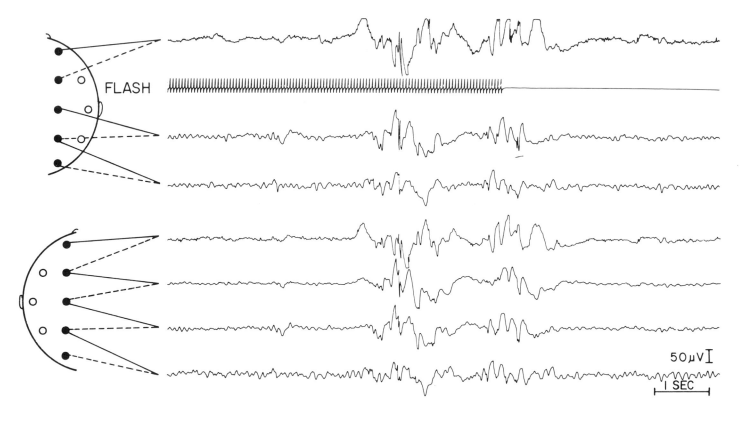

FLASH

50 μV

1 SEC

Fig. 14.5. Photoconvulsive response. Repetitive flash stimulation, monitored in channel 2, elicits no driving; rather, a paroxysm of irregular spikes, sharp and slow waves appears suddenly and in a wide distribution. The generalized epileptiform activity outlasts the end of photic stimulation. Similar paroxysms were elicited repeatedly with similar stimuli in other parts of the same recording. This 23-year-old woman had a generalized tonic-clonic seizure one day before the EEG recording. The seizure began while the patient looked at a television screen showing horizontal bars which turned over vertically.

on the right side, even a 2-fold difference of amplitude of photic driving on either side is not definitely abnormal. High frequency components of the response may be so prominent as to form spikes as part of a normal photic driving response.

The incidence and prominence of photic responses depends on the frequency, intensity, color and pattern of the stimulus, and on the alertness and attention of the subject. Flashes given while the eyes are closed often elicit a response of higher amplitude and different configuration than flashes given while the eyes are open. Responses may appear, change and disappear during continued stimulation. Many subjects show photic driving only at some stimulus frequencies, usually in the range of 8–15 Hz. Driving at high rates is rare in young infants and old persons. Driving cannot be elicited in newborns. Photic responses may be entirely absent in normal subjects even though they can be demonstrated in virtually all subjects of any age by computer averaging of evoked potentials (7.6.1).

14.3.2 *Photomyoclonic or photomyogenic responses* consist of brief muscle contractions triggered in a few susceptible subjects by flashes given while the eyes are closed. The contractions involve mainly the eyelids but may extend into other muscles of the head, neck and body and lead to rather violent twitching (Fig. 14.3).

14.3.3 *Abnormalities of photic responses* consist of extreme variations of response amplitude, or of photoparoxysmal responses.

As an isolated finding, an asymmetric driving response is not clinically significant. If it is associated with other abnormal findings in a consistent fashion, then it is appropriate to consider it as an additional abnormality (Fig. 14.4). The question of whether the higher or the lower amplitude indicates the abnormal side can often be answered if the recording also contains unilateral slow waves or spikes and sharp waves indicating the abnormal side.

A marked bilateral increase or decrease of amplitude, established by comparison with a control recording obtained from the same subject under the same recording and stimulating conditions, raises the suspicion of an abnormality. However, a single recording showing the extremes of either very high amplitude or complete absence of responses is not abnormal.

Photoconvulsive or photoparoxysmal responses consist of spikes and other epileptiform activity (25.5.2). While normal photic responses may contain sharp waves and spikes which repeat at the stimulus rate, remain maximal in the posterior head regions and end with the cessation of stimulation, photoconvulsive responses usually show no clear relationship to the stimulus frequency, often involve the entire head and may outlast the end of stimulation.

Indeed, those which are maximal over the frontal and central head regions and which outlast the duration of the photic stimulus are most often associated with seizure disorders (Fig. 14.5). Photic stimulation rarely evokes a focal epileptiform response and is therefore most useful when a primarily generalized seizure disorder is suspected.

14.4 OTHER STIMULI

Other activation procedures may be used in cases where episodic symptoms or signs suggest a convulsive disorder triggered by known stimuli and where a diagnosis is wanting. These procedures should be used with caution and with the intention of inducing EEG abnormalities while avoiding precipitation of a seizure. The benefits of the diagnostic information obtainable by activation of EEG discharges must be weighed against the risk of inducing a seizure. Great care should be taken to precisely reproduce the triggering conditions which are suspected to bring on seizures in the patient under study. Many of these triggering conditions consist of very specific visual, auditory or other sensory stimuli.

14.4.1 *Pattern sensitivity* is characterized by paroxysmal discharges, similar to photoconvulsive responses, which can be induced in the EEG while a patient looks at an image containing visual detail. The triggering mechanism can be further analyzed in terms of visual content and manner of looking. A patient may be sensitive to stripes of a certain width, direction, brightness, contrast and color, but may be insensitive to other, slightly different, patterns. The pattern may be effective only when the patient keeps scanning it, when he switches from looking at the pattern to looking at a blank surface or vice versa, when he opens or closes his eyes while facing the pattern, etc. While the effective stimulus condition remains constant in some patients, responsiveness varies in others. Some patients have seizures while watching television. This may be due to one or more mechanisms, including the appearance of effective patterns. In some cases, television becomes an effective stimulus only when the television set malfunctions so as to produce a flickering stimulus.

14.4.2 *Auditory stimuli* of several different kinds may trigger paroxysmal discharges in the EEG and seizures. In some patients, a sudden loud noise may be more effective than other startling stimuli. Other patients require more specific auditory stimuli such as a certain sound, a tune, a tune in a certain instrumentation, or a tune played by a certain orchestra ('musicogenic epilepsy'). Certain stimuli may have an emotional impact on the patient, and this may be at least as important for the triggering as the sensory quality of the stimulus. This is probably true of some rare triggering mechanisms such as the hearing of a particular word or sentence or the confrontation with the need to make a decision.

14.4.3 *Reading* may induce paroxysms through one of two mechanisms.
   Primary reading epilepsy, also called 'intrinsic' or 'perceptive', is characterized by paroxysmal abnormalities which appear only with reading. Paroxysms occur

after a period of reading, have a maximum in the parieto-occipital regions, and are often associated with jaw jerking or clicking preceding a generalized seizure.

Secondary reading epilepsy, also called 'extrinsic' or 'sensorial', is characterized by paroxysmal discharges which appear not only with reading but also under other conditions. This form of reading epilepsy may be associated with pattern sensitivity, photoconvulsive and photomyoclonic responses, suggesting that the abnormal responses depend not on the deciphering of the written text but on the photic stimulation resulting from the scanning eye movements during reading.

14.4.4 *Tactile stimulation* of certain parts of the body may induce or abolish paroxysmal EEG discharges and seizures in some patients.

14.5   PENTYLENE TETRAZOL, BEMEGRIDE AND OTHER CONVULSANT DRUGS

When given in sufficient doses, these drugs can induce generalized seizures in anyone. The addition of photic stimulation during administration of pentylene tetrazol ('photometrazol test') often brings out paroxysms and seizures at slightly lower drug doses. Because the effective doses for the production of seizures and of epileptiform EEG discharges under either condition are not clearly different for persons with and without epilepsy, convulsant drugs cannot be used to establish the diagnosis of epilepsy.

In the past convulsant drugs were used only in patients with medically refractory seizures as part of the evaluation for epilepsy surgery. These agents were used to: (1) determine the precise location of the epileptogenic zone by triggering the patient's typical seizure during EEG recording, and (2) to exclude the existence of additional epileptogenic foci which could continue to produce seizures after surgery. These agents are rarely used today since it is now known that they may evoke seizures from ectopic foci producing misleading localizing information. Instead seizure localization is accomplished by recording the patient's typical seizures during long-term monitoring and by obtaining indirect localizing evidence through neuroimaging procedures.

REFERENCES

Ahuja, G.K., Mohandas, S. and Narayanaswamy, A.S. (1980) Eating epilepsy. Epilepsia 21: 85–89.

Anderson, N.E. and Wallis, W.E. (1986) Activation of epileptiform activity by mental arithmetic. Arch. Neurol. 43: 624–626.

Bancaud, J. (1976) EEG activation by metrazol and megimide in the diagnosis of epilepsy. In: Rémond, A. (Ed.), Handbook of Electroencephalography and Clinical Neurophysiology, Elsevier, Amsterdam.

Bickford, R.G., Whelan, J.L., Klass, D.W. and Corbin, K.B. (1956) Reading epilepsy: Clinical and electroencephalographic studies of a new syndrome. Trans. Amer. Neurol. Assn. 81: 100–102.

Bickford, R.G. (1979) Activation procedures and special electrodes. In: Klass, D.W. and Daly, D.D. (Eds.), Current Practice of Clinical Electroencephalography, Raven, New York, pp. 269–306.

Binnie, C.D., Coles, P.A. and Margerison, J.H. (1969) The influence of end-tidal carbon dioxide tension on EEG changes during routine hyperventilation in different age groups. Electroenceph. clin. Neurophysiol. 27: 304–306.

Binnie, C.D., Rowan, A.J. and Gutter, T. (1982) A Manual of Electroencephalographic Technology, Cambridge University Press, Cambridge.

Bostem, F. (1976) Section II. Hyperventilation. In: Rémond, A. (Ed.), Handbook of Electroenceph. clin. Neurophysiol., Vol. 3D, pp. 74–88.

Chatrian, G.E. and Perez-Borja, C. (1964) Depth electrographic observations in two cases of photo-oculoclonic responses. Electroenceph. clin. Neurophysiol. 17: 71–75.

Coull, B.M. and Pedley, T.A. (1978) Intermittent photic stimulation. Clinical usefulness of nonconvulsive responses. Electroenceph. clin. Neurophysiol. 44: 353–363.

DeMarco, P. and Tassinari, C.A. (1981) Extreme somatosensory evoked potentials (EPSEP): An EEG sign forecasting the possible occurrence of seizures in children. Epilepsia 22: 569–575.

Ellingson, R.J., Wilken, K. and Bennett, D.R. (1984) Efficacy of sleep deprivation as an activation procedure in epilepsy patients. J. clin. Neurophysiol. 1: 83–102.

Engel, J. (1974) Selective photoconvulsive responses to intermittent diffuse and patterned photic stimulation. Electroenceph. clin. Neurophysiol. 37: 283–292.

Fisch, B.J., Hauser, W.A., Brust, J.C.M., Gupta, G.S., Lubin, R., Tawfik, G. and Hyacinthe, J.C. (1989) The EEG response to diffuse and patterned photic stimulation during acute untreated alcohol withdrawal. Neurology 39: 434–436.

Forster, F.M. (1977) Reflex Epilepsy, Behavioral Therapy and Conditional Reflexes. C.C. Thomas, Springfield.

Gabor, A.J. and Seyal, M. (1986) Effect of sleep on the electroencephalographic manifestations of epilepsy. J. clin. Neurophysiol. 3: 23–38.

Gloor, P. (1976) Section V. Intracarotid amobarbital and pentylenetetrazol activation. In: Rémond, A. (Ed.), Handbook of Electroenceph. clin. Neurophysiol., Vol. 3D, Elsevier, Amsterdam, pp. 121–151.

Harden, A., Pampiglione, G. and Picton-Robinson, N. (1973) Electroretinogram and visual evoked response in a form of 'neuronal lipidosis' with diagnostic EEG features. J. Neurol. Neurosurg. Psychiat. 36: 61.

Hiraga, H., Aoki, Y. and Kodama, N. (1980) Electroencephalographic findings in moyamoya disease: Its diagnostic value and classification. Clin. EEG (Okasaka) 22: 513–526.

Holmes, G.L., Blair, S., Eisenberg, E., Scheebaum, R., Margraf, J. and Zimmerman, A.W. (1982) Tooth-brushing induced epilepsy. Epilepsia 23: 657–661.

Jeavons, P.M. and Harding, G.F.A. (1975) Photosensitive Epilepsy. A Review of the Literature and a Study of 460 Patients. Heinemann, London.

Klass, D.W. and Fischer-Williams, M. (1976) Section I. Sensory stimulation, sleep and sleep deprivation. In: Rémond, A. (Ed.), Handbook of Electroenceph. clin. Neurophysiol., Vol. 3D, Elsevier, Amsterdam, pp. 5–73.

Lesser, R.P. (1985) Psychogenic seizures. In: Pedley, T.A. and Meldrum, B.S. (Eds.), Recent Advances in Epilepsy, Vol. 2, Churchill/Livingstone, Edinburgh, pp. 273–296.

Matsuoka, H., Takahashi, T., Hasegawa, T. and Okuma, T. (1983) The role of psychic tension in the precipitation of epileptic seizures, with special reference to the findings obtained from neuropsychological EEG activation. J. Jpn. Epil. Soc. 1: 128–138.

Meier-Ewert, K. and Broughton, R.J. (1967) Photomyoclonic response of epileptic and non-epileptic subjects during wakefulness, sleep and arousal. Electroenceph. clin. Neurophysiol. 23: 142–151.

Mesri, J.C. and Pagano, M.A. (1987) Reading epilepsy. Epilepsia 28: 301–304.

Newmark, M.E. and Penry, J.K. (1979) Photosensitivity and Epilepsy. A Review. Raven, New York.

Panayiotopoulos, C.P. (1974) Effectiveness of photic stimulation on various eye-states in photosensitive epilepsy. J. neurol. Sci. 23: 165–173.

Patel, V.M. and Maulsby, R.L. (1987) How hyperventilation alters the electroencephalogram: A review of controversial viewpoints emphasizing neurophysiological mechanisms. J. clin. Neurophysiol. 4: 101–120.

Paulson, O.B. and Sharbrough, F.W. (1974) Physiologic and pathophysiologic relationship between the electroencephalogram and the regional cerebral blood flow. Acta neurol. scand. 50: 194–220.

Takahashi, T. (1987) Activation methods. In: Niedermeyer, E. and Lopes da Silva, F. (Eds.), Electroencephalography: Basic Principles, Clinical Applications, and Related Fields. Urban and Schwarzenberg, Baltimore, pp. 209–228.

Reilly, E.L. and Peters, J.F. (1973) Relationship of some varieties of electroencephalographic photosensitivity to clinical convulsive disorders. Neurology 23: 1050–1057.

Sperling, M.R. (1984) Hypoglycemic activation of focal abnormalities in the EEG of patients considered for temporal lobectomy. Electroenceph. clin. Neurophysiol. 58: 506–512.

Sunder, T.R., Erwin, C.W. and Dubois, P.J. (1980) Hyperventilation induced abnormalities in the electroencephalogram of children with moyamoya disease. Electroenceph. clin. Neurophysiol. 49: 414–420.

Sutherling, W.W., Hershman, L.M., Miller, J.Q. and Lee, S.I. (1980) Seizures induced by playing music. Neurology 30: 1001–1004.

Tyner, F.S., Knott, J.R. and Mayer Jr., W.B. (1983) Fundamentals of EEG Technology. Vol. 1: Basic Concepts and Methods, Raven, New York, pp. 267–279.

Vignaendra, V., Thian Ghee, L., Chong Lee, L. and Siew Tin, C. (1976) Epileptic discharges triggered by blinking and eye closure. Electroenceph. clin. Neurophysiol. 40: 491–498.

Wiebers, D.O., Westmorland, B.F. and Klass, D.W. (1979) EEG activation and mathematical calculation. Neurology 29: 1499–1503.

Wilkins, A.J., Darby, C.E., Binnie, C.D., Stafansson, S.B., Jeavons, P.M. and Harding, G.F.A. (1979) Television epilepsy. The role of pattern. Electroenceph. clin. Neurophysiol. 47: 163–171.

Wilkins, A. and Lindsay, J. (1985) Common forms of reflex epilepsy: Physiological mechanisms and techniques for treatment. In: Pedley, T.A. and Mcldrum, B.S. (Eds.), Recent Advances in Epilepsy, Vol. 2, Churchill/Livingstone, Edinburgh, pp. 239–272.

Wyler, A.R., Richey, E.T., Atkinson, R.A. and Hermann, B.P. (1987) Methohexital activation of epileptogenic foci during acute electrocorticography. Epilepsia 28: 490–494.

Part C
The abnormal EEG

Abnormal EEG patterns, correlation with underlying cerebral lesions and neurological diseases

15

SUMMARY

(15.1)   An EEG is usually called abnormal not because it lacks normal patterns but because it contains: A. Epileptiform activity, B. Slow waves, C. Abnormalities of amplitude, or D. Deviations from normal patterns. These abnormalities can be subdivided into a few basic abnormal EEG patterns.

(15.2)   The basic abnormal EEG patterns correspond fairly well with a few kinds of cerebral lesions.

(15.3)   However, the basic abnormal EEG patterns do not correlate directly with specific neurological diseases because similar cerebral lesions, and thus similar EEG patterns, may be produced by a great variety of neurological diseases. Moreover, many diseases may produce more than one abnormal pattern. The EEG therefore cannot make a clinical diagnosis but can help to select one of several possible diagnoses.

15.1   DEFINITION OF THE ABNORMAL EEG

An EEG is abnormal if it contains A. epileptiform activity, B. slow waves, C. amplitude abnormalities, or D. certain patterns resembling normal activity but deviating from it in frequency, reactivity, distribution or other features. In most abnormal EEGs, the abnormal patterns do not entirely replace normal activity: they appear only intermittently, only in some channels, or only superimposed on a normal background.

The most important EEG abnormalities can be divided into the following basic abnormal EEG patterns which are discussed in the subsequent chapters.

A. Epileptiform activity
    1. Localized epileptiform activity
    2. Generalized epileptiform activity

3. Special epileptiform patterns
B. Slow waves
1. Localized slow waves
2. Generalized asynchronous slow waves
3. Bilaterally synchronous slow waves
C. Amplitude abnormalities
1. Localized amplitude changes: Asymmetries
2. Generalized amplitude changes
D. Deviations from normal patterns.

15.2 CORRELATION BETWEEN ABNORMAL EEG PATTERNS, GENERAL CEREBRAL
PATHOLOGY AND SPECIFIC NEUROLOGICAL DISEASES

Each of the basic abnormal EEG patterns listed above can be caused by one or a few
types of cerebral abnormalities. The abnormalities are characterized by their irritative or destructive character and by their cortical, subcortical and epicortical
location. The correlation between EEG patterns, cerebral pathology and specific
diseases is summarized in a series of tables and discussed in the subsequent chapters.
The four major categories of abnormal EEG patterns are the subject of Table 15.1
– Basic epileptiform patterns, 15.2 – Basic patterns of slow wave abnormalities,
15.3 – Basic patterns of abnormal amplitude and 25.1 – Deviations from normal
patterns. The epileptiform patterns listed in Table 15.1 are further detailed in Tables
17.1, 18.1, 19.1, 19.2, 19.3 and 19.4; the patterns of abnormal amplitude listed in
Table 15.3 are shown in more detail in Tables 23.1 and 24.1

15.2.1 *Epileptiform activity* is outlined in Table 15.1. Local epileptiform activity is
usually due to a focal irritative lesion of the cerebral cortex; in infants, such activity

TABLE 15.1
Basic epileptiform patterns: Pathological and clinical correlates

Basic patterns	General pathological correlates	Examples of specific diseases
1. *Local epileptiform activity* (Table 17.1)	(1) Chronic local cortical lesions	Cortical scars after strokes and injuries, tumors; with or without recurring partial seizures: symptomatic epilepsy
	(2) Acute local cortical lesions	Acute strokes, head injuries; with or without acute partial seizures
	(3) In young infants (a) Widespread structural damage	Perinatal injury, anoxia, ischemia; with or without partial, uni- or bilateral seizures
	(b) Toxic, metabolic, electrolytic abnormalities	Hypoglycemia, pyridoxine deficiency, phenylketonuria; with or without seizures as above
	(4) Children without detectable lesion	Benign epilepsy of childhood with partial seizures
2. *Generalized epileptiform activity* (Table 18.1)	(1) No detectable abnormality	Idiopathic epilepsy with primary generalized seizures
	(2) Diffuse cortical and subcortical disorders: (a) Structural (aa) Acute damage	Acute anoxia, head injury, encephalitis; with or without primary generalized seizures
	(bb) Chronic diseases	Postanoxic and posttraumatic generalized cerebral damage, myoclonus epilepsy; with or without primary generalized seizures
	(b) Toxic, metabolic, endocrine, electrolytic disorders	Hypoglycemia, renal encephalopathy, alcohol withdrawal; with or without primary generalized seizures during the disorder
3. *Special epileptiform patterns* 3.1 Infantile and juvenile patterns of multifocal and generalized spikes (Table 19.1)	Widespread structural or metabolic cerebral disease; patterns are more specific for age than for cause	Pre-, peri- and postnatal injury, cerebromacular degeneration, tuberous sclerosis, phenylketonuria, leukodystrophies; with or without partial or generalized seizures
3.2 Periodic complexes (Table 19.2)	Acute or subacute, fairly widespread cerebral damage or metabolic derangements	Fresh cerebral infarcts, Jakob-Creutzfeldt disease, subacute sclerosing panencephalitis, barbiturate intoxication, herpes simplex encephalitis, metabolic encephalopathies; with or without myoclonus
3.3 Ictal patterns without spikes and sharp waves (Table 19.3)	No common pathological correlate	Certain partial complex seizures, tonic seizures, neonatal seizures, absence seizures, epilepsia partialis continua
3.4 Epileptiform patterns without known pathological correlates and without seizures (Table 19.4)	No detectable abnormality	No known diseases or seizures

may be the result of widespread lesions or of toxic, metabolic or electrolytic abnormalities whereas some children have local spikes without any detectable cerebral lesions. Generalized epileptiform activity is either not associated with demonstrable lesions or associated with a variety of conditions which increase the excitability of subcortical centers, of wide parts of the cerebral cortex, or of both. Special epileptiform patterns have a great variety of pathological correlates.

15.2.2 *Slow wave abnormalities* and their correlates are shown in Table 15.2.

Table 15.2
Basic patterns of slow wave abnormalities: Pathological and clinical correlates

Basic patterns	General pathological correlates	Examples of specific diseases
1. Local slow waves	(1) Local structural damage of	
	(a) Subcortical white matter	Strokes, tumors, abscesses
	(b) Thalamus	As above
	(2) Local disorders of cerebral blood flow or metabolism	Transient ischemic attacks, migraine, postictal condition
2. Generalized asynchronous slow waves	(1) No detectable abnormality in some cases of mild or moderate slow waves	No known disease, in 10–15% of normal adults
	(2) Widespread structural damage including subcortical white matter	Widespread degenerative and cerebrovascular disease
	(3) Generalized disorders of cerebral function	Acute anoxia, syncope, coma, postictal condition
3. Bilaterally synchronous slow waves	Deep midline grey matter involvement by	
	(1) Diffuse diseases damaging subcortical and cortical grey matter more than white matter	Presenile dementia, progressive supranuclear palsy
	(2) Local structural lesions which directly involve or compress, distort or render ischemic deep midline structures of the mesencephalon, diencephalon, mesial and orbital parts of frontal lobe	Tumors, strokes at or near the bottom of the anterior, middle or posterior fossa
	(3) Metabolic, toxic, and endocrine encephalopathies	Hepatic, renal, hypoparathyroid encephalopathies

Local slow waves are often due to circumscribed damage of the white matter of the hemispheres with or without involvement of the cortex. Generalized asynchronous slow waves suggest a widespread disturbance of cerebral function, often due to greater involvement of subcortical white matter than of the cerebral cortex. Bisynchronous slow waves are often due to widespread involvement of subcortical and cortical grey matter or to local involvement of deep midline structures; this may be due to structural damage or to metabolic, toxic or endocrine disorders.

15.2.3 *Amplitude changes* are described in Table 15.3. Local reductions of amplitude are often due either to superficial lesions which reduce the electrical potentials generated in the cortex or to material that is interposed between cortex

TABLE 15.3
Basic patterns of abnormal amplitude: Pathological and clinical correlates

Basic patterns	General pathological correlates	Examples of specific diseases
1. Local differences of amplitude (asymmetries) (Table 23.1)	(1) Locally decreased EEG production	
	(a) Structural cortical damage	Cortical infarct, contusion
	(b) Disorder of cortical function	Cortical transient ischemia, migraine
	(2) Local change of media between cortex and recording electrode	
	(a) Increase	Subdural hematoma, subgaleal hematoma
	(b) Decrease	Surgical skull defect
2. Generalized changes of amplitude (Table 24.1)	(1) Generally decreased EEG production	
	(a) No detectable abnormality in some cases of mild or moderate reduction	No known disease, in 5–10% of normal adults
	(b) Structural diseases of cerebral cortex	Huntington's chorea, postanoxic encephalopathy
	(c) Disorders of cortical function	Hypothyroidism, acute anoxia, hypothermia, intoxications, anxiety, postictal
	(2) Bilateral increase of media between cortex and recording electrodes	Subdural hematoma

275

and recording electrodes and interferes with the electrical conduction of cortical potentials to the recording electrodes; a local increase of amplitude often results from skull defects. Generalized reductions of amplitude are due either to a widespread decrease of the production of electrocortical potentials or to a generalized increase of the conducting media between cortex and recording electrodes.

15.2.4 *Deviations from normal patterns* are listed in Table 25.1. These patterns resemble normal patterns but deviate from them in specific regards, for instance in frequency, reactivity or distribution; some of them correlate with particular cerebral abnormalities.

Each cerebral lesion can be caused by many different neurological diseases. Examples are listed in the right columns of the tables. It is obvious that not any one EEG pattern is specific for any one disease: each pattern can be caused by several diseases. The correlation between patterns and diseases is further weakened by several facts. (a) Many diseases cause more than one type of cerebral lesion and, therefore, more than one pattern. (b) Not all cases of a neurological disease cause an EEG abnormality; the EEG may be normal especially if the cerebral lesion is small, chronic or located deeply in the brain. A disease may also produce EEG abnormalities which are intermittent and so rare that they do not appear during the period of a routine EEG recording. (c) The EEG may be abnormal in some persons who show no other evidence for a disease; for instance, the EEG abnormality may precede or outlast all other signs of a disease.

Because each abnormal EEG pattern can be caused by more than one disease and because some diseases cause more than one abnormal EEG pattern, the EEG alone cannot be used to make a specific clinical diagnosis but can only suggest a set of possible diagnoses. Even so, the EEG can become a powerful diagnostic tool when it is applied to the specific clinical presentation of a case. Like other laboratory tests, the EEG can limit the differential diagnosis and thereby lead to the selection of the correct diagnosis. For example, in an alcoholic patient in coma who is suspected of having either a subdural hematoma or a hepatic encephalopathy, focal slow waves or depression of amplitude would clearly favor the former diagnosis and bisynchronous generalized triphasic waves the latter even though each of these diseases can cause many other EEG patterns and even though each of these EEG patterns occurs in many other diseases.

Even in cases where the clinical options are wider, the EEG may select some of them as being more likely. For instance, an elderly patient with increasing episodes of confusion may have spikes in the temporal lobe suggesting that he suffers from complex partial seizures; he may show focal slow waves over a frontal area and suffer from a structural lesion such as a frontal lobe tumor; he may have an EEG of very low amplitude and suffer from Huntington's chorea, hypothyroidism, bilateral subdural hematomas or postanoxic encephalopathy; or he may have a normal EEG or an exaggeration of the EEG changes normally appearing with advancing age and suffer from presenile dementia.

In general, the EEG reflects changes of cerebral function more directly and reliably than it detects structural lesions, especially if the structural lesions are not discrete and localized near the surface of the hemispheres. As a result, the EEG has been found to be more useful in the differential diagnosis of some disorders than in that of others. The indication for ordering an EEG therefore depends on the diagnoses entertained in each case. The *diagnostic value* of an EEG is likely to be:

(a) *High* in sudden and rapidly progressive disorders of the hemispheres and of midline diencephalic and mesencephalic structures, for instance in: (1) Seizure disorders; (2) Toxic-metabolic encephalopathies; (3) Coma of undetermined cause;

(4) Suspected cerebral death; (5) Reduction of cerebral blood flow during carotid endarterectomy; (6) Encephalitis; (7) Jakob-Creutzfeldt disease, Huntington's chorea.

(b) *Moderate* in recent or progressive focal mass lesions of the hemispheres or of midline diencephalic and mesencephalic structures; although these lesions are usually more precisely localized by M.R.I. and computerized tomographic brain scans, in some cases they may be recognized earlier or only by EEG. Examples are: (1) Brain tumor; (2) Strokes; (3) Head injury; (4) Chronic subdural hematoma; (5) Cerebral abscesses.

(c) *Low* in lesions below the hemispheres and not impinging upon midline diencephalic and mesencephalic structures, and in mild, old stationary or slowly progressive generalized disorders of the hemispheres, namely in: (1) Cerebellar diseases and lesions; (2) Brainstem lesions involving cranial nerves and long tracts but not the reticular core; (3) Psychiatric diseases; (4) Alzheimer's disease, Parkinson's disease, Wilson's disease, spinocerebellar degenerations; (5) Chronic headaches of undetermined cause.

Even though the diagnostic value of the EEG is generally low in certain diseases, the EEG may be of value in many cases of these diseases by excluding other diagnostic possibilities; for instance, although the EEG in Alzheimer's disease may show only mild generalized slow waves, the finding of such slow waves may help to rule out other possible causes of dementia such as a frontal tumor or hypothyroid encephalopathy. The EEG is often also useful in monitoring the progress of a patient's disease or the effect of treatment. This is true for a wide variety of acute and subacute disorders of cerebral structure and function. For instance, the EEG may help to demonstrate recovery from postanoxic coma, intoxications, metabolic encephalopathy or status epilepticus. It is very important to obtain a baseline recording early in the course of these disorders and before the beginning of any treatment.

REFERENCES

Goldensohn, E.S. and Koehle, R. (1975) EEG Interpretation: Problems of Overreading. Futura, Mount Kisco.

Kiloh, L.G., McComas, A.J., Osselton, J.W. and Upton, A.R.M. (1981) Clinical Electroencephalography, Appleton-Century-Crofts, New York.

Klass, D.W. (1987) Identifying the abnormal EEG. In: Halliday, A.M., Butler, S.R. and Paul, R. (Eds.), A Textbook of Clinical Neurophysiology, Wiley, Chichester, pp. 189–200.

Kooi, K.A., Tucker, R.P. and Marshall, R.E. (1978) Fundamentals of Electroencephalography. Harper and Row, Hagerstown.

Maulsby, R.L. (1979) EEG patterns of uncertain diagnostic significance. In: Klass, D.W. and Daly, D.D. (Eds.), Current Practice of Clinical Electroencephalography, Raven, New York, pp. 411–420.

Rémond, A., Ed. (1971–1978) Handbook of Electroencephalography and Clinical Neurophysiology, Elsevier, Amsterdam, Vols. 1–16.

Rowan, A.J. and French, J.A. (1988) The role of the electroencephalogram in the diagnosis and management of epilepsy. In: Pedley, T.A. and Meldrum, B.S. (Eds.), Recent Advances in Epilepsy, Churchill/Livingstone, London, pp. 63–92.

Salinsky, M., Kanter, R. and Dashieff, R.M. (1987) Effectiveness of multiple EEGs in supporting the diagnosis of epilepsy: An operational curve. Epilepsia 28: 331–334.

Sharbrough, F.W. (1987) Nonspecific abnormal EEG patterns. In: Niedermeyer, E. and Lopes da Silva, F. (Eds.), Electroencephalography: Basic Principles, Clinical Applications and Related Fields, Urban and Schwarzenberg, Baltimore, pp. 163–182.

Werner, S., Stockard, J.E. and Bickford, R.G. (1977) Atlas of Neonatal Electroencephalography. Raven, New York.

Williams, G.W., Luders, H.O., Brickner, A., Goormastic, M. and Klass, D.W. (1985) Interobserver variability in EEG interpretation. Neurology 35: 1714–1719.

Classification of seizures

16

SUMMARY

This chapter differs from those which follow in that it deals more with the clinical and behavioral aspects of seizures than with EEG patterns. This is done in order to prepare the reader for the clinical correlates of epileptiform EEG patterns.

(16.1)   *Definitions: Seizures* are episodes of sudden disturbances of mental, motor, sensory or autonomic activity caused by a paroxysmal cerebral malfunction. *Convulsions* are seizures consisting of violent involuntary contractions of somatic muscles. *Seizures disorder and convulsive disorder* are terms describing the condition of patients who have had one or more seizures or convulsions. *Epilepsy* is defined clinically as a chronic recurrent seizure; the cause may be known ('symptomatic epilepsy') or unknown ('idiopathic epilepsy' or 'cryptogenic epilepsy'). *Status epilepticus* is the recurrence of seizure episodes at intervals too short to allow recovery of the pre-seizure condition. *Epilepsia partials continua* consists of repetitive seizure manifestations, usually rhythmical twitching of a limb, persisting for several days or weeks and not forming discrete seizure episodes.

(16.2)   *The international classification of epileptic seizures* divides seizures by their clinical manifestations as shown in Table 16.1.

16.1   DEFINITIONS

16.1.1   *Seizures*, in neurological terms, are episodes of sudden disturbances of consciousness, mental functions, motor, sensory and autonomic activity, caused by a paroxysmal malfunction of cerebral nerve cells. Seizures are discrete episodes lasting only one or a few minutes and involving either only a part of the brain or the entire brain. Most seizures show varying manifestations during their course. They may progressively involve different parts of the body to the other, and they may produce one manifestation, for instance a sustained tonic contraction, before another manifestation, for instance a rhythmical, clonic contraction. Seizures are often followed by a transient paralysis of that function which had been hyperactive during the seizure ('Todd's paralysis'). Seizures occurring in the same person usually resemble each other closely. These characteristics in most instances clearly distinguish seizures from other conditions producing an episodic loss of consciousness or changes in behavior (such as syncope, transient ischemic attacks or psychiatric disturbances).

16.1.2 *Convulsions* are violent involuntary contractions of the body musculature. In neurology, this term is usually limited to contractions produced by cerebral seizure activity.

16.1.3 *Seizure disorder* and *convulsive disorder* are terms used to describe the condition of patients who have had one or more seizures or convulsions.

16.1.4 *Epilepsy* describes the condition of patients who have recurring seizures due to some lasting cerebral abnormality. Patients who have had only one seizure or who have recurrent seizures due to transient cerebral abnormalities or to abnormalities primarily outside the brain such as alcohol withdrawal, hypoglycemia or fever are not usually said to have epilepsy.

16.1.5 *Status epilepticus* describes the recurrence of seizures at intervals too short to allow recovery of the condition which existed before the onset of the seizures. Usually more than two or three seizures occur and form cycles of discrete seizure episodes separated from each other by only brief pauses. The seizure episodes consist of constant or progressively changing manifestations, each episode usually resembling the others. This repetition of discrete episodes distinguishes focal status epilepticus from epilepsia partialis continua.

16.1.6 *Epilepsia partialis continua* is a continuous and rather stereotyped repetition of one, fairly constant, type of epileptic activity, usually rhythmical jerking of a limb or of part of a limb; alertness is usually reduced. This activity may last for weeks or months. Sometimes, it may be interrupted by discrete partial or generalized seizures or may become less violent or more restricted and even disappear intermittently.

16.1.7 *Reflex epilepsy* denotes seizures triggered by sensory stimuli and other mechanisms specific for each patient (14.4; 25.5.2). Many patients with reflex epilepsy also have seizures which are not triggered by these mechanisms.

16.2a   CLASSIFICATION OF SEIZURES – GENERAL

The most widely used and generally accepted classification of epileptic seizures is that proposed by the Commission on Classification and Terminology of the International League Against Epilepsy. Unlike previous classifications, it defines seizure types only in terms of clinical manifestations and EEG findings. It also differs from previous classifications because it is based on the study of videotape recordings of simultaneously recorded EEG and clinical epileptic seizures. The classification is divided into four major categories as shown in Table 16.1. *Partial Seizures*, the first major category, are those in which the first clinical and electrographic changes indicate the initial involvement of a group of neurons limited to part of one cerebral hemisphere. If consciousness is not impaired during the attack, then the seizure is classified as a *simple partial seizure*. If consciousness is impaired, then the seizure

TABLE 16.1
Proposal for revised seizure classification*

I. Partial (focal, local) seizures

Partial seizures can be classified into one of the following three fundamental groups:

A. Simple partial seizures
B. Complex partial seizures
    1. With impairment of consciousness at onset
    2. Simple partial onset followed by impairment of consciousness
C. Partial seizures evolving to generalized tonic-clonic convulsions (GTC)
    1. Simple evolving to GTC
    2. Complex evolving to GTC (including those with simple partial onset)

Clinical seizure type	EEG seizure type	EEG interictal expression
A. *Simple partial seizures* (consciousness not impaired)	Local contralateral discharge starting over the corresponding area of cortical representation (not always recorded on the scalp)	Local contralateral discharge

1. With motor signs
    (a) Focal motor without march
    (b) Focal motor with march (Jacksonian)
    (c) Versive
    (d) Postural
    (e) Phonatory (vocalization or arrest of speech)

2. With somatosensory or special-sensory symptoms (simple hallucinations, e.g., tingling, light flashes, buzzing)
    (a) Somatosensory
    (b) Visual
    (c) Auditory
    (d) Olfactory
    (e) Gustatory
    (f) Vertiginous

* Adapted from Epilepsia, 22: 498–501, 1981.

TABLE 16.1 *(continued)*

Clinical seizure type	EEG seizure type	EEG interictal expression

3. With autonomic symptoms or signs (including epigastric sensation, pallor, sweating, flushing, piloerection and pupillary dilatation)

4. With psychic symptoms (disturbance of higher cerebral function). These symptoms rarely occur without impairment of consciousness and are much more commonly experienced as complex partial seizures
   (a) Dysphasic
   (b) Dysmnesic (e.g., déjà-vu)
   (c) Cognitive (e.g., dreamy states, distortions of time sense)
   (d) Affective (fear, anger, etc.)
   (e) Illusions (e.g., macropsia)
   (f) Structured hallucinations (e.g., music, scenes)

B. *Complex partial seizures*

Clinical seizure type	EEG seizure type	EEG interictal expression

(with impairment of consciousness; may sometimes begin with simple symptomatology)
1. Simple partial onset followed by impairment of consciousness
  (a) With simple partial features (A.1.–A.4.) followed by impaired consciousness
  (b) With automatisms
2. With impairment of consciousness at onset
	Unilateral or frequently bilateral discharge, diffuse or focal in temporal or frontotemporal regions	Unilateral or bilateral generally asynchronous focus; usually in the temporal or frontal regions

TABLE 16.1 *(continued)*

Clinical seizure type	EEG seizure type	EEG interictal expression
(a) With impairment of consciousness only		
(b) With automatisms		
C. *Partial seizures evolving to secondarily generalized seizures* (This may be generalized tonic-clonic, tonic, or clonic)	Above discharges become secondarily and rapidly generalized	
1. Simple partial seizures (A) evolving to generalized seizures		
2. Complex partial seizures (B) evolving to generalized seizures		
3. Simple partial seizures evolving to complex partial seizures evolving to generalized seizures		

II. Generalized seizures (convulsive or nonconvulsive)

Clinical seizure type	EEG seizure type	EEG interictal expression
A. 1. *Absence seizures*	Usually regular and symmetrical 3 Hz but may be 2–4 Hz spike-and-slow-wave complexes and may have multiple spike-and-slow-wave complexes. Abnormalities are bilateral	Background activity usually normal although paroxysmal activity (such as spikes or spike-and-slow-wave complexes) may occur. This activity is usually regular and symmetrical
(a) Impairment of consciousness only		

TABLE 16.1 *(continued)*

Clinical seizure type	EEG seizure type	EEG interictal expression
(b) With mild clonic components (c) With atonic components (d) With tonic components (e) With automatisms (f) With autonomic components (b through f may be used alone or in combination)		
2. *Atypical absence*	EEG more heterogeneous; may include irregular spike-and-slow-wave complexes, fast activity or other paroxysmal activity. Abnormalities are bilateral but often irregular and asymmetrical	Background usually abnormal; paroxysmal activity (such as spikes or spike-and-slow-wave complexes) frequently irregular and asymmetrical
May have: (a) Changes in tone that are more pronounced than in A.1 (b) Onset and/or cessation that is not abrupt		
B. *Myoclonic seizures* Myoclonic jerks (single or multiple)	Polyspike and wave, or sometimes spike and wave or sharp and slow waves	Same as ictal
C. *Clonic seizures*	Fast activity (10 c/sec or more) and slow waves; occasional spike-and-wave patterns	Spike-and-wave or polyspike-and-wave discharges

TABLE 16.1 *(continued)*

Clinical seizure type	EEG seizure type	EEG interictal expression
D. *Tonic seizures*	Low voltage, fast activity or a fast rhythm of 9–10 c/sec or more decreasing in frequency and increasing in amplitude	More or less rhythmic discharges of sharp and slow waves, sometimes asymmetrical. Background is often abnormal for age
E. *Tonic-clonic seizures*	Rhythm at 10 or more c/sec decreasing in frequency and increasing in amplitude during tonic phase, interrupted by slow waves during clonic phase	Polyspike and waves or spike and wave, or, sometimes, sharp and slow wave discharges
F. *Atonic seizures* (Astatic) (combinations of the above may occur, e.g., B and F, B and D)	Polyspikes and wave or flattening or low-voltage fast activity	Polyspikes and slow wave

III. Unclassified epileptic seizures

Includes all seizures that cannot be classified because of inadequate or incomplete data and some that defy classification in hitherto described categories. This includes some neonatal seizures, e.g., rhythmic eye movements, chewing, and swimming movements.

IV. Addendum

Repeated epileptic seizures occur under a variety of circumstances:

1. as fortuitous attacks, coming unexpectedly and without any apparent provocation; 2. as cyclic attacks, at more or less regular intervals (e.g., in relation to the menstrual cycle, or the sleep-waking cycle); 3. as attacks provoked by: (a) nonsensory factors (fatigue, alcohol, emotion, etc.), or (b) sensory factors, sometimes referred to as 'reflex seizures'.

Prolonged or repetitive seizures (status epilepticus). The term 'status epilepticus' is used whenever a seizure persists for a sufficient length of time or is repeated frequently enough that recovery between attacks does not occur. Status epilepticus may be divided into partial (e.g., Jacksonian), or generalized (e.g., absence status or tonic-clonic status). When very localized motor status occurs, it is referred to as epilepsia partialis continua.

is classified as a *complex partial seizure*. *Simple partial seizures* often involve only one hemisphere electrographically, whereas *complex partial seizures* frequently involve both hemispheres in routine recordings. *Simple partial seizures may not show any electrographic changes, whereas complex partial seizures always produce some change in routine scalp recordings. Simple partial seizures* can be further categorized according to accompanying symptoms and signs as listed in Table 16.1. *Generalized Seizures*, the second major category, are those in which the first clinical and electrographic changes indicate initial involvement of both hemispheres. They usually produce loss of consciousness, bilateral motor activity, or both.

The third category, *Unclassified Epileptic Seizures*, is included because certain kinds of seizures cannot yet be properly characterized due to either a lack of data or a concensus of opinion among investigators. This category includes certain forms of neonatal seizures. The fourth category emphasizes circumstances that influence the occurrence of seizures, such as the sleep-waking cycle or specific triggering stimuli associated with certain forms of reflex epilepsy, and includes definitions of the terms *status epilepticus* and *epilepsia partialis continua*.

Each of the terms used in the classification have been defined by the Commission on Classification and Terminology of the International League Against Epilepsy and can be found in Appendix III. The reader is strongly encouraged to carefully study Table 16.1 and Appendix III. The electroencephalographic ictal and interictal patterns associated with specific types of seizures will be presented in subsequent chapters.

It is important to recognize that efforts are under way to revise the current classification of seizures according to new clinical and laboratory data. One aspect of this revision will concern the way in which a given seizure may evolve. The current classification already recognizes that a *simple partial seizure* may progress to *a complex partial seizure* or to *a generalized tonic-clonic seizure*, or that a *complex partial seizure* may evolve into a *generalized tonic-clonic seizure*. However, the classification does not provide for the occurrence of other known patterns of seizure evolution, such as absence seizures that evolve to tonic-clonic seizures or tonic-clonic seizures that begin with myoclonic or clonic activity (so-called clonic-tonic-clonic seizures).

In addition to the International Classification of Epileptic Seizures, there is also an International Classification of the Epilepsies. The classification of the epilepsies attempts to classify chronic, recurrent seizure disorders into specific syndromes or clinical categories. The categories are organized according to: (1) whether the seizures are partial or generalized and, (2) whether they are idiopathic or symptomatic of an identifiable underlying abnormality. The classification of the epilepsies will not be described in detail here since it is not essential for the correct identification of clinical seizures by behavioral or EEG criteria. Special, well established epileptic syndromes with characteristic EEG patterns will be described in the following chapters. Those readers interested in the classification of the epilepsies are referred to the bibliography referenced at the end of this chapter.

16.2b CLASSIFICATION OF SEIZURES – SPECIFIC

I. *Partial seizures*

These seizures are restricted to part of the brain and produce symptoms in those body parts or mental functions which are represented in the cerebral areas involved by the seizure.

A. *Simple partial seizures*

These seizures produce focal motor, sensory, autonomic, mixed or psychic symptoms without change of consciousness.

    1. *Partial seizures with motor symptoms*:
(i) *Focal motor seizures* consist of sustained tonic contractions or intermittent clonic

290

contractions, or of a sequence of tonic and clonic movements. They involve the face, one part of a limb, an entire limb or half of the body.

(ii) *Jacksonian seizures* are focal motor seizures which successively involve adjacent parts on one side of the body during a seizure. This march is due to the spread of the seizure activity over adjacent parts of the motor cortex.

(iii) *Versive seizures* cause turning of the body, usually in a direction away from the side of the seizure discharge. They are also called 'adversive' or 'contraversive' seizures.

(iv) *Postural seizures* consist of involuntary changes of body posture.

(v) *Inhibitory motor seizures* may cause a paroxysmal cessation of all muscle tone in a part of the body.

(vi) *Aphasic seizures* are characterized by expressive, receptive or global loss of language. They result from seizure activity in speech areas.

(vii) *Phonatory seizures* consist of vocalization or of speech arrest.

2. *Partial seizures with special sensory and somatosensory symptoms*:

(i) *Somatosensory seizures* produce sudden sensations such as tingling, heaviness, numbness or burning which, like motor symptoms, either remain in one part of the body or march over part, or all, of the side of the body opposite to the seizure discharge in the somatosensory area of the brain.

(ii) *Visual seizures* produce hallucinations of white or colored simple shapes, for instance stars and flashes or alterations of visual perception or highly structured visual images.

(iii) *Auditory seizures* cause hallucinations of simple sounds or structured, recognizable sounds.

(iv) *Olfactory seizures* produce hallucinations of odors; they often precede complex partial seizures.

(v) *Gustatory seizures* consist of hallucinations of taste.

(vi) *Vertiginous* seizures cause transient vertigo; unless associated with other seizure.

291

manifestations, these rare seizures may be difficult to distinguish from vertigo of other causes.

3. *Partial seizures with autonomic symptoms* are rarely seen in isolation, but autonomic symptoms are often part of other partial seizures. The seizure symptoms consist of salivation, perspiration, changes in pupillary size, heart beat, respiration or skin color, sexual symptoms, urination, epigastric discomfort or increased gastrointestinal activity. Abdominal epilepsy is a rare cause of periumbilical pain and may be associated with symptoms of complex partial seizures, but this diagnosis requires strict exclusion of local abdominal abnormalities as a cause of the paroxysmal pain. The autonomic symptoms seem to depend on seizure discharges in the insula, the depth of the Sylvian fissure or the mesial frontal areas.

4. *Partial seizures with psychic symptoms* include:

(i) *Partial seizures with cognitive symptoms* may lead to disturbances of memory. Some patients feel and act as though in a dream ('dreamy state'). Other patients become conscious of a lack of memory while some feel that they have seen, heard, or lived through the same situation before ('déjà-vu', 'déjà-entendu', 'déjà-vécu') or that they are strangely unfamiliar with their situation ('jamais vu'). Ideational symptoms include the appearance and persistence of an idea or a thought which is out of context and seems to be forced upon the mind ('forced thinking') during the seizure.

(ii) *Partial seizures with affective symptoms* may cause sudden, unprompted and seemingly inappropriate changes of affect. Most common is a display of fear. Less common are laughing and crying. Rage is not usually a primary seizure manifestation but may be induced as a reaction to restraining environmental factors. Patients with partial complex seizures are not capable of volitionally directed violent behavior; they may commit violent acts by accident, not by intention.

B. Compex partial seizures

These seizures have often been called 'temporal lobe seizures' because they usually arise from foci in the mesial and inferior part of the temporal lobe or adjacent parts of the frontal lobe. The complex symptoms consist primarily of changes of the content of consciousness which reduce the ability of patients to interact with their surroundings; complete loss of consciousness is not a primary symptom. A variety of other mental symptoms may also occur. Patients have no recollection or only incomplete memory of events which occur during the seizure although they may remember simple symptoms at the onset of the seizure such as an awareness of a bad odor. Such olfactory hallucinations presumably arise from the uncus of the temporal lobe and are called 'uncinate fits'.

1. *Partial seizures with impaired consciousness only* are associated with a reduction of awareness which is manifested by confusion.

2. *Partial seizures with automatisms* consist of repetitive movements which seem purposeful in themselves although they serve no obvious purpose in the actual situation; these movements may seem automatic ('automatism'). Simple movements may consist of scratching, patting, chewing, swallowing, mumbling and lip smacking. More highly organized symptoms include facial, gestural and verbal expressions.

C. *Partial seizures secondarily generalized*

These seizures begin like other partial seizures. They then evolve into a generalized seizure either suddenly or after gradually spreading to larger areas. Secondary generalized seizures are usually symmetrical and tonic-clonic, but may be asymmetrical and tonic or clonic. The partial onset of the generalized seizure may be remembered by the patient or observed by witnesses; it may, however, be too short to produce any clinical manifestations. A focal onset may be suggested by the EEG in some cases of apparently primary generalized seizures, but it remains an open question whether some, many or all apparently primary generalized seizures are really secondary generalizations from clinically and electroencephalographically undetected foci.

II. *Generalized seizures*

These seizures involve the entire brain and produce bilateral and fairly symmetrical motor changes; autonomic manifestations may be pronounced. Most generalized seizures begin and remain associated with loss of consciousness. In general, any type of seizure may occur in children; infants do not usually have bilaterally synchronous and symmetrical seizures whereas adults rarely have generalized seizures other than bilateral massive epileptic myoclonus or tonic-clonic seizures.

1. *Absences ('petit mal' seizures)*

Absence attacks, formerly called 'petit mal' seizures, usually occur in childhood and rarely persist into adulthood. In most cases they are an idiopathic form of epilepsy and not associated with clinical or EEG abnormalities except during the attacks ('typical absences' or 'typical petit mal'). However, in some cases, absence attacks are associated with a wide variety of diseases acquired early in life and manifested by various EEG and clinical abnormalities which persist independent of attacks ('atypical absence' or 'petit mal variant').

(a) *Typical absence attacks* consist of impairment of consciousness without loss of muscle tone and posture. They often manifest as a momentary apparent inattentiveness, an empty stave, or an interruption of speech or motion. However, automatisms, myoclonic, and clonic (3 Hz) activity also occur frequently. Usually the interrupted activity is promptly resumed after the attack and the patient has no memory of the lapse of awareness. Some patients retain a limited degree of awareness and continue simple repetitive movements. Attacks may go unnoticed unless they interrupt some motor activity or unless a lapse of awareness or memory can be demonstrated (5.1). Attacks are often triggered by hyperventilation and photic stimulation.

Absences may follow each other closely or continue without noticeable pause so that the patient remains confused or stuporous. This form of status epilepticus, sometimes called 'absence status' occurs usually in children. However, a similar condition may appear in patients over 60 years of age, especially in women, who have not previously had absence attacks (Fig. 18.4).

(b) *Atypical absence attacks* are characterized by a combination of impaired consciousness and motor or autonomic changes, and usually pronounced changes in tone. Atypical absence seizures usually have more gradual onset and cessation than typical absence seizures. Examples of atypical absence seizures include:

(i) *Retropulsive absences* are associated with a sudden increase of postural tone causing the patient to move backward;

(ii) *Atonic absences* are combined with a decrease of postural tone producing drop attacks similar to those occurring in brief atonic seizures; and

(iii) *Mixed forms* of absences may contain more than one of the components listed above.

2. *Bilateral massive epileptic myoclonus (myoclonic jerks)*

Bilateral massive epileptic myoclonus or myoclonic jerks are brief contractions which involve mainly flexor muscles on both sides of the body and may vary in distribution. The contractions may recur at irregular or regular intervals. In some cases, they are precipitated by photic stimulation. This type of generalized seizure is so brief that a loss of consciousness cannot usually be detected. Epileptic myoclonus, in contrast to nonepileptic myoclonic contractions, is associated with brief epileptiform activity in the EEG. Thus, epileptic myoclonus precipitated by photic stimuli differs from the more common photomyoclonic response (25.5.3).

3. *Infantile spasms*

Infantile spasms are brief sudden contractions mainly of flexor muscles of the limb girdle producing quick nodding or jack-knife movements of the body. The contractions may last for several seconds and they may recur irregularly for several minutes. Akinesia and reduced responsiveness follow the spasms in some instances and are the only seizure manifestation in others.

4. *Clonic seizures*

Clonic seizures consist of generalized rhythmical myoclonic movements which last for a minute or more and are associated with loss of consciousness. These seizures commonly occur as febrile seizures in childhood.

5. *Tonic seizures*

Tonic seizures consist of contractions of the axial musculature of the entire body and produce flexor positions. They last up to one minute and are associated with loss of consciousness.

6. *Tonic-clonic seizures ('grand mal' seizures)*

Tonic-clonic seizures, formerly called 'grand mal', are the most severe form of generalized seizures and are the most common type of generalized seizures in adults. They begin suddenly with loss of consciousness, sometimes preceded by a shrill cry. Few patients have vague premonitions up to a few hours or days before a seizure, but well-described symptoms preceding the loss of consciousness ('aura') raise the suspicion of a partial seizure with secondary generalization. During the initial tonic phase, most muscles of the body contract intensely, causing stiffening and occasional quivering of the entire body, respiratory arrest with cyanosis, increased heart rate and blood pressure, pupillary dilatation, and perspiration. After 10–20 seconds, the tonic muscle contraction gives way to rhythmic twitching which builds up to violent, generalized and bilaterally synchronous jerking movements of the entire body. This clonic phase may result in injury, tongue biting, irregular respiration and foaming at the mouth. The clonic phase stops in about 30 seconds and leaves the patient in deep coma from which he gradually recovers after passing through the stages of sleep, somnolence and confusion. Urinary and fecal incontinence may occur in this stage.

7. *Atonic seizures*

Atonic seizures consist of sudden loss of muscle tone. They may be associated with myoclonic jerks to form myoclonic-atonic seizures.

(a) *Brief atonic seizures or epileptic drop attacks* lead to sudden falls; the attacks usually last one or two seconds.

(b) *Long atonic seizures* cause patients to suddenly lose consciousness, fall to the floor and remain completely flaccid for one or several minutes.

REFERENCES

Aicardi, J. (1988) Epileptic syndromes in childhood. Epilepsia 29 (Suppl. 3): S1–5.
Commission on Classification and Terminology of the International League Against Epilepsy. (1985) Proposal for Classification of Epilepsies and Epileptic Syndromes. Epilepsia 26: 268–278.
Commission on Classification and Terminology of the International League Against Epilepsy. (1981) Proposal for revised clinical and electrographic classification of epileptic seizures. Epilepsia 22: 489–501.
Dreifuss, F.E. (1987) The different types of epileptic seizures, and the international classification of epileptic seizures and of the epilepsies. In: Hopkins, A. (Ed.), Epilepsy, Demos, New York, pp. 169–200.
Gastaut, H. and Broughton, R. (1972) Epileptic Seizures. Clinical and Electrographic Features, Diagnosis and Treatment. Thomas, Springfield.
Holmes, G. (1987) Neonatal seizures. In: Diagnosis and Management of Seizures in Children, Saunders, Philadelphia, pp. 237–261.
Masland, R.L. (1974) The classification of the epilepsies. A historical review. In: Vinken, P.J. and Bruyn, G.W. (Eds.), Handbook of Clinical Neurology. North-Holland, Amsterdam, pp. 1–29.
Mizrahi, E.M. (1987) Neonatal seizures: Problems in diagnosis and classification. Epilepsia 28: Suppl. 1: S46–55.
Porter, R.J. (1987) The classification of epileptic seizures and epileptic syndromes. In: Luders, H. and Lesser, R. (Eds.), Epilepsy: Electroclinical Syndromes, Springer, New York, pp. 1–12.

Swartz, B.E. and Delgado-Escueta, A.V. (1987) Complex partial seizures of extratemporal origin: 'The evidence for'. In: Wieser, H.G., Speckman, E.J. and Engel Jr., J. (Eds.), The Epileptic Focus, Current Problems in Epilepsy, John Libbey, London, pp. 137–174.

Wolf, P. (1985) The classification of seizures and the epilepsies. In: Porter, R.J. and Morselli, P.L. (Eds.), The Epilepsies, Butterworth, London, pp. 106–124.

Localized epileptiform patterns

17

SUMMARY

(17.1)   The *patterns* of localized epileptiform activity consist of single or multiple focal spikes or sharp waves often in combination with slow waves. Although the spikes and sharp waves may have multiple phases, the polarity of the highest voltage phase is almost always electronegative. Epileptiform activity occurring between seizures is referred to as *interictal epileptiform activity*. Interictal epileptiform activity is usually brief in duration (typically lasting less than 1 second) and almost always exceeds the amplitude of the surrounding background activity. Localized *ictal epileptiform activity* (also referred to as *electrographic seizure activity*) usually persists for more than several seconds, begins abruptly, and consists of repetitive, rhythmic waveforms that tend to vary in form, frequency and topography throughout the seizure. Scalp recorded EEG changes during focal seizures may also be absent or so subtle that they appear as only a mild attenuation in amplitude or as other minor changes in the ongoing background activity. Subtle EEG alterations require correlation with simultaneous behavioral changes to be correctly identified as ictal events. More clearly identifiable ictal EEG patterns that occur in the absence of clinical seizure manifestations are referred to as *subclinical* ictal or electrographic seizure activity. Interictal localized activity is usually restricted to one or a few electrodes, while ictal activity often produces changes in a more widespread distribution or rapidly involves both hemispheres in an asymmetric fashion.

(17.2.1)   *Clinical correlates* of localized epileptiform activity are partial seizures. The type of partial seizure depends on the location of the ictal discharges in the brain. Local discharges in motor and sensory areas generally cause partial seizures with elementary motor and sensory symptoms. Local discharges in the temporal areas are likely to cause partial seizures with psychic or special sensory symptoms. The correlation between the appearance of epileptiform discharges and clinical seizures is not perfect. Some patients suffer from seizures but show no epileptiform activity during the EEG recording, whereas a few patients show epileptiform activity without ever having had a seizure.

(17.2.2)   *Causes* of focal epileptiform activity in adults are acute or chronic lesions which produce partial damage in a circumscribed cortical area. It is not known why some lesions cause epileptiform activity while other, similar, lesions do not. In infants and children, single or multiple foci may be the result of fairly widespread cortical damage; such foci tend to shift in distribution and have little localizing value. In some patients with focal epileptiform activity, no underlying structural lesion can be demonstrated.

(17.3) *Other EEG abnormalities* associated with focal epileptiform activity may suggest specific clinical correlates and causes.

(17.4) *Mechanisms* underlying focal epileptiform activity are thought to involve paroxysmal depolarizing shifts of the membrane potential of a group of cells synchronized by a few pacemaker neurons ('epileptic neurons', 'epileptic neuronal aggregate'). The depolarizing shifts are limited in time and space by hyperpolarizing mechanisms except during seizures when the depolarization becomes repetitive and may spread in distribution.

(17.5) *Specific disorders* causing focal epileptiform activity are mainly cerebral injuries, tumors and strokes, but also include a wide variety of degenerative, developmental, metabolic, and infectious diseases.

17.1 DESCRIPTION OF PATTERNS

17.1.1 *Focal epileptiform activity* consists of spikes or sharp waves which appear at one or a few neighboring electrodes. Focal epileptiform activity is divided into interictal and ictal activity (9.1). Abnormal interictal focal (and generalized) epileptiform waveforms are distinguished from non-epileptiform sharp transients and other paroxysmal waveforms by the following criteria:

(1) Epileptiform spikes and sharp waves are usually asymmetric. The initial half of the wave (from the baseline to peak) often has a shorter duration than the second half of the wave (from the peak to baseline). In contrast, non-epileptiform transients are often approximately symmetric (e.g., wicket spikes). *p.49 Epstein*

(2) Epileptiform spikes and sharp waves may be followed by a slow wave. The slow wave is not sharply contoured and it has a longer duration than the predominant background waveforms.

(3) Epileptiform spikes and sharp waves have more than one phase (usually 2 or 3), and the duration of each phase differs from the durations of the phases of the surrounding background waveforms.

(4) Epileptiform spikes and sharp waves do not appear as simply an abrupt in-

300

also POSTS

crease in the amplitude of sharply contoured waveforms that are part of the ongoing background activity. (spiky alpha)

(5) Epileptiform activity often interrupts the ongoing background beyond the duration of the spike or sharp wave due to the presence of an aftergoing slow wave or surrounding irregular slower waveforms that may preceed or follow the spike or sharp wave.

(6) Sharply contoured waveforms that are recorded from only one electrode may be non-cerebral in origin. Therefore, epileptiform activity should always be detected at more than one electrode site. When activity is only detected at one electrode, the impedance of that electrode should be tested and one or more additional recording electrodes should be placed near the active electrode.

In practice interictal epileptiform activity often lacks some of the aforementioned features. Similarly, sharp transients and other non-epileptiform paroxysmal events may demonstrate some of these features (Fig. 17.1). Therefore, the correct identification of interictal epileptiform activity often depends largely on the experience and judgment of the electroencephalographer. However, the likelihood of correct interpretation increases according to the number of these criteria that are fulfilled.

Interictal and ictal activity differ in: (1) wave shape; (2) distribution; and (3) duration (Table 17.1).

(1) *The wave shape* of interictal activity consists of spikes or sharp waves which are sometimes followed by a slow wave; these discharges are usually intermittent but may repeat briefly with little or no variation of shape. In contrast, ictal activity consists of paroxysmal rhythmical waves which continue to change in shape, frequency and amplitude during the discharge. Ictal discharges often contain components other than spikes and sharp waves. The interictal activity of a patient usually consists of waveforms which differ from those of his ictal patterns. Although the shapes of interictal and ictal patterns differ between patients, most adult patients have only one or a few interictal and ictal patterns; infants and

301

TABLE 17.1
Localized epileptiform activity

Interictal epileptiform pattern	Ictal epileptiform pattern	Clinical seizure type	Underlying brain lesion
Intermittent focal spikes, sharp waves, spike-and-waves, rarely repetitive	Episodes of repetitive epileptiform activity, usually different from interictal patterns	Partial seizures	
A. *Located usually outside of temporal and fronto-temporal areas, in:* 1. Motor cortex 2. Sensory cortex 3. Insula, sylvian fissure, mesial frontal cortex 4. Cortex of more than one area	*Located usually in similar distribution as interictal patterns, but may occupy wider area*	*Simple partial seizures* ('focal seizures') 1. With motor symptoms 2. With sensory symptoms 3. With autonomic symptoms 4. Compound forms	Often history or clinical findings consistent with a recent or old local cortical lesion
	Patterns include: Fast waves of increasing amplitude and decreasing frequency; paroxysmal theta, delta or alpha activity; no EEG change;		
B. *Located usually in temporal or fronto-temporal areas*	*Located usually in similar distribution as interictal patterns but may occupy wider and bilateral areas*	*Complex partial seizures and simple partial seizures with psychic symptoms* 1. With impaired consciousness 2. With cognitive symptoms 3. With affective symptoms 4. With illusions and hallucinations 5. With automatisms ('psychomotor seizures') 6. Compound forms	Often no history or clinical evidence for a lesion
	Patterns include those in A. above; 4–6 Hz unilateral or bisynchronous waves; bilateral 14–20 Hz waves; flattening of EEG		
C. *Followed by generalized epileptiform activity* As in A. and B., occasionally followed by generalized epileptiform activity	*Ictal discharges* begin as above in A. and B., then involve the entire brain	*Partial seizures secondarily generalized* Begin as above in A. and B., followed by generalized seizure	As above in A. and B.

children show a much greater variety of patterns and often have several interictal and ictal patterns. Both interictal and ictal activity may occur in the same recording, but interictal activity is seen much more commonly.

(2) *The distribution* of interictal discharges is usually limited to one or a few electrodes over an area which is often called a 'spike focus', 'sharp wave focus' or 'epileptogenic focus'. Ictal discharges often have a wider distribution; they may start at the focus of interictal activity and gradually extend to a larger area or they may initially appear in such a larger area which includes the focus of interictal activity.

(3) *Duration.* It is important to recognize that the terms *ictal* and *interictal* epileptiform activity are electrographic descriptors, whose interpretation and clinical implications may be modified by clinical circumstances. For example, brief epileptiform activity most often occurs as an interictal phenomenon. Therefore, it is interpreted as interictal unless an associated behavioral change is observed. If an abnormal behavioral change or impairment of consciousness occurs at the time of the activity, then even if it has a brief duration and characteristic interictal appearance, it should be interpreted as an ictal event. Conversely, some discharges having a long duration and other EEG features usually associated with seizures may occur in the absence of apparent behavioral changes. If such activity occurs in individuals with abnormally impaired consciousness or those whose repetoir of behavioral responses limits behavioral testing (e.g., patients with severe encephalopathies or neonates), then the EEG pattern may be referred to as an *electrographic* or *subclinical* seizure discharge.

17.1.2 *Specific interictal patterns* consist of spikes or sharp waves (Figs. 17.4, 20.4) which may combine with slow waves to form spike-and-wave complexes or sharp-and-slow wave complexes (Figs. 17.3, 17.4). The major component of most spikes and sharp waves has negative electrical polarity and therefore causes upgoing

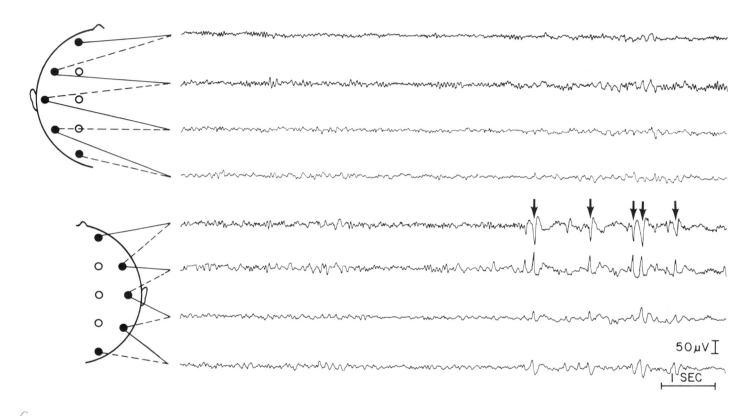

Fig. 17.1. Focal sharp waves in the right anterior temporal region (arrows). The patient is a 30-year-old man with a history of birth injury; for 15 years he has had partial seizures characterized by confusion and automatic behavior. Despite this history these wave forms recorded during wakefulness probably represent wicket spikes.

304

pen deflections in channels connected to an electrode near the focus through input 1, and downgoing pen deflections in channels connected to such an electrode through input 2 (4.1). Focal epileptiform activity is usually intermittent and rarely repeats to form polyspikes and repetitive spike-and-wave or polyspike-and-wave complexes; the repetition of these elements is often irregular in contrast to that of most generalized epileptiform activity. Some types of focal epileptiform activity which repeat periodically are described under 'special epileptiform patterns' (19.2).

The location of foci remains fixed in many adults but may vary slightly in some. More than one focus may occur in the same patient and the shape of the discharges from each focus may be different. Pairs of foci are often located in corresponding parts of the hemispheres, especially in the temporal areas; they are often called 'mirror foci'. One focus may fire only when the other one fires suggesting that it is triggered by the other, or both foci may fire independently of each other. Multiple foci which shift location from moment to moment are common in infants (18.2.3) and young children. Foci in older children are slightly more stable in location but may change location between different recordings made at fairly short intervals. Slight shifts in the location of foci are more common up to the age of adolescence than during adulthood (17.5.6).

17.1.3 *Specific ictal patterns* consist of repetitive waves which, in many instances, change configuration and, or distribution as the discharge progresses (Fig. 17.2). They often contain spikes or sharp waves mixed with slow waves and form a variety of patterns. Many ictal discharges begin with low amplitude rhythmical activity which increases in amplitude and decreases in frequency. Less often, the pattern may evolve from a slower to a faster frequency discharge. Only some ictal discharges begin with spikes of the interictal type and only rarely do ictal discharges consist of a repetition of interictal discharges. Ictal discharges end abruptly or with a few intermittent bursts and may be followed first by a generalized depression of all activity and then by slow waves in the distribution of the discharge.

305

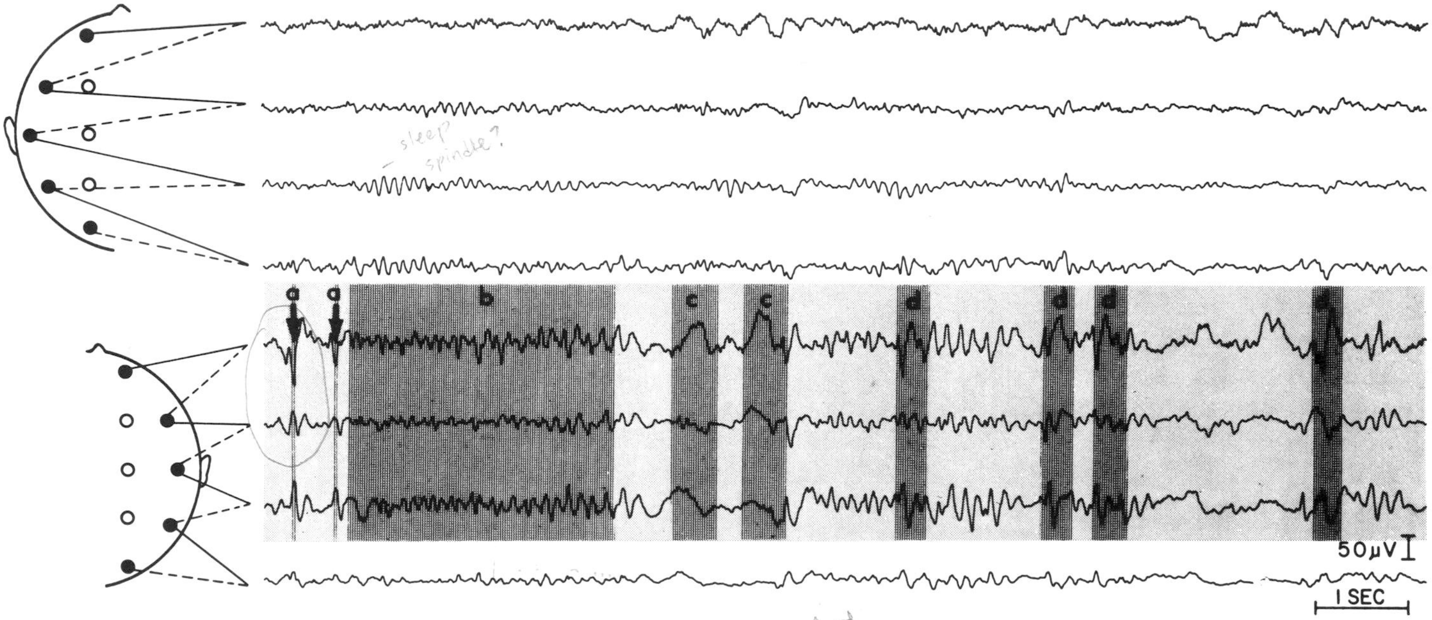

Fig. 17.2. Focal ictal discharge in the right anterior temporal region, consisting of initial intermittent spikes (a) followed by a rhythm of 10 Hz of increasing amplitude and decreasing frequency (b) which is interrupted by slow waves (c) and forms irregular spike-and-wave complexes (d). This short ictal discharge, occurring during light sleep, was not associated with any clinical manifestations. This 57-year-old man had a series of generalized convulsions three days before the EEG recording.

In routine scalp recordings in adults localized ictal discharges may occasionally ↓ be quite subtle compared to direct cortical or depth electrode recordings. Less often routine surface recordings may show no electrographic changes. In other cases the discharge may be clearly epileptiform but falsely localizing. These variations are largely due to: (1) the attenuation and dispersion of electrical activity caused by the skull and intervening tissues (particularly the dura and cerebrospinal fluid); (2) the orientation and location of the discharge in relation to the recording electrodes; and (3) the secondary activation of cortical structures at a distance from the site where the discharge actually began. Ictal events in scalp recordings may therefore only appear as varying degrees of localized background attenuation, slowing or disorganization. Such nonspecific patterns should not be considered as electrographic evidence for a possible seizure unless clearly correlated with typical ictal behavioral changes.

17.2 CLINICAL SIGNIFICANCE OF FOCAL EPILEPTIFORM ACTIVITY

17.2.1 *Association with seizures.* Many patients who show local epileptiform activity in their EEG have a history of partial or generalized seizures, and many patients with such a history show local epileptiform EEG activity. However, some patients showing epileptiform activity in their EEG never have a seizure, and many patients with a history of seizures do not show epileptiform activity in an EEG recording. This limited correlation between epileptiform activity and clinical seizures holds true especially for interictal epileptiform activity which is much more commonly recorded than ictal activity in routine EEGs; ictal activity is usually associated with clinical manifestations at the time of the recording.

Epileptiform activity in patients with seizure history. In adults, the location of the epileptiform activity usually correlates with the seizure type. This correlation is fairly good for interictal discharges and very good for ictal discharges, especially those outside the temporal and frontotemporal areas. Focal discharges in the motor area are associated with partial seizures with motor symptoms, while focal discharges in sensory and other areas outside the temporal and frontotemporal regions are associated with partial seizures with the corresponding simple symptoms (16.2). Some patients with focal epileptiform activity have seizures that appear to be clinically generalized from the start. Although these seizures are usually due to the secondary generalization of a focal discharge, only a few of these patients show transitions between focal and generalized discharges (17.3.2) in their EEG between seizures (Fig. 17.3). Patients with secondarily generalized seizures may present with a history of seizures that appear to be generalized from onset.

In a few patients, focal epileptiform discharges with or without seizure manifestations can be precipitated during the recording by activating procedures including special sensory stimuli (14.4).

Recurrent local ictal discharges are usually seen in status epilepticus but occasionally occur in patients not having clinical seizure manifestations; these patients are said to be in subclinical electrographic status epilepticus. Periodic discharges of focal epileptiform activity (19.2) or of slow waves (19.3.2) are seen in patients with epilepsia partialis continua; in some cases, the periodic discharges are interrupted by episodes of focal seizure discharges.

The EEG can be of great value in the diagnosis of seizure disorders because clinical symptoms similar to those seen during some seizures can be caused by other conditions, namely syncope, hyperventilation, transient cerebral ischemia and psychiatric disorders. The EEG can make the diagnosis of a seizure disorder likely if it reveals epileptiform activity. The likelihood that a patient's symptoms are manifestations of seizures is further increased if the location of the focal epileptiform activity corresponds with the clinical manifestations of a patient's seizures. A positive identification of clinical symptoms as seizure manifestations can be made on those rare occasions when both an ictal discharge and the clinical manifestations of a seizure occur together during an EEG recording. Conversely, if the clinical symptoms occur during an EEG recording without being associated with epileptiform activity, it is very unlikely that they are due to a convulsive disorder. Individuals with simple partial seizures occasionally do not demonstrate epileptiform activity or other definite EEG changes during the seizure (Table 16.1).

Epileptiform activity in persons without seizure history. Focal interictal epileptiform activity similar to that seen in patients with epilepsy may rarely be found in the EEGs of individuals who have no history of seizures (less than 2%). In general, this is more likely if the epileptiform activity is localized to the parietal or occipital head regions than the anterior temporal, frontal or central head regions. Indeed, visual system defects are frequently associated with the development of occipital spikes in children who never develop seizures. In some cases interictal epileptiform activity may arise from epileptogenic lesions which have remained below a threshold for the production of clinical seizures. In neonates and infants in particular, focal epileptiform activity is the expression of a great variety of pathological conditions which do not produce seizures. It is possible that this abnormal EEG activity represents epileptogenic lesions which have remained below a threshold for the production of clinical seizures. In infants and children in particular, focal epileptiform acitivity is the expression of a great variety of pathological conditions which do not produce seizures.

Patients with a history of seizures but without epileptiform EEG activity. Recordings between seizures may contain no epileptiform activity in approximately 20–40% of patients with a history of seizures even if the recordings include the activation procedures of hyperventilation, photic stimulation and sleep. Both longer recording periods and repeated sampling increase the likelihood of recording epileptiform activity. In separate studies it has been shown that approximately 50–60% of patients who will show interictal epileptiform do so on the first recording. Each subsequent recording yields approximately half as many new patients

309

*30%

with interictal epileptiform activity as the previous one. Thus, there is usually little to be gained by performing additional routine recordings if 3 separate recordings with sleep, wakefulness, hyperventilation and photic stimulation have failed to show epileptiform changes. The likelihood of recording epileptiform activity does not directly depend on anticonvulsant medication (except in the case of ethosuximide and typical generalized 3 Hz spike and wave activity) although it may decrease as anticonvulsants reduce the frequency of seizures. The incidence of interictal epileptiform activity varies little with the type of underlying lesion except that metastatic brain tumors are less likely to produce epileptiform activity between seizures than are other lesions producing seizures of similar frequency. Interictal focal epileptiform activity may fail to appear in the scalp EEG if the focus is small, is located deeply in the brain, or has an unusual spatial orientation with respect to the recording electrodes.

17.2.2 *Underlying cerebral abnormalities. Adults and adolescents* develop focal epileptiform activity often as the result of acute or chronic damage to a circumscribed area of the cerebral cortex. *Acute* damage causes epileptiform activity which usually lasts only for a few days. *Chronic* epileptogenic lesions either are stationary, for instance scars resulting from head injuries or strokes, or are gradually progressive, as in cases of slowly growing tumors. In stationary lesions, epileptiform activity may not develop until after a period of several months or years, even in patients who have briefly shown epileptiform activity during the few days after an acute cerebral injury. Lesions in the temporal and frontal lobes are more likely than lesions in the parietal and occipital cortical areas to produce epileptogenic foci. In some patients with chronic recurrent epileptiform activity, no historical, clinical or laboratory evidence for a lesion can be found. It is, however, reasonable to assume that in such cases microanatomical lesions are present.

Infants and children react with focal discharges to acute damage which is often more widespread than that which produces focal epileptiform discharges in adults. The widespread involvement of the brain is probably one reason why focal discharges in children may shift from moment to moment and do not reliably indicate a focus of circumscribed damage. Although foci do not shift so rapidly after infancy, the fact that they change location gradually and that many of them disappear before puberty would indicate that focal epileptiform activity at an early age often does not have the same significance in indicating an underlying lesion as it does in adults.

17.3 OTHER EEG ABNORMALITIES ASSOCIATED WITH FOCAL EPILEPTIFORM ACTIVITY

17.3.1 *Focal sharp transients,* which have less distinct and more variable shapes than do spikes and sharp waves (9.1), may be seen in recordings which also contain focal spikes and sharp waves in the same distribution. However, sharp transients unassociated with spikes and sharp waves, although suggesting some local hyperexcitability, are not a definite indicator of an established epileptogenic focus.

17.3.2 *Generalized interictal epileptiform activity*, i.e., epileptiform activity which by routine visual inspection appears simultaneously on both sides, is sometimes produced by a focal epileptogenic lesion. This may occur by a process referred to as *secondary bilateral synchrony* in which an epileptic focus is thought to trigger a central pacemaker which in turn produces a bilaterally synchronous epileptiform pattern (18.4.1). In such cases the interictal and ictal epileptiform patterns may be generalized all or most of the time. Since *primary* and *secondary bilateral synchrony* have quite different clinical implications, it is important for the electroencephalographer to be familiar with those features that are sometimes helpful in distinguishing one from the other.

311

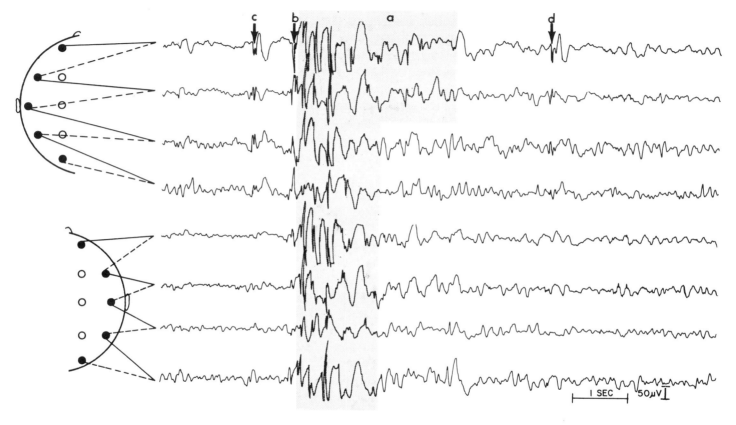

Fig. 17.3. Generalized spike-and-wave discharges (a) preceded by focal left temporal spike discharge (b). Focal left temporal spikes also appear before (c) and after (d) the generalized discharge. This 22-year-old man was hit on the head with a garbage can and passed out briefly five months before the recording; he began to have attacks of being dazed for 10–15 seconds 6 weeks before the recording and had a generalized seizure on the day of the recording.

The interictal discharges due to secondary bilateral synchrony are distinguished by the following features: (1) they are most often less than 3 Hz when rhythmic; (2) they may demonstrate considerable morphological variability from complex to complex; (3) they usually contain a single site of phase reversal in transverse bipolar montages; (4) they may be consistently asymmetrical; and (5) consistently focal epileptiform spikes or sharp waves may be present (Fig. 17.3). Other EEG findings that suggest the presence of secondary bilateral synchrony are those typically associated with cerebral lesions, particularly focal slowing or focal background attenuation. In contrast, the discharges of primary bilateral synchrony are most often rhythmical with a repetition rate of 2.5 Hz or greater, show approximately the same morphology with each occurrence, often have more than one phase reversal in transverse bipolar montages, and are usually symmetrical. In general, when it is difficult to distinguish between primary and secondary bilateral synchrony, a prolonged recording often provides additional distinguishing features.

17.3.3 *Unilateral epileptiform activity* may develop gradually or suddenly from focal interictal and ictal epileptiform activity. This unilateral form of generalization occurs practically only in infants and young children and is one of the EEG correlates of unilateral seizures.

17.3.4 *Local slow waves* may be the result of epileptogenic cerebral damage (Fig. 20.4) or of focal epileptiform activity itself.

17.3.5 *Local reduction of amplitude* of the background in the area of the focal discharge has similar connotations as do focal slow waves except that postictal depression of amplitude usually persists for only a few seconds or minutes after the end of the ictal discharge.

313

17.3.6 *Generalized asynchronous and bisynchronous slow waves* may be due either to a recent secondarily generalized seizure, to a condition giving rise to both epileptiform and slow wave activity, or to unrelated causes.

17.4 MECHANISMS UNDERLYING FOCAL EPILEPTIFORM ACTIVITY

17.4.1 *Interictal focal epileptiform discharges* are the reflection of synchronized and abnormally intense fluctuations of membrane potentials of neurons in the epileptogenic focus. Microelectrode recordings from neurons within a focus suggest (a) that the abnormal synchronization is accomplished by a small group of neurons ('epileptic neurons' or 'epileptic neuronal aggregate') which send intermittent bursts of action potentials to many neurons in the focus, and (b) that the abnormally intense membrane fluctuation consists of a powerful paroxysmal depolarizing shift (which is probably triggered by an excitatory input) followed by a transient hyperpolarization.

17.4.2 *Ictal focal epileptiform discharges* occur when, for reasons not yet understood, the hyperpolarization following each paroxysmal depolarizing shift weakens and is overwhelmed by depolarization. This leads to repetitive depolarizations manifested by rhythmical membrane fluctuations of neurons in the focus and by rhythmical ictal patterns in the EEG. Subcortical structures connected to the cortical focus may become involved in the seizure activity and probably serve to sustain it. Failure of surrounding inhibition can lead to the spread of focal ictal discharges to adjacent parts of the cortex.

17.4.3 *Acute focal epileptiform activity* is produced by various kinds of cerebral lesions. It can be explained by several mechanisms all of which reduce the level of the neuronal membrane potential and thereby increase the tendency of the neuron to

314

depolarize and to fire repetitively. Some of these mechanisms are: Mechanical deformation of neuronal membrane, changes of membrane permeability resulting in abnormal ion exchanges; changes of ion concentrations, especially increase of potassium and decrease of calcium in the extracellular space; ischemia, hypoxia and toxic products paralyzing the cellular metabolism needed to maintain the neuronal membrane potential.

17.4.4 *Chronic focal epileptiform activity* in adults is usually due to lasting structural change. Because spikes and ictal discharges in a chronic focus usually do not vary much in shape, it can be assumed that the sequence of the underlying neuronal events in the established focus is very stereotyped, i.e. that the epileptiform neuronal aggregate is rigidly organized. The long delay of several months or years between cerebral damage and the establishment of a discharging focus suggests that extensive reorganization of local circuitry takes place during this period. Pathological studies of foci usually show scars of astrocytic gliosis at the site of the chronic epileptogenic focus. However, anatomical, histological, biochemical and other techniques have not so far been able to distinguish between lesions which produce epileptiform activity and those which do not.

The mechanisms immediately responsible for the production of epileptiform activity in the chronic focus include those listed for the acute focus. In addition, several other mechanisms have been considered important in the case of chronic focal activity. Partial deafferentation of cortical neurons may lead to altered sensitivity to synaptic transmitters. Reorganiztion of synaptic connections and collateral sprouting of axon terminals after injury may lead to increased excitation or decreased inhibition of neurons in the focus. Chronic foci unassociated with gross structural abnormalities may result from excessive afferent stimulation, for instance by repeated abnormal input from distant epileptogenic zones (17.1.2). The secondarily activated area is then referred to as a *secondary focus*. A contralateral homotopic secondary focus is referred to as a *mirror focus*. Currently, in humans there is only limited evidence to suggest that a secondary focus can actually generate seizures and sustain itself in the absence of a primary focus. That abnormal input alone can generate such a focus is suggested by the experimental phenomenon of *kindling* in animals: Periodic electrical stimulation that is too low in intensity to actually trigger a seizure will eventually produce epileptiform activity and clinical seizures if applied repeatedly to certain susceptible parts of the brain (e.g., the amygdaloid nucleus). If the intermittent application of this initially subthreshold stimulus is continued, then ultimately seizures will occur spontaneously in the absence of electrical stimulation. However, the more phylogenetically advanced the animal is, the more difficult it is to produce the kindling phenomenon. For this reason, and because it has not been unequivocally demonstrated in humans, the relevance of kindling to human epilepsy remains unclear.

17.5 SPECIFIC DISORDERS CAUSING FOCAL EPILEPTIFORM ACTIVITY

17.5.1 *Degenerative, developmental and demyelinating diseases*:

(1) *Senile and presenile dementia (Alzheimer's disease)* in some patients leads to sharp transients in the same distribution as the intermittent left temporal slow waves characteristically seen in normal older persons. The sharp transients often form complexes with the slow waves. These patients generally do not have seizures.

(2) *Jakob-Creutzfeldt disease* is associated with periodic sharp wave complexes in many cases (Fig. 19.10). The sharp waves may be localized to one part of the brain for several days before they become generalized. They are usually associated with myoclonic twitching.

(3) *Tuberous sclerosis* often presents with single or multiple spike foci in addition to single or multiple slow wave foci and generalized asynchronous slow waves,

316

especially in children and adults with mental deficiency and epilepsy. Infants with tuberous sclerosis often show hypsarrhythmia (19.2.1) or multifocal independent spikes (19.2.3).

(4) *Sturge-Weber syndrome* is associated with epileptiform activity in about one-half of all cases. Local reductions of amplitude are very common. The epileptiform discharges may arise from one focus, from several foci near the involved area, or from the entire area. They may secondarily generalize or be generalized from the start.

(5) *Porencephaly, microgyria, pachygyria, agyria, holoprosencephaly and hydrocephaly of various causes* all can cause focal spikes although they more characteristically cause focal slow waves.

(6) *Bilateral optic neuritis* in children, if causing significant visual loss, may lead to occipital spikes unassociated with seizures (19.4.6).

17.5.2 *Metabolic and toxic encephalopathies*:

(1) *Acute metabolic encephalopathies* such as those produced by hypoglycemia, hypoxia, hyperosmolar nonketotic hyperglycemia, hypoparathyroidism and acute porphyria are most commonly characterized by generalized bisynchronous (22.6.2) and asynchronous (21.6.2) slow waves. Generalized epileptiform activity is common while focal spikes or sharp waves are less common and may be due to the activation of a chronic abnormality caused by earlier damage.

(2) *Cerebral lipidoses* may produce focal spikes, usually of the multifocal type (19.1). The late infantile form of ceroid lipofuscinosis (also referred to as the Beilschowsky–Jansky form) is specifically associated with excessively high amplitude occipital spikes that occur in a time locked fashion in response to slow rates of photic stimulation.

17.5.3 *Cerebrovascular diseases*:

(1) *Acute strokes* due to arterial thrombosis, embolism, intracerebral hemorrhage

317

and subarachnoid hemorrhage extending into the brain may cause focal epileptiform discharges, usually associated with focal slow waves, generalized slow waves and amplitude asymmetries indicating recent structural damage. The focal epileptiform discharges are of the interictal and ictal types. Interictal epileptiform activity in the first week following ischemic stroke correlates highly with the occurrence of seizures. The predictive value of such activity for the occurrence of late seizures, months or years after the stroke, is uncertain. Periodic lateralizing epileptiform discharges (19.3.1) occur acutely in 1–2% of individuals with non-hemorrhagic strokes involving cortical structures. Single or repetitive partial seizures, status epilepticus and epilepsia partialis continua may occur at the time of the acute damage.

(2) *Basilar artery migraine* has been noted to occur in association with posterior epileptiform activity or slow waves during or even between attacks.

(3) *Old strokes* can lead to the production of chronic epileptogenic foci several months or years after the acute event. This development is slightly more likely in patients who showed focal epileptiform activity at the time of the acute event. The background of the EEG and the clinical condition of the patient may show little or no residual evidence of the stroke when the chronic focus appears.

(4) *Chronic subdural hematoma* rarely causes focal epileptiform activity in the area of focal slow waves or amplitude reduction; such activity and partial seizures may, however, develop after surgical evacuation of the hematoma.

17.5.4 *Cerebral trauma*:

(1) *'Traumatic seizures' or 'early posttraumatic seizures'* may occur during the first 1 or 2 weeks after head injuries of sufficient strength to produce cortical damage. The EEG may show focal spikes and sharp waves which are practically always associated with other EEG abnormalities. Similar abnormalities may occur after brain surgery. In children, early posttraumatic epileptiform activity is more

common, more dramatic and more persistent than in adults; multiple shifting or stationary foci (19.1) are a common indicator of cerebral damage in infants and young children.

(2) *'Posttraumatic epilepsy' or 'late traumatic epilepsy'* may develop several months or years after severe head injuries, especially after injuries which penetrate into the brain. Spike foci develop not only in patients with this form of epilepsy but also in some patients with similar head injuries which do not lead to posttraumatic epilepsy. Focal epileptiform EEG discharges and epilepsy may also develop after brain surgery, especially after operations associated with major cortical damage; however, both abnormalities may occur after operations producing only minor cortical damage, for instance the insertion of a ventricular shunt or of stereotaxic probes, although they occur more often after major cortical damage. Skull defects may enhance the local sharp activity (23.4.2).

Posttraumatic, postoperative and other spike foci may require surgical excision if they generate a disabling seizure disorder which cannot be controlled medically. Before surgery, activation with convulsant drugs (14.5) and special recording methods are often used to evaluate the role of a focus in the production of seizures. During surgery, recordings from electrodes on the cortical surface can guide the excision of spike foci.

17.5.5. *Brain tumors.* *Supratentorial tumors* are most likely to produce a focus of epileptiform activity if they grow slowly and near the cortex. Spike foci are therefore most common in oligodendrogliomas and angiomas, fairly common in astrocytomas and meningiomas, and least common in the faster growing glioblastomas and metastases. Spike foci due to tumors are not always associated with clinical seizures; the association also depends on the type of tumor. While seizures are most common in oligodendrogliomas and angiomas, they are also fairly common in meningiomas and metastases and least common in astrocytomas and glioblastomas.

319

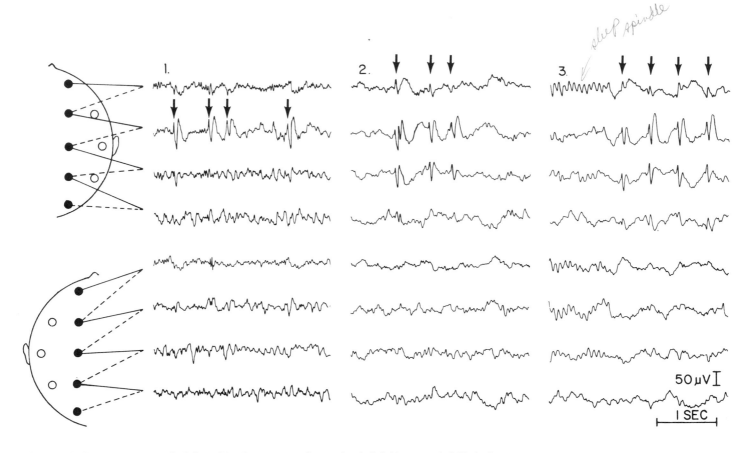

sleep spindle

Fig. 17.4. Spikes (arrows), usually followed by slow waves and repeating in brief bursts at 1–2 Hz in the right fronto-central regions ('Rolandic spikes'). 1. Awake: Spikes limited to the area between frontal and central electrode; 2. Light sleep: Slightly wider distribution and occasional polyphasic spikes; 3. Deeper sleep: Widest distribution. This 6-year-old girl had her first seizure a few hours before the EEG recording. The seizure began in the left side of the face and then generalized. History, clinical examination and other test results were normal.

Although epileptiform activity caused by tumors is usually localized to the site of the tumor, it may also appear in a bilaterally symmetric and synchronous or asynchronous fashion, or at a distance from the tumor. Thus, spike foci caused by tumors, even when unilateral, do not have the same localizing value as continuous focal slowing or localized background attenuation.

17.5.6. *Focal epileptiform activity in seizure disorders without known underlying diseases and in normal persons:*

(1) *Benign childhood epilepsy with centro-temporal spikes*, also referred to as 'Rolandic epilepsy' is a fairly distinct and common convulsive disorder of childhood with onset between 2 and 12 years of age. It is benign in the majority of cases in that it typically disappears between the ages of 15 and 18 years. The history, clinical findings and laboratory tests give no evidence of a local brain lesion in spite of the clearly focal origin of the epileptiform activity and seizures. The EEG contains spikes which frequently have a characteristic morphology and are often followed by slow waves. The spikes are sometimes grouped together in short runs with a repetition rate of 1.5–3 Hz (Fig. 17.4). They are located predominantly in the central or temporal areas and may demonstrate a slightly shifting distribution. They may also occur unilaterally (in approximately 70% of patients with a single recording) or bilaterally with varying degrees of interhemispheric synchrony. The individual spikes sometimes have the field distribution of horizontal dipoles (also referred to as parallel generators) with a single spike showing a phase reversal in ear reference recordings and more than one phase reversal in longitudinal bipolar recordings. Drowsiness and light sleep activate the discharges, although occasionally they are abundant during wakefulness. Apart from the background disturbance related to the epileptiform activity, the EEG is normal. Children with rolandic spikes most often have simple partial seizures with motor symptoms. The motor activity may be tonic or clonic, limited to one side of the face, and associated with speech arrest or

pharyngeal manifestations. Because the seizures typically occur at night they may go unnoticed. It is important to recognize, however, that only 50–70% of children with typical centro-temporal spikes actually have seizures. The seizure disorder, as well as the electrographic findings, are inherited in an autosomal dominant pattern with incomplete and age dependent penetrance.

(2) *Childhood epilepsy with occipital paroxysms* is a more recently described syndrome of idiopathic epilepsy in which seizures begin in childhood and usually cease by adulthood. The seizures typically begin with visual symptoms and may be followed by a postictal migrainous headache. The interictal EEG shows prominent occipital spikes or sharp waves that may occur in a semi-rhythmic pattern at 1–3 Hz. The discharges attenuate or disappear with eye opening and are not activated by photic stimulation. EEG background activity is usually normal. Onset between ages 2 and 8 and predominantly nocturnal seizures with deviation of the eyes and vomiting are thought to be favorable prognostic features.

Several factors combine to make this syndrome less well defined than the more common syndrome of Rolandic epilepsy: (1) the prognosis is more variable, (2) a similar EEG pattern may be seen in individuals with underlying structural abnormalities, (3) headaches may precede or follow a variety of seizure types, and (4) there may be some overlap with Rolandic epilepsy since it has been reported that some children with rolandic spikes may initially have epileptiform activity localized to the occipital head regions. For these reasons, further observations are needed to better define this constellation of electrographic and clinical findings as a distinct epileptic syndrome.

(3) *Landau–Kleffner syndrome of acquired epileptic aphasia* is a rare disorder that usually occurs in children and is characterized by seizures and a progressive disturbance of language function. The language disturbance may initially be limited to difficulty with comprehension and then progress to include speech. The seizures may precede or follow the onset of the language disturbance. Interictal epileptiform

322

+ benign occipital epilepsy of childhood (?)

activity typically consists of moderate to high amplitude spikes or spike-and-wave complexes that are localized to the temporal head regions. The discharges may be strictly unilateral, but more often show either shifting lateralization or appear in a bilaterally independent fashion. They often become more abundant with the onset of sleep. Epileptic seizures in some cases are benign in that they are easily controlled with anticonvulsant medication and do not persist throughout life. A number of cases have also been described in which only epileptiform activity and language dysfunction are present without any evidence of clinical seizures. Although mild gliotic cortical changes have been described the etiology is unknown. Because this disorder is so rare and there are few reports of long term follow-up, the prognosis is also uncertain.

(4) *Normal individuals* may show certain EEG patterns which resemble epileptiform activity but have no clearly proven pathological significance. These so-called pseudoepileptiform patterns must therefore be distinguished from true epileptiform activity (19.5).

17.5.7. *Infectious diseases:*

(1) *Meningitis and encephalitis* produce focal spikes only rarely in adults. Because infants are likely to react to widespread cerebral damage with focal spikes, such spikes may be seen in neonatal meningitis, syphilis and cytomegalic inclusion body disease; they may be associated with partial, unilateral or generalized seizures.

(2) *Cerebral abscesses* rarely produce interictal or ictal focal epileptiform abnormalities in adults.

(3) *Thrombophlebitis* of the cerebral venous sinus systems can produce focal or unilateral spikes in addition to decreased amplitude and slow waves. Septic phlebitis of the lateral or cavernous sinus may lead to the syndrome of hemiconvulsions, hemiplegia and epilepsy (HHE syndrome) in children. The acute phase of this syndrome is characterized by long-lasting and repetitive seizures of unilateral onset;

this phase may be followed by epilepsy with partial complex seizures at a later age.

(4) *Herpes simplex encephalitis* often leads to periodic sharp waves in the temporal regions (19.3.1).

(5) *Subacute sclerosing panencephalitis* is usually associated with periodic sharp wave complexes which may begin locally (19.3.3).

17.5.8 *Psychiatric diseases. Behavior disorders and episodic psychotic or psychopathic behavior in children* have been found in association with focal spikes, especially in the temporal lobes, in many patients with these disorders. However, because the relationship between spike foci and the psychiatric abnormalities is unclear, focal cerebral lesions must be searched for in these patients.

REFERENCES

Aicardi, J. and Newton, R. (1987) Clinical findings in children with occipital spike wave complexes suppressed by eye opening. In: Andermann, F. and Lugaresi, E. (Eds.), Migraine and Epilepsy, Butterworth, Boston, pp. 111–124.

Ajmone Marsan, C. and Zivin, L.S. (1970) Factors related to the occurrence of typical paroxysmal abnormalities in the EEG records of epileptic patients. Epilepsia 11: 361–381.

Beaussart, M. (1972) Benign epilepsy of children with Rolandic (centro-temporal) paroxysmal foci. A clinical entity. Study of 221 cases. Epilepsia 13: 795–811.

Binnie, C.D., Batchelor, B.G., Gainsborough, A.J., Lloyd, D.S.L., Smith, D.M. and Smith, G.F. (1979) Visual and computer-assisted assessment of the EEG in epilepsy of late onset. Electroenceph. clin. Neurophysiol. 47: 102–107.

Binnie, C.D. (1987) Electroencephalography and epilepsy. In: Hopkins, A. (Ed.), Epilepsy, Demos, New York, pp. 169–200.

Cole, A.J., Andermann, F., Taylor, L., Olivier, A., Rasmussen, T., Robitaille, Y. and Spire, J.-P. (1988) The Landau–Kleffner syndrome of acquired epileptic aphasia: Unusual clinical outcome, surgical experience, and absence of encephalitis. Neurology 38: 31–38.

Cole, A.J., Gloor, P. and Kaplan, R. (1987) Transient global amnesia: The electroencephalogram at onset. Ann. Neurol. 22: 771–772.

Fisch, B.J., Rosenstein, R., Ramirez-Lassepas, M. and Hauser, W.A. (1986) The electroencephalogram as a predictor of epilepsy following occlusive cerebrovascular insult. Epilepsia 27: 615.

Gastaut, H., Poirier, F., Payan, H., Salamon, G., Toga, M. and Vigouroux, M. (1960) H.H.E. syndrome: Hemiconvulsions, hemiplegia, epilepsy. Epilepsia 1: 418–447.

Gastaut, H. and Zifkin, B.G. (1987) Benign epilepsy of childhood with occipital spike and wave complexes. In: Andermann, F. and Lugaresi, E. (Eds.), Migraine and Epilepsy, Butterworth, Boston, pp. 47–82.

Geier, S., Bancaud, J., Talairach, J., Bonis, A., Szikla, G. and Enjelvin, M. (1977) The seizures of frontal lobe epilepsy. A study of clinical manifestations. Neurology 27: 951–958.

Geiger, L.R. and Harner, R.N. (1978) EEG patterns at the time of focal seizure onset. Arch. Neurol. 35: 276–286.

Gotman, J. and Marciani, M.G. (1985) Electroencephalographic spiking activity, drug levels, and seizure occurrence in epileptic patients. Ann. Neurol. 17: 597–603.

Hughes, J.R. and Zak, S.M. (1987) EEG and clinical changes in patients with chronic seizures associated with slowly growing brain tumors. Arch. Neurol. 44: 540–543.

Hughes, J.R. (1989) The significance of the interictal spike discharge: A review. J. clin. Neurophysiol. 6: 207–226.

Jennett, B. (1975) Epilepsy After Non-Missile Head Injuries. 2nd Ed., William Heinemann Medical Books, Chicago.

Jensen, I. and Klinken, L. (1976) Temporal lobe epilepsy and neuropathology. Acta Neurol. Scand. 54: 391–414.

Kellaway, P. (1981) The incidence, significance and natural history of spike foci in children. In: Henry, C.E. (Ed.), Current Clinical Neurophysiology, Elsevier, Amsterdam, pp. 151–175.

King, D.W. and Ajmone Marsan, C. (1977) Clinical features and ictal patterns in epileptic patients with EEG temporal lobe foci. Ann. Neurol. 2: 138–147.

Klass, D.W. (1975) Electroencephalographic manifestations of complex partial seizures. In: Penry, J.K. and Daly, D.D. (Eds.), Advances in Neurology, Vol. 11, Raven, New York, pp. 113–140.

Kuzniecky, R. and Rosenblatt, B. (1987) Benign occipital epilepsy: A family study. Epilepsia 28: 346–350.

Lerman, P. and Kivity, S. (1975) Benign focal epilepsy of childhood. Arch. Neurol. 32: 261–264.

Loiseau, P., Duche, B., Cordova, S., Dartigues, J.F. and Cohadon, S. (1988) Prognosis of benign childhood epilepsy with centrotemporal spikes: A follow-up study of 168 patients. Epilepsia 29: 229–235.

Loiseau, P. and Duche, B. (1989) Benign childhood epilepsy with centromidtemporal spikes. Cleveland Clin. J. Med. 56 (Suppl. 1): S17–22.

Luders, H., Lesser, R.P., Dinner, D.S. and Morris, H.H. (1987) Benign focal epilepsy of childhood. In: Luders, H. and Lesser, R.P. (Eds.), Epilepsy: Electroclinical Syndromes, Springer, New York, pp. 279–302.

Ludwig, B.I. and Ajmone Marsan, C. (1975) Clinical ictal patterns in epileptic patients with occipital electroencephalographic foci. Neurology 25: 463–471.

Ludwig, B.I., Ajmone Marsan, C. and Van Buren, J. (1976) Depth and direct cortical recording in seizure disorders of extratemporal origin. Neurology 26: 1085–1099.

Markand, O.N., Wheeler, G.L. and Pollack, S.L. (1978) Complex partial status epilepticus (psychomotor status). Neurology 28: 189–196.

McLachlan, R.S. and Girvin, J.P. (1989) Electroencephalographic features of midline spikes in the cat penicillin focus and in human epilepsy. Electroenceph. clin. Neurophysiol. 72: 140–146.

Michel, B., Gastaut, J.L. and Bianchi, L. (1979) Electroencephalographic cranial computerized tomographic correlates in brain abscess. Electroenceph. clin. Neurophysiol. 46: 256–273.

Miller, J.W., Yanagihara, T., Peterwen, R.C. and Klass, D.W. (1987) Transient global amnesia and epilepsy. Arch. Neurology 44: 629–633.

Niedermeyer, E. (1987) Epileptic seizure disorders. In: Niedermeyer, E. and Lopes da Silva, F. (Eds.), Electroencephalography: Basic Principles, Clinical Applications and Related Fields, Urban and Schwarzenberg, Baltimore, pp. 405–510.

Pampiglione, G. and Harden, A. (1977) So-called neuronal ceroid lipofuscinosis. Neurophysiological studies in 60 children. J. Neurol. Neurosurg. Psychiatr. 40: 323–330.

Panayiotopoulos, C.P. (1989) Benign childhood epilepsy with occipital paroxysms: A 15-year prospective study. Ann. Neurol. 26: 51–56.

Pedley, T.A., Tharp, B.R. and Herman, K. (1981) Clinical and electroencephalographic characteristics of midline parasagittal foci. Ann. Neurol. 9: 142–149.

Pedley, T.A. (1987) Epilepsy. In: Halliday, A.M., Butler, S.R. and Paul, R. (Eds.), A Textbook of Clinical Neurophysiology, Wiley, Chichester, pp. 231–267.

Quesney, L.F. (1986) Seizures of frontal lobe origin. In: Pedley, T.A. and Meldrum, B.S. (Eds.), Recent Advances in Epilepsy, Churchill/Livingstone, London, pp. 81–110.

Robertson, R., Langill, L., Wong, P.K.H. and Ho, H.H. (1988) Rett syndrome: EEG presentation. Electroenceph. clin. Neurophysiol. 70: 388–395.

Salinsky, M., Kanter, R. and Dasheiff, R.M. (1987) Effectiveness of multiple EEGs in supporting the diagnosis of epilepsy: An operational curve. Epilepsia 28: 331–334.

Sammaritano, M., De Lothiniere, A., Andermann, F., Olivier, A., Gloor, P. and Quesney, L.F. (1987) False lateralization by surface EEG of seizure onset in patients with temporal lobe epilepsy and gross focal cerebral lesions. Ann. Neurol. 21: 361–369.

Sawhney, I.M.S., Suresh, N., Dhand, U.K. and Chopra, J.S. (1988) Acquired aphasia with epilepsy – Landa–Kleffner syndrome. Epilepsia 29: 283–287.

Schwartzkroin, P.A. and Wyler, A.R. (1980) Mechanisms underlying epileptiform burst discharge. Ann. Neurol. 7: 95–107.

Sharbrough, F.W. (1987) Complex partial seizures. In: Luders, H. and Lesser, R.P. (Eds.), Epilepsy: Electroclinical Syndromes, Springer, New York, pp. 279–302.

Swanson, J.W. and Vick, N.A. (1978) Basilar artery migraine. Neurology 28: 782–786.

Shewmon, D.A. and Erwin, R.J. (1988) The effect of focal interictal spikes on perception and reaction time. I. General considerations. Electroenceph. clin. Neurophysiol. 69: 319–337.

Shewmon, D.A. and Erwin, R.J. (1988) The effect of focal interictal spikes on perception and reaction time. II. Neuroanatomic specificity. Electroenceph. clin. Neurophysiol. 69: 338–352.

Spencer, S.S., Williamson, P.D., Bridgers, S.L., Mattson, R.H., Cicchetti, D.V. and Spencer, D.D. (1985) Reliability and accuracy of localization by scalp ictal EEG. Neurology 35: 1567–1575.

Swanson, J.W. and Vick, N.A. (1978) Basilar artery migraine. Neurology 28: 782–786.

Theodore, W.H., Sato, S. and Porter, R.J. (1984) Serial EEG in intractable epilepsy. Neurology 34: 863–867.

Thomas, J.E., Reagan, T.J. and Klass, D.W. (1977) Epilepsia partialis continua: A review of 32 cases. Arch. Neurol. 34: 266–275.

Trojaborg, W. (1968) Changes of spike foci in children. In: Kellaway, P. and Petersén, I. (Eds.), Clinical Electroencephalography of Children. Stockholm, Almqvist and Wiksell, pp. 213–225.

Westmoreland, B.F. and Sharbrough, F.W. (1978) The EEG in cerebromacular degeneration. Electroenceph. clin. Neurophysiol. 45: 28P–29P.

Westmoreland, B.F. (1985) The electroencephalogram in patients with epilepsy. In: Aminoff, M.J. (Ed.), Electrodiagnosis, Neurologic Clinics, W.B. Saunders, Philadelphia, pp. 599–614.

Zivin, L. and Ajmone-Marsan, C. (1968) Incidence and prognostic significance of 'epileptiform' activity in the EEG of non-epileptic subjects. Brain 91: 751–778.

Generalized epileptiform patterns

18

SUMMARY

(18.1)   *The patterns* of generalized epileptiform activity (Table 18.1) differ from those of focal epileptiform activity in that they appear over most or all parts of both hemispheres and usually have similar shape, amplitude and timing in corresponding areas. Generalized discharges resemble focal ones in that they consist of sharp waves, spikes, polyspikes and their combinations with slow waves. Generalized interictal discharges, more commonly than local interictal discharges, consist of brief repetitive discharges, often of spike-and-wave complexes, at regular intervals. Generalized ictal patterns consist either of longer repetitions of interictal patterns, or of patterns containing different, progressively changing elements. *(as in focal seizures)*

(18.2.1)   *Clinical correlates* of generalized epileptiform activity (Table 18.1) are generalized seizures. There is some correspondence between the type of seizure and the type of ictal discharge. Like patients with partial seizures and focal epileptiform discharges, many patients with a history of generalized seizures have normal EEGs whereas others have generalized epileptiform activity in their EEG without having had any seizures.

(18.2.2)   *Causes* of generalized epileptiform activity cannot be found in a large portion of patients, especially those who have symmetrical and synchronous epileptiform activity and no other EEG and clinical abnormalities; such patients are said to have idiopathic epilepsy. Other patients have epilepsy as a manifestation of widespread, lasting cerebral diseases which cause other clinical and EEG abnormalities as well. Another group of patients, not usually said to have epilepsy, have generalized epileptiform discharges, with or without generalized seizures, as a result of transient cerebral diseases or as the result of toxic, metabolic or other primary extracerebral disorders.

(18.3)   *Other EEG abnormalities* do not usually occur in patients with idiopathic epilepsy. The appearance of other EEG abnormalities may therefore indicate underlying cerebral or extracerebral pathology.

(18.4)   *Mechanisms* producing generalized interictal epileptiform discharges currently include *corticoreticular activation* for primarily generalized seizures and *secondary generalization* and *secondary bilateral synchrony* for partial or secondarily generalized seizures. An increased familial incidence of epilepsy in patients with primarily generalized seizures and no evidence of other cerebral or systemic abnormalities suggests a hereditary predisposition. The widespread and bilaterally synchronous appearance of epileptiform activity may be secondary to the interaction of a central, subcortical pacemaker with a diffusely and abnormally reactive cortex (the corticoreticular theory of primarily generalized seizures) or result from an extremely rapid spread of epileptiform activity via interhemispheric pathways from a focal epileptogenic cortical zone.

(18.5) *Specific disorders* causing generalized epileptiform activity include degenerative, metabolic, toxic, vascular and inflammatory disorders which involve large areas of the brain.

18.1 DESCRIPTION OF PATTERNS

18.1.1 *Generalized epileptiform activity* differs from focal epileptiform activity mainly in distribution and slightly in configuration. It appears over corresponding parts of both hemispheres or the entire head. The waveforms usually have similar configuration, symmetrical amplitude, simultaneous onset and synchronous timing in corresponding parts of the two hemispheres, but may differ slightly in different parts of the same hemisphere. In many patients, the epileptiform discharges at some times have a higher amplitude or are apparent only in one area of the brain, but discharges with local predominance are usually transient and may be followed by discharges having greater prominence in other areas. In other patients, generalized discharges begin consistently in the same area and often have higher amplitude and greater persistence in that area. These generalized discharges with focal emphasis suggest a focal origin of the generalized discharges, but this remains unproven unless focal discharges either consistently precede the generalized discharges or appear independent of the generalized discharges.

Like localized epileptiform activity, generalized discharges usually contain spikes and sharp waves, often in combination with slow waves, and can be divided into interictal activity lasting less than a few seconds and ictal activity which lasts longer (Table 18.1). Generalized interictal discharges, in contrast to localized interictal discharges, often consist of spike-and-wave and other complexes which repeat at regular rates. Generalized ictal discharges, more often than focal ictal discharges, consist of long repetitions of interictal patterns. The shape of generalized ictal

330

Table 18.1
Generalized epileptiform activity

Interictal epileptiform pattern	Ictal epileptiform pattern	Clinical seizure type	Underlying brain lesion
Usually complexes of spike-and-waves or polyspike-and-waves, often repetitive; rarely single spikes and sharp waves	Episodes of prolonged activity of interictal type or of progressively changing activity	Generalized seizures	Unknown ('idiopathic') or widespread structural or metabolic diseases
1. Three hertz spike-and-waves or polyspike-and-waves, symmetrical and synchronous	Same as interictal pattern, but longer	*Absences* ('petit mal seizures')[a]	Unknown
2. Polyspike-and-waves, spike-and-waves, mono- and polyphasic sharp waves	Same as interictal, but repetitive	Bilateral massive epileptic myoclonus[a,c]	Unknown or widespread structural or metabolic diseases
3. Hypsarrhythmia and other patterns (Table 19.1)	(Table 19.1)	Infantile spasms[b]	As above
4. Spike-and-waves or polyspike-and-waves	Mixture of fast waves of over 10 Hz and slow waves with occasional spike-and-wave patterns	Clonic seizures[a]	As above
5. Slow spike-and-waves and other patterns (Table 19.1)	Rhythm of 10 Hz or more with increasing amplitude and decreasing frequency	Tonic seizures[b]	As above
6. Spike-and-waves or polyspike-and-waves	Rhythm of 10 Hz or more with increasing amplitude and decreasing frequency, later interrupted by slow waves	*Tonic-clonic seizures*[a] ('grand mal seizures')	As above
7a. Polyspike-and-waves or spike-and-waves	Polyspike-and-waves	Brief atonic seizures (epileptic drop attacks)	As above
7b. Polyspike-and-waves, spike-and-waves	Mixed fast and slow waves with occasional spike-and-wave patterns	Long atonic seizures[a] (incl. atonic absences)	As above
8. Polyspike-and-waves	Mixed fast and slow waves with occasional spike-and-wave patterns	Akinetic seizures[a]	As above

[a] Also occur with special infantile patterns (Table 19.1).
[b] Usually occur with special infantile patterns (Table 19.1).
[c] Also occur with periodic complexes (Table 19.2).

331

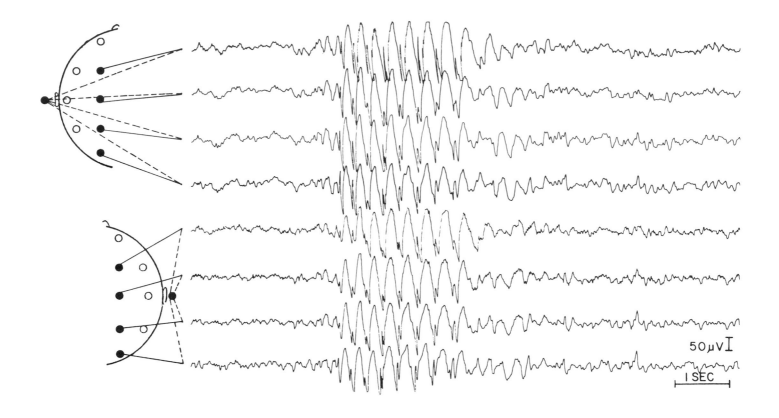

Fig. 18.1. Interictal generalized 3 Hz spike-and-wave discharge, unassociated with clinical manifestations; the patient remembered a test word given during the discharge. This 22-year-old woman has a history of absence attacks since age 12 and of generalized tonic-clonic seizures since age 18.

patterns is of greater clinical importance than that of localized ictal patterns because it correlates fairly well with clinical seizure type (see also 17.1.1).

18.1.2 *Interictal patterns:*

(1) *Three Hz spike and wave complexes*, also called *typical spike and wave complexes*, consist of a spike of high amplitude followed by a slow wave of similar or sometimes greater amplitude. The spike and wave complexes repeat at a frequency of about 3 Hz (Fig. 18.1). The slow wave immediately follows the spike, or the spike may appear to be superimposed on the beginning or end of the slow wave. The time relation between the spike and wave may differ in different derivations and may shift during the same discharge. In many instances 2 or 3 spikes appear with each slow wave. This is more likely to be observed if recording derivations with long interelectrode distances are employed. Although the frequency is often constant, some bursts begin at rates of 3–4 Hz and end at 2–3 Hz.

The discharges typically have a frontal maximum, showing phase reversals in both longitudinal and transverse bipolar montages. At other times the background may contain bisynchronous slow wave bursts at 3 Hz resembling the 3-Hz spike-and-wave complexes without the spikes. There may also be brief runs of 3-Hz slow waves that are maximal over the occipital head regions. This occipitally dominant pattern is not specifically related to epilepsy, but in approximately one-third of individuals in which it occurs, the typical 3-Hz spike-and-wave pattern may also be seen. The 3-Hz spike-and-wave pattern is readily detected in routine recordings (>98%) that include hyperventilation unless the patient is receiving anticonvulsant medication.

The sleep record regularly shows complexes of multiple spikes which are separated from each other by smaller slow waves than those in the waking epileptiform pattern (Fig. 18.2); these complexes may or may not repeat at 3 Hz. During wakefulness brief (less than 1 sec) generalized or lateralized irregular epileptiform activity or bursts of theta and delta waves may also occasionally coexist with the

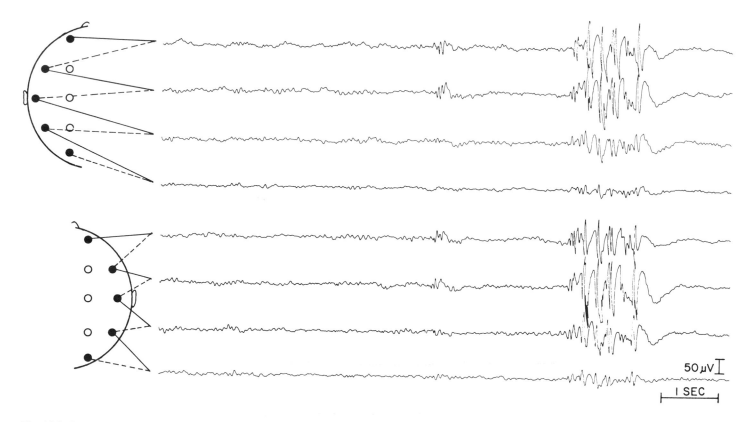

50 μV

1 SEC

Fig. 18.2. Paroxysm of generalized 3–4 Hz spike-and-wave and polyspike-and-wave complexes during light sleep. Same patient as in Fig. 18.1.

typical 3-Hz spike-and-wave pattern. Other abnormalities of the background are very uncommon. Three hertz spike-and-wave discharges are usually facilitated by hyperventilation and often precipitated by photic stimulation.

(2) *Atypical spike and wave complexes* differ from the typical spike and wave pattern by either being less rhythmical or having a faster repetition rate. The frequency of spikes may vary in a burst or between bursts (Fig. 18.3). If the frequency reaches 6 Hz (Fig. 18.3, Part 2), these complexes must be distinguished from 6 Hz spike-and-slow-wave discharges (19.5.1) which are typically smaller, shorter lasting and usually not as widely distributed (Fig. 19.13). - p. 387 ↳ tiny

(3) *Slow spike-and-wave discharges* (Fig. 19.6) are similar to the 3 Hz spike-and-wave complexes except that (a) they repeat at rates of less than 3 Hz, usually at 1.5−2.5 Hz; (b) the first component may be a sharp wave rather than a spike in which case the discharges are called 'sharp-and-slow-wave complexes'; (c) the discharges may have focal preponderance or consistently focal onset in one area; (d) they are usually not facilitated by hyperventilation. The pattern of slow spike-and-wave discharges is discussed in the next chapter (19.2).

(4) *Hypsarrhythmia* is described in the next chapter (19.2).

(5) *Intermittent spikes, polyspikes and sharp waves* occur either sporadically as rudiments of other interictal patterns or periodically as elements of periodic complexes (19.3). These elements are seen much less often as interictal generalized epileptiform activity than as interictal focal epileptiform activity.

(6) *Generalized paroxysmal fast activity* is an infrequently encountered pattern that consists of runs of rapid spikes or sharply contoured waveforms in the beta frequency range. It usually appears during sleep with maximal amplitude over the frontal or frontocentral head regions. The discharge typically lasts 2−4 sec, but has been observed to last up to 18 sec. Although it is occasionally seen in individuals with normal intelligence, it is far more common in those with mental retardation. Most patients with this pattern have tonic-clonic and absence seizures, but other types of generalized seizures (e.g., tonic or clonic) may also occur.

335

* phantom

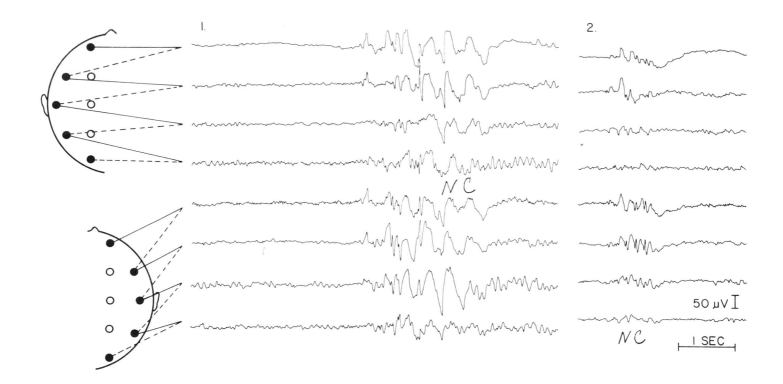

Fig. 18.3. Interictal generalized spike-and-wave discharges. 1. Irregular discharges during drowsiness; 2. Regular discharges at 6 Hz during light sleep. This 24-year-old woman has a history of generalized tonic-clonic seizures since the age of 4.

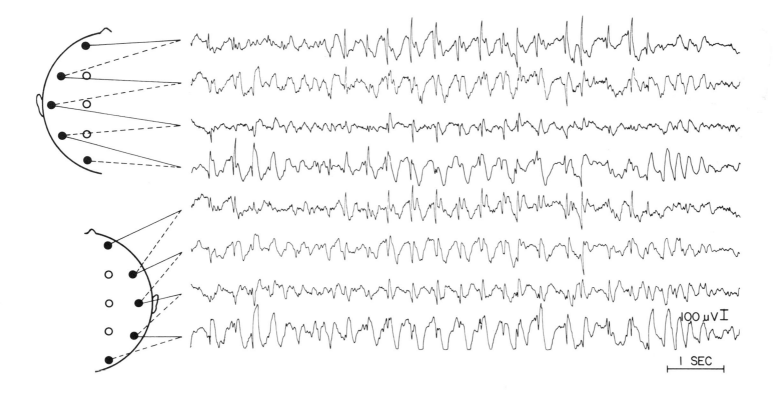

Fig. 18.4. Ictal generalized spike-and-wave discharges at 2–3 Hz. This 60-year-old woman has a history of generalized tonic-clonic seizures since childhood with sudden onset of absence status two days before this recording.

18.1.3 *Ictal patterns* are of many different types (Table 18.1). Some of the more common patterns have fairly reliable associations with clinical seizure types. The most common ictal patterns are described below.

(1) *3 Hz spike-and-wave discharges* are repetitions of the interictal 3 Hz spike-and-wave pattern and last more than a few seconds. Most patients with this ictal pattern have the same interictal pattern, but not all patients with interictal 3 Hz spike-and-wave discharges show this ictal pattern. Patients with petit mal epilepsy (absence epilepsy) who are in absence status may show prolonged runs of typical 3-Hz spike-and-wave (so called Petit Mal Status). In other patients with generalized non-convulsive status (also referred to as absence status) who have no history of typical absence seizures (petit mal seizures), less regular spike and wave complexes (e.g., multiple spike and wave complexes) are present continually with a variable repetition rate; this pattern is particularly common in adults and elderly individuals who may suddenly develop absence status with or without having had a history of prior seizures (Fig. 18.4).

(2) *Slow spike-and-wave discharges and sharp-and-slow-wave discharges* are repetitions of the corresponding interictal patterns. They are often associated with atypical absence attacks. They are related to infantile patterns and are further described in the next chapter (19.2).

(3) *A rhythm of 10 Hz or more* increases in amplitude and decreases in frequency to form repetitive spikes which are occasionally interrupted by slow waves before the discharge ends. A discharge of this kind forms the first of the two phases associated with generalized tonic-clonic seizures (Fig. 18.5). A similar discharge is often associated with tonic seizures (Fig. 19.4) and appears mainly in patients with interictal patterns described in the next chapter (19.2).

(4) *Polyspike-and-wave discharges and spike-and-wave discharges* which are usually less regular than the 3 Hz spike-and-wave discharges appear in patients who often have interictal discharges of similar shape and suffer from a variety of

338

different seizures. Similar discharges form the second phase of the diphasic discharge associated with generalized tonic-clonic seizures (Figs. 18.5–18.7).

(5) *A biphasic discharge,* often associated with tonic-clonic seizures, consists of a sequence of the two last-described patterns (Figs. 18.5–18.7). A rhythm of 10 Hz or more which increases in amplitude and decreases in frequency corresponds with the tonic phase of the seizure; it lasts about 10–20 seconds. At the end, it may be interrupted by slow waves which appear at regular intervals and lead to a gradual development of the second phase. This clonic phase is characterized by high amplitude spike-and-wave or polyspike-and-wave complexes which repeat at 1–4 Hz for about 30 seconds, having a faster rate initially and then becoming slower. When they stop, the record usually shows no distinguishable activity for many seconds or a few minutes before slow waves of low amplitude begin to appear. The waves gradually increase amplitude and frequency until pre-ictal patterns eventually reappear. Postictal bilateral slow waves may very rarely remain as a residual EEG abnormality for up to several days following a single generalized tonic-clonic seizure. Far more often the EEG returns to baseline with minutes. However, if more than one generalized convulsive seizure occurs, then the duration of postictal slowing is increased.

Most patients with this ictal pattern have interictal patterns of spike-and wave complexes of any frequency although some patients show no interictal abnormalities at all.

(6) *A sudden transient decrease of amplitude* of all activity or a paroxysmal appearance of *generalized fast waves* are ictal patterns mainly seen in infants and very young children (19.2).

18.2 CLINICAL SIGNIFICANCE OF GENERALIZED EPILEPTIFORM ACTIVITY

18.2.1 *Association with seizures and epilepsy*

Epileptiform activity associated with seizures. Most patients with generalized

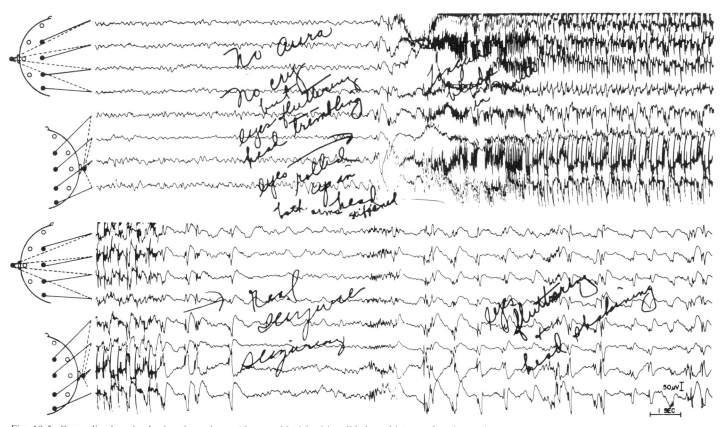

Fig. 18.5. Generalized tonic-clonic seizure in an 18-year-old girl with a life-long history of major and minor generalized seizures. *Top*: Pattern of slight drowsiness, suddenly interrupted by intermittent spikes and movement artifacts at the onset of a rhythm of generalized repetitive spikes of increasing amplitude and decreasing frequency which lasts about 10 seconds. Technician's comments read: 'No aura, no cry, but eyes fluttering, head trembling, eyes rolled up in head, both arms stiffened. Tongue blade in mouth'. This represents the tonic phase of the tonic-clonic seizure. *Bottom*: Spikes begin to be interrupted by slow waves. This signals the beginning of the clonic phase which starts with rhythmical high amplitude polyspike-and-wave and spike-and-wave complexes at about 1 Hz. Technician's notes read: 'Real seizure, seizuring. Eyes fluttering + head shaking'.

340

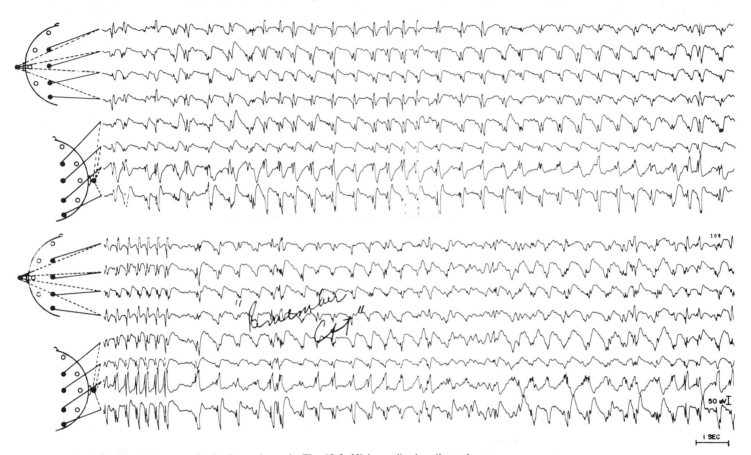

Fig. 18.6. Continuation of the generalized seizure shown in Fig. 18.5. High amplitude spike-and-wave discharges continue during the clonic phase. Top part is continuous with the bottom part of Fig. 18.5. Technician's note reads: 'Remember Cat', indicating that the technician was testing the patient's ability to remember a test word; the patient later did not recall anything.

341

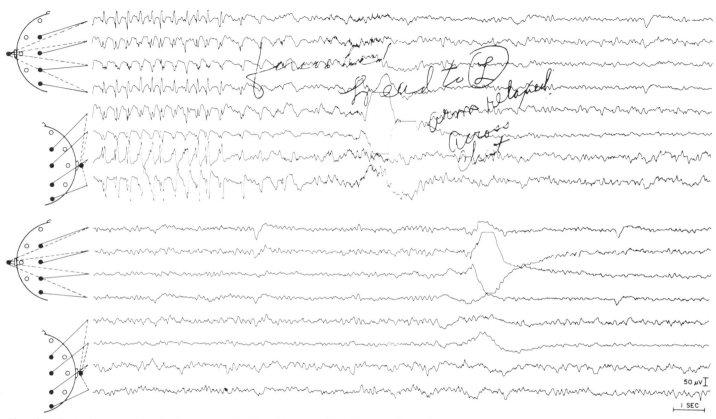

Fig. 18.7. End of the generalized seizure shown in Figs. 18.5. and 18.6. Top part is continuous with bottom part of Fig. 18.6. The end of the high amplitude generalized bisynchronous spike-and-wave complexes represents the end of the clonic phase of the seizure. This is followed by slow waves, movement artifacts and gradual return of normal background activity. Technician's notes read: 'Head to left, arms relaxed across chest'. This was a mild generalized seizure. More violent seizures are usually followed by postictal depression of amplitude and longer lasting slow waves of lower frequency. Violent seizures can usually not be recorded completely because the recording electrodes become dislodged.

epileptiform EEG activity, similar to patients with focal epileptiform activity, have a history of seizures, and many patients with a history of seizures show generalized epileptiform activity in the EEG. Generalized electrographic seizures are almost always accompanied by obvious clinical seizure manifestations except in cases where the responses of the patient are limited (e.g., patients in coma or patients with severe, chronic encephalopathy). Rarely, generalized non-convulsive status (absence status) may be accompanied by a very mild impairment of mentation. In some patients, generalized epileptiform activity and seizure manifestations are precipitated by specific external sensory stimuli, mental tasks, or other factors. In contrast to patients with precipitated focal discharges and partial seizures, patients with precipitated generalized seizures are more susceptible to simple stimuli. The response often varies with stimulus intensity and has a short latency from the time of the stimulus presentation.

The occurrence of an interictal typical 3-Hz spike-and-wave pattern strongly suggests the presence of absence seizures. *In every recording in which this or any other generalized epileptiform pattern occurs, clinical response testing should be performed during the discharge to determine if there is an associated impairment of consciousness.* If an impairment is clearly documented, then the pattern is considered an ictal event, regardless of its duration. The presence of the typical spike and wave pattern does not necessarily mean that the patient with seizures has only absence seizures. Indeed, the majority of patients with typical absence seizures will eventually experience one or more tonic-clonic seizures. To the extent that the interictal pattern deviates from the classical 3-Hz spike-and-wave pattern the likelihood of absence seizures becomes more uncertain and the likelihood of other kinds of generalized seizures becomes more likely.

The presence or absence of the typical 3-Hz spike-and-wave interictal pattern in patients with idiopathic absence seizures can be used as a measure of the efficacy of therapeutic intervention. *In this regard the typical spike and wave pattern differs from all other known focal or generalized interictal patterns.* If anticonvulsant treatment is completely effective, then there is usually a dramatic, if not complete, suppression of 3-Hz spike-and-wave discharges at rest and during hyperventilation.

Epileptiform activity without seizures. Like patients with localized epileptiform activity, some patients with generalized epileptiform activity have no evidence of seizures. This is commonly encountered in family members of patients with idiopathic primarily generalized seizures and occasionally in some patients with seizures precipitated by metabolic/toxic encephalopathies. The bilateral benign epileptiform (or 'pseudo-epileptiform') patterns of 6-Hz phantom spike and wave, 14 and 6 per second positive spikes, paroxysmal hypnogogic hypersynchrony, and subclinical rhythmic EEG discharges of adults (SREDA) also have no proven relation to seizures.

Epilepsy and seizures without obvious epileptiform activity may occur for several reasons. EEG recordings made between seizures may fail to show epileptiform activity for reasons discussed in connection with localized epileptiform activity. Patients with generalized seizures due to transient disorders such as drug withdrawal or toxic and metabolic encephalopathies are unlikely to show epileptiform activity after the disorder is resolved or at times other than during the periods of heightened susceptibility to seizures. Generalized seizures that produce an impairment of consciousness always show epileptiform activity (unless obscured by artifact) or prominent background changes with or without postictal slowing. Epileptiform activity during generalized convulsive ('tonic-clonic') seizures is often obscured by artifact, but postictal slowing always occurs and is usually easily discerned.

18.2.2 *Underlying cerebral abnormality in adults and adolescents. No demonstrable lesion* is found in the majority of adults and adolescents with primary generalized epileptiform activity, especially in those who have bilaterally synchronous and symmetrical epileptiform patterns and no other EEG abnormalities. There

344

is no historical, clinical or laboratory evidence of cerebral damage. These patients have idiopathic epilepsy.

Widespread lasting structural damage is present in some patients with generalized epileptiform activity. Most patients in this group have a history, clinical signs or laboratory findings pointing to the cause of the lesions; they may have suffered widespread cerebral injury, anoxia or encephalitis. The EEG may show other abnormalities in addition to generalized epileptiform discharges. These discharges are generally less symmetrical and synchronous than those of patients without obvious cerebral lesions.

Transient conditions that can cause seizures and generalized epileptiform activity are legion. Far more often these disorders occur without interictal generalized epileptiform activity. Some of the more common transient conditions associated with generalized epileptiform patterns and seizures include acute anoxia, recent severe head injury, hypoglycemia, withdrawal from chronic use of alcohol, barbiturates and other CNS depressant drugs and renal, hepatic or other metabolic encephalopathies. However, the EEG in these conditions more often shows other nonspecific background abnormalities than epileptiform activity. If the underlying transient abnormality resolves without residual cerebral dysfunction, then the EEG returns to baseline.

18.3 OTHER EEG ABNORMALITIES ASSOCIATED WITH GENERALIZED EPILEPTIFORM
ACTIVITY

18.3.1 *Focal epileptiform discharges* in a record also showing generalized epileptiform discharges strongly suggest that the generalized epileptiform activity is triggered by a focal discharge. This is supported if generalized discharges consistently follow the focal discharges (17.3.2).

18.3.2 *Focal slow waves* or a *local decrease of background amplitude* may suggest a focal brain lesion related to the generalized epileptiform discharges.

18.3.3 *Generalized asynchronous and bisynchronous slow waves and generalized decrease of amplitude* may indicate a generalized cerebral abnormality giving rise to generalized epileptiform discharges (e.g. metabolic encephalopathy, postanoxic myoclonus, Jakob-Creutzfeldt disease). However, similar abnormalities may be the result of a generalized seizure discharge; mild postictal slow waves may persist for several days after a seizure.

18.4 MECHANISMS UNDERLYING GENERALIZED EPILEPTIFORM ACTIVITY

18.4.1 *The involvement of intact cortex* by bilateral and approximately symmetrical and synchronous epileptiform activity distinguishes primarily generalized from secondarily generalized epileptiform activity. In secondarily generalized interictal epileptiform activity there is a focal cortical epileptogenic disturbance that gives rise to a generalized epileptiform pattern. One mechanism by which this occurs is commonly referred to as *secondary bilateral synchrony* and is discussed in section 17.3.2. Cortical lesions giving rise to secondary bilateral synchrony are classically located in the mesial frontal cortex, but other cortical areas, including the temporal lobe, may be involved. Mesial frontal foci are best detected with transverse bipolar montages. Additional electrodes placed between the routine 10–20 electrode positions are often helpful since the critical finding is a single phase reversal that is lateralized to the left or right of the midline.

In 1954 Penfield and Jasper proposed the first modern theory of primarily generalized seizure propagation. They suggested that the epileptogenic discharge originated in a 'central integrating system of the higher brainstem'. Subsequently, such seizures were called *centrencephalic seizures* in accord with their postulated site

346

of origin. Observations that supported the theory of centrencephalic seizures included the following: (1) the apparently bisynchronous onset of epileptiform activity involving every area of the cortex simultaneously seemed to require a subcortical generator; (2) Dempsey and Morison (1942) had demonstrated the existence of a diffuse nonspecific projection system of thalamocortical connections by which medial and intralaminar thalamic nuclei could induce widespread cortical rhythmic activity; and (3) an electrographic pattern approximating 3-Hz spike and slow-wave complexes could be produced in anesthetized or brainstem transected cats by electrical stimulation of the medial intralaminar region of the thalamus.

The centrencephalic theory has been considerably modified largely through the work of Gloor and colleagues who propose that the cortex also plays a primary role in the propagation of primarily generalized seizures. This now generally accepted mechanism for primarily generalized seizures is referred to as the *corticoreticular* theory. Support for the corticoreticular theory includes the following experimental observations: (1) high dose parenteral penicillin induces bilaterally synchronous bursts of 3–5 Hz spike and wave discharges that appear first in cortex, not in the thalamus or brainstem; (2) generalized spike-and-wave activity can also be produced by the direct application of penicillin to the cortex, application to the thalamus is ineffective in producing epileptiform discharges; (3) thalamic input appears to be the triggering event since thalamic stimulation which would normally induce sleep spindles or recruiting responses elicits spike and wave activity in the penicillin model; (4) thalamic function and thalamocortical connections are prerequisites since depression of thalamic function by potassium chloride or thalamectomy abolishes spike-and-wave discharges; and (5) the brainstem reticular formation appears to modulate spike-wave activity by altering the level of cortical excitability.

Hereditary predisposition also plays an important role in the genesis of epilepsy in individuals with primarily generalized seizures since: (1) the incidence of epilepsy in family members is significantly higher than in the general population and, (2) the incidence of epileptiform activity is also increased in unaffected family members. This familial tendency is most apparent among individuals with the least evidence of cerebral disease, as in those with petit mal epilepsy with typical absence seizures.

18.5.1 *Degenerative, developmental and demyelinating diseases:*

(1) *Unverricht-Lundborg's myoclonus epilepsy* is associated with interictal multiple spikes or bursts of spike-and-waves at 3–6 Hz which last for 1–2 seconds. The background contains theta and delta activity with superimposed beta waves. Photic stimulation may elicit multiple generalized spikes and waves with or without myoclonic jerks.

(2) *Lafora's inclusion body epilepsy* may show spikes, polyspikes and spike-and-wave complexes with focal or bilaterally synchronous distribution and with limited correlation to myoclonic jerks. The background may show diffuse asynchronous and bisynchronous delta waves of high amplitude.

(3) *Jakob-Creutzfeldt disease* often shows generalized periodic sharp waves (19.3).

(4) *Ramsey Hunt's syndrome of dyssynergia cerebellaris myoclonica* may be associated with spikes, spike-and-waves, polyspike-and-waves at 4–6 Hz, with an anterior maximum. Photic stimulation often elicits a paroxysmal response with jerks. Focal spikes may appear in sleep. Seizures are tonic-clonic or only clonic.

(5) *Sturge-Weber syndrome* may show bilateral spikes although it is often associated with local reduction of amplitude and local spikes.

(6) *Riley-Day's familial dysautonomia* may be associated with generalized epileptiform activity.

(7) *Microgyria, agyria and holoprosencephaly* may show generalized spikes, spike-and-waves as well as focal slow waves, focal spikes, hypsarrhythmia and multifocal spikes (19.2).

18.5.2 *Metabolic and toxic encephalopathies.* Generalized spikes or sharp waves occur in many of these encephalopathies, usually on a background of widespread bisynchronous and asynchronous slow waves. Generalized epileptiform discharges occasionally repeat at regular intervals, and may form complexes resembling spike-and-wave discharges. Regular, organized and sustained spike-and-wave patterns are rarely seen in adults except in some cases of dialysis encephalopathy. In infants and children, metabolic encephalopathies may be associated with multifocal or generalized epileptiform discharges of special types (19.1).

infants and children, metabolic encephalopathies may be associated with multifocal or generalized epileptiform discharges of special types (19.1).

The following metabolic and endocrine encephalopathies may be associated with generalized epileptiform activity: Addison's disease, dialysis encephalopathy, hyperglycemia without ketoacidosis, hypoglycemia, hypocalcemia due to hypoparathyroidism of pseudohypoparathyroidism, hyponatremia, acute intermittent porphyria, pyridoxine deficiency and uremia (Table 22.1).

A very great number of toxic agents are capable of producing generalized epileptiform activity. Among the more common agents are high doses of therapeutic agents, such as phenothiazines, haloperidol, rauwolfia derivatives, INH, tricyclic antidepressants, environmental agents and organic solvents such as methyl bromide and chloride, pesticides, DDT, lead and mercury.

Withdrawal from chronic use of drugs depressing central nervous function can induce generalized epileptiform activity for a few days after withdrawal; photoconvulsive responses are often seen in this condition. The most common agents are barbiturates. └ i.e. alcohol

Hyperthermia can induce or precipitate generalized epileptiform activity, especially in young children who tend to have seizures during febrile illnesses. These *febrile seizures* are usually tonic or clonic. Most of these children show no epileptiform EEG activity between seizures, but some of them develop such activity, and recurring generalized seizures, independent of fever.

349

18.5.3 *Cerebrovascular diseases:*

(1) *Postanoxic encephalopathy* may produce generalized epileptiform activity among many other EEG abnormalities. A special form of this activity consists of periodic sharp waves which are seen in cases of postanoxic myoclonus (19.3).

(2) Cerebral infarction rarely causes generalized epileptiform activity unless both hemispheres are affected, as for example in sickle cell disease or malaria. In such cases synchronous or asynchronous bilateral periodic lateralizing discharges (PLEDs) may occur (19.3). If epileptiform activity occurs as a result of cerebral infarction it is almost always focal or lateralized.

18.5.4 *Cerebral trauma.* Severe head injuries can lead to generalized epileptiform activity and seizures. Like focal epileptiform abnormalities, the generalized abnormalities may appear soon after the injury or with a delay. The effects of cerebral injury on the EEG are especially pronounced in infants and young children who may react with special epileptiform patterns (19.1).

18.5.5 *Brain tumors.* The incidence of generalized epileptiform activity may be increased very slightly compared with that encountered in the general population.

18.5.6 *Generalized epileptiform activity in seizure disorders without known underlying diseases and in normal persons.* *Idiopathic epilepsy* is the diagnosis of many cases of generalized epileptiform seizures without known cause, especially in cases of typical absence attacks associated with interictal and ictal 3 Hz spike-and-wave patterns, and in cases of generalized tonic-clonic seizures.

In practice, this diagnosis requires exclusion of organic disorders known to cause generalized seizures. Organic lesions must be suspected in patients who have (a) EEG findings of asynchronous and asymmetrical generalized epileptiform activity and of abnormal background activity; (b) a history of cerebral injuries or diseases at any time from before birth to before the onset of seizures; (c) abnormal findings on neurological examination; (d) a general medical condition capable of causing generalized seizures. *Normal subjects* may show specific patterns of generalized epileptiform activity (18.2.1; 18.4).

18.5.7 *Infectious diseases* produce generalized epileptiform activity only rarely and then mainly in the form of periodic complexes seen in subacute sclerosing panencephalitis, Jakob-Creutzfeldt diseases and herpes simplex (19.3) or of infantile patterns (19.2).

18.5.8 *Psychiatric diseases* are not characterized by generalized epileptiform activity although widespread interictal discharges have been reported in small fractions of large groups of patients with various diseases. The possibility of causes other than non-organic psychiatric disorders must be evaluated in every case.

REFERENCES

Ajmone-Marsan, C. and Zivin, L.S. (1970) Factors related to the occurrence of typical paroxysmal abnormalities in the EEG records of epileptic patients. Epilepsia 11: 361–381.
Bancaud, J., Talairach, J., Morel, P., Bresson, M., Bonis, A., Geier, S., Hemon, E. and Buser, P. (1974) 'Generalized' epileptic seizures elicited by electrical stimulation of the frontal lobe in man. Electroenceph. clin. Neurophysiol. 37: 275–282.
Binnie, C.D. (1987) Electroencephalography and epilepsy. In: Hopkins, A. (Ed.), Epilepsy, Demos, New York, pp. 169–200.
Brenner, R.P. and Atkinson, R. (1982) Generalized paroxysmal fast activity: Electroencephalographic and clinical features. Ann. Neurol. 11: 386–390.
Blume, W.T. and Lemieux, J.F. (1988) Morphology of spikes in spike-and-wave complexes. Electroenceph. clin. Neurophysiol. 69: 508–515.
Dieter, J. (1989) Juvenile myoclonic epilepsy. Cleveland Clin. J. Med. 56 (Suppl. 1): S23–33.
Ellis, J.M. and Lee, S.I. (1978) Acute prolonged confusion in later life as an ictal state. Epilepsia 19: 119–128.

Fisch, B.J. and Pedley, T.A. (1987) Generalized Tonic-Clonic Epilepsies. In: Luders, H. and Lesser, R.P. (Eds.), Epilepsy: Electroclinical Syndromes. Springer, New York, pp. 151–187.

Forster, F.M. (1977) Reflex Epilepsy, Behavioral Therapy and Conditional Reflexes. Thomas, Springfield.

Fromm, G.H. (1987) The brain stem and seizures: Summary and synthesis. In: Fromm, G.H., Faingold, C.L., Browning, R.A. and Burning, W.M. (Eds.), Epilepsy and the Reticular Formation. Liss, New York, pp. 203–218.

Gloor, P. (1979) Generalized epilepsy with spike-and-wave discharge: A reinterpretation of its electrographic and clinical manifestations. Epilepsia 20: 571–588.

Gomez, M.R. and Westmoreland, B.F. (1987) Absence seizures. In: Luders, H. and Lesser, R. (Eds.), Epilepsy: Electroclinical Syndromes. Springer, London, pp. 105–129.

Guberman, A., Cantu-Reyna, G., Stuss, D. and Broughton, R. (1986) Nonconvulsive generalized status epilepticus: Clinical features, neuropsychological testing, and long-term follow-up. Neurology 36: 1284–1291.

Loiseau, P., Pestre, M., Dartigues, J.F., Commenges, D., Barberger-Gateau, C. and Cohadon, S. (1983) Long-term prognosis in two forms of childhood epilepsy: Typical absence seizures and epilepsy with rolandic (centrotemporal) EEG foci. Ann. Neurol. 13: 642–648.

Lombroso, C.T. and Erba, G. (1970) Primary and secondary bilateral synchrony in epilepsy. Arch. Neurol. 22: 321–334.

Luders, H., Lesser, R.P., Dinner, D.S. and Morris, H.H. (1984) Generalized epilepsies: A review. Cleve. Clin. Q., 51: 205–226.

Mancardi, G.L., Primavera, A., Leonardi, A., De Martini, I., Salvarani, S. and Bugiani, O. (1979) Tendency to periodic recurrence of EEG changes in Lafora's disease. Eur. Neurol. 18: 129–135.

Niedermeyer, E., Fineyre, F., Riley, T. and Uematsu, S. (1979) Absence status (petit mal status) with focal characteristics. Arch. Neurol. 36: 417–421.

Niedermeyer, E. (1987) Epileptic seizure disorders. In: Niedermeyer, E. and Lopes da Silva, F. (Eds.), Electroencephalography: Basic Principles, Clinical Applications and Related Fields. Urban and Schwarzenberg, Baltimore, pp. 405–510.

Noriega-Sanchez, A., Martinez-Maldonado, M. and Haiffe, R.M. (1978) Clinical and electroencephalographic changes in progressive uremic encephalopathy. Neurology 28: 667–669.

Pedley, T.A. (1987) Epilepsy. In: Halliday, A.M., Butler, S.R. and Paul, R. (Eds.), A Textbook of Clinical Neurophysiology. Wiley, Chichester, pp. 231–267.

Penry, J.K., Porter, R.J. and Dreifuss, F.E. (1975) Simultaneous recording of absence seizures with video tape and electroencephalography. A study of 374 seizures in 48 patients. Brain 98: 427–440.

Rodin, E., Smid, N. and Mason, K. (1976) The grand mal pattern of Gibbs, Gibbs and Lennox. Electroenceph. clin. Neurophysiol. 40: 401–406.

Salinsky, M., Kanter, R. and Dasheiff, R.M. (1987) Effectiveness of multiple EEGs in supporting the diagnosis of epilepsy: an operational curve. Epilepsia 28: 331–334.

Theodore, W.H., Sato, S. and Porter, R.J. (1984) Serial EEG in intractable epilepsy. Neurology 34: 863–867.

Tükel, K. and Jasper, H. (1952) The electroencephalogram in parasagittal lesions. Electroenceph. clin. Neurophysiol. 4: 481–494.

Westmoreland, B.F. (1985) The electroencephalogram in patients with epilepsy. In: Aminoff, M.J. (Ed.), Electrodiagnosis, Neurologic Clinics, W.B. Saunders, Philadelphia, pp. 599–614.

Zivin, L. and Ajmone-Marsan, C. (1968) Incidence and prognostic significance of epileptiform activity in the EEG of non-epileptic subjects. Brain 91: 751–778.

Special epileptiform patterns

19

SUMMARY

This chapter joins several groups of interictal and ictal patterns which are clearly distinguished from the epileptiform patterns described in the preceding chapters.

(19.1)   *Ictal patterns in neonates* are almost always focal or multifocal and often consist of rhythmical activity often without spike or sharp wave components. Ictal patterns in neonates frequently occur without obvious clinical manifestations.

(19.2)   *Hypsarrhythmia, slow spike and wave complexes and multifocal independent spikes* have features of both focal and generalized epileptiform activity and appear at slightly different ages in infants and young children as the result of a great variety of organic brain disorders.

(19.3)   *Periodic complexes* are characterized by the fairly regular recurrence of paroxysmal activity of various forms.

(19.4)   *Ictal patterns without spikes and sharp waves* occur in patients with various focal and generalized interictal patterns which have been described in other sections.

(19.5)   *Pseudo-epileptogenic patterns* contain epileptiform activity but have no proven relation to epilepsy and seizures.

19.1   NEONATAL SEIZURES

19.1.1   In neonates spike or sharp wave abnormalities consist mainly of: (1) an increase in the number of multifocal sharp transients (MSTs) beyond that normally expected for a particular conceptual age; (2) persistent and frequent focal spikes involving a single head region in any state at any age; and (3) positive rolandic sharp waves. In order to avoid 'overreading' epileptiform activity in neonatal EEGs it is important to recognize that similar shaped waveforms are normal at certain conceptual ages depending on their distribution, frequency of occurrence, and correlation with behavioral state (10.1).

An abnormal increase in the abundance of MSTs represents a nonspecific

TABLE 19.1
Special infantile and juvenile epileptiform patterns

Interictal epileptiform pattern	Ictal epileptiform pattern	Clinical seizure type	Underlying brain lesion
A. *Hypsarrhythmia:* Multiple spikes with shifting foci, on high amplitude, generalized asynchronous and bisynchronous slow waves	1. Sudden attenuation of amplitude, often preceded by a large slow wave or a sharp-and-slow-wave complex 2. A sharp-and-slow-wave complex or large slow wave only 3. Fast activity during amplitude attenuation	Infantile spasms Tonic seizures	*Prenatal* Prematurity Complicated pregnancy Meningocele Encephalocele Hydrocephalus Microcephaly Tuberous sclerosis Toxoplasmosis
B. *Slow spike-and-wave* ('Petit mal variant'): Spike-and-wave or sharp-and-slow-wave at 1.5–2.5 Hz; synchronous and symmetrical or not	1. Long slow-spike-and-wave discharge 2. Low voltage fast 3. Rhythmic 10 Hz discharge with increasing amplitude and decreasing frequency 4. Mixed fast and slow 5. Flattening 6. Slow waves 7. Pattern as in tonic-clonic seizures (Table 18.1)	Absences Bilateral massive epileptic myoclonus Tonic seizures Long atonic seizures Akinetic seizures Tonic-clonic seizures	Cerebromacular degeneration Phenylketonuria Sturge-Weber *Perinatal* Birth injury Anoxia Ischemia Hypoglycemia
C. *Independent multifocal spikes:* Spikes from more than two foci of constant location	Focal or generalized seizure discharges similar to those of adults (Tables 17.1, 18.1)	Partial simple seizures Partial complex seizures Generalized tonic, clonic, tonic-clonic seizures	*Postnatal* Infections Head injuries Cerebrovascular disease Metachromatic leukodystrophy Pyridoxine deficiency

response to any encephalopathic process and does not specifically suggest the presence of a seizure disorder. If it is the only abnormal finding, then it should be considered a mild abnormality.

Persistent focal spikes may be associated with seizures or underlying structural abnormalities, particularly when accompanied by focal background slowing. Occasional spikes that occur in any location during wakefulness or active sleep after 42 weeks CA are abnormal, but are not specifically related to seizures.

Positive sharp waves (spikes with positive polarity) that: (1) occur over the rolandic and parasagittal head regions; (2) clearly stand out from both the ongoing background activity and other sharp transients; and (3) are accompanied by other EEG abnormalities, are thought to be specifically associated with periventricular encephalomalacia (usually a consequence of intraventricular hemorrhage).

19.1.2 *Neonatal ictal patterns* are almost always focal or lateralized in onset. It is thought that generalized patterns are rarely seen because intra- and interhemispheric cortical pathways are not sufficiently developed to allow for more widespread seizure propagation. The morphology of neonatal ictal patterns consists of either rhythmical, monomorphic waveforms or repetitive spikes or sharp waves (Fig. 19.1). Electrographic seizures are usually characterized by a buildup of activity that evolves in repetition rate and morphology. The duration of neonatal electrographic seizures may be less than 10 sec or more than 30 min, but the majority last less than 1 min.

There is, in general, a poor correlation between specific ictal neonatal EEG patterns and clinical manifestations. Although it has been suggested that some patterns are correlated with certain behaviors, such as rhythmic delta waves during tonic seizures and rhythmic alpha waves during apneic seizures, such correlations are not well established.

Neonatal electrographic seizures are frequently multifocal, often involve more

357

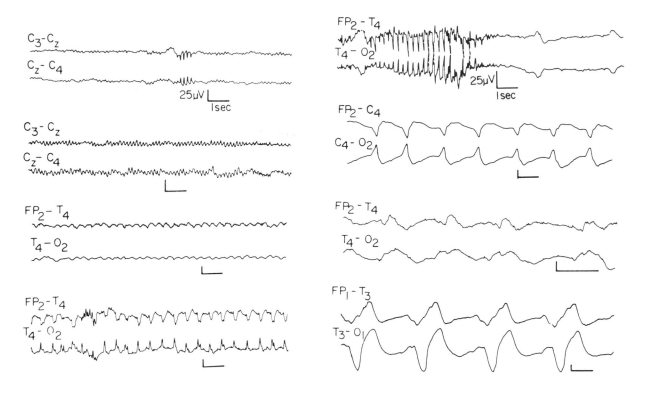

Fig. 19.1. Typical ictal patterns in premature and full term infants. Except where otherwise indicated, calibration: 50 μV; 1 sec. Courtesy B.R. Tharp, Electrodiagnosis in Clinical Neurology, 1986.

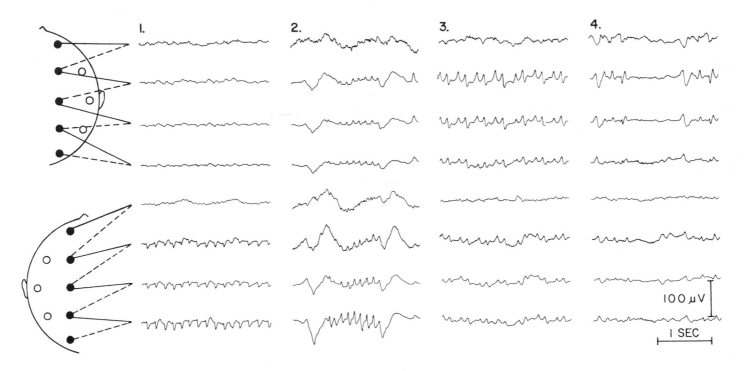

Fig. 19.2. Neonatal status epilepticus with seizure discharges on alternating sides in a 1-day-old full-term infant following an anoxic episode at birth. 1. Seizure discharge of rhythmical waves of 6–7 Hz, mainly on the left side; 2. One minute later, the left-sided seizure discharge consists of polyspikes, separated by high amplitude slow waves; similar discharges of lower amplitude appear on the right side; 3. Two minutes later, the seizure discharge on the left side abates and seizure discharges on the right side are at their height; 4. One minute later, the seizure discharge on the right side diminishes.

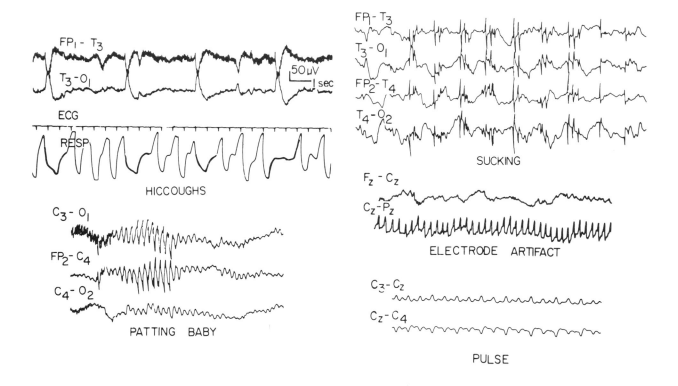

Fig. 19.3. Rhythmic artifacts which can be confused with ictal patterns. Calibration 50 μV; 1 sec. Courtesy B.R. Tharp, Electrodiagnosis in Clinical Neurology, 1986.

than one hemisphere, and may overlap in time. A distinctive feature of neonatal electrographic seizures is the tendency for some to remain focal but gradually change location in the same hemisphere as the seizure progresses. In other cases the discharge may begin in one hemisphere and gradually move to the opposite hemisphere (Fig. 19.2).

Neonatal seizures are typically highly focal and may appear to involve only one electrode. Prominent changes restricted to one electrode and abrupt rhythmic patterns involving one or more electrodes should always raise the question of noncerebral activity. Certain rhythmical artifacts are characteristic findings in neonatal recordings and others occur commonly. Examples of artifacts that could be confused with neonatal electrographic seizures are shown in Fig. 19.3.

Neonatal electrographic seizures may occur in the absence of clinical manifestations (*occult or subclinical seizures*). Alternatively, the clinical change may be overlooked because it does not represent an obvious departure from the neonate's baseline behavior. However, if the patient is carefully inspected during the electrographic seizure, then subtle clinical changes are usually detected. If clinical changes are not seen despite careful inspection, then the prognosis for normal development is currently thought to be poor.

Subclinical seizures have been shown to occur frequently in patients with or without any obvious impairment of consciousness. In general, if neonatal seizures are present, they occur frequently, with interictal periods usually lasting less than 10 min. Therefore, a typical neonatal recording (45–60 min in duration) is almost always sufficient to screen for the presence of seizures. Also, since EEG recording is the most sensitive technique for detecting neonatal seizures, it should be liberally employed in all cases of suspected seizures. Once electrographic seizures are observed repeat recordings should be performed to monitor the efficacy of treatment.

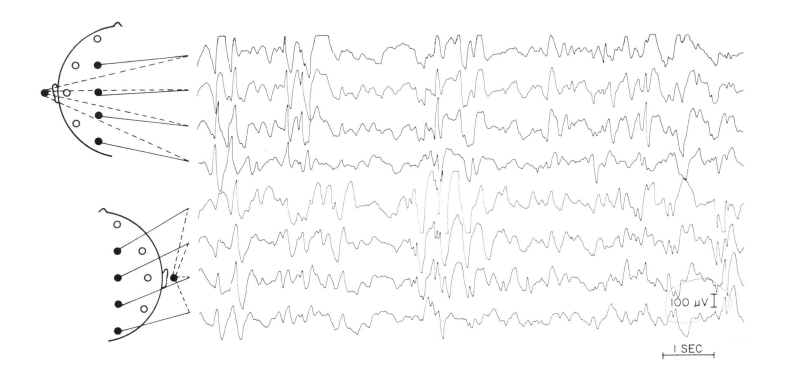

Fig. 19.4. Pattern of hypsarrhythmia. Interictal continuous spikes and slow waves of high amplitude in a shifting distribution. The patient is a 6-month-old infant with dysplasia of the left posterior fossa, hypotonia and infantile spasms.

These patterns (Table 19.1) are similar to each other in that (1) they usually have some focal or multifocal interictal features even though many of their ictal patterns are generalized from the start; (2) they are often associated with neurological abnormalities in the form of mental retardation and seizures; (3) they are the result of a great variety of prenatal, perinatal and postnatal pathological conditions most of which produce widespread or multifocal cerebral damage; (4) they depend more on the age of the patient and the severity of the underlying condition than on the particular type of the lesion. Hypsarrhythmia begins between the ages of 6 months to 2 years and may be replaced by one of the other patterns. The slow spike-and-wave pattern begins at the age of 2 to 4 years and may continue through early childhood. The pattern of multifocal independent spikes may develop from either one of the other patterns, or appear at the same ages as the other patterns in which case it usually represents less severe damage.

19.2.1 *Hypsarrhythmia.* Hypsarrhythmia is a term derived from the words 'hypselos', a Greek word which means 'high', and the word 'arrhythmia'. It thus describes a continuously irregular, high voltage pattern that cannot be recorded at routine sensitivity settings. The pattern consists of a largely chaotic admixture of spikes, sharp waves, and slow waves (Fig. 19.4).

The classical pattern of hypsarrhythmia differs from other patterns of multifocal epileptiform discharges in that the locations of the focal spikes-and-sharp waves are not constant but shift from moment to moment. In addition, the spikes-and-sharp waves are often greatest in amplitude over the posterior head regions (a point which is sometimes helpful in distinguishing hypsarrhythmia from the early onset of the Lennox-Gastaut syndrome; 19.2.2).

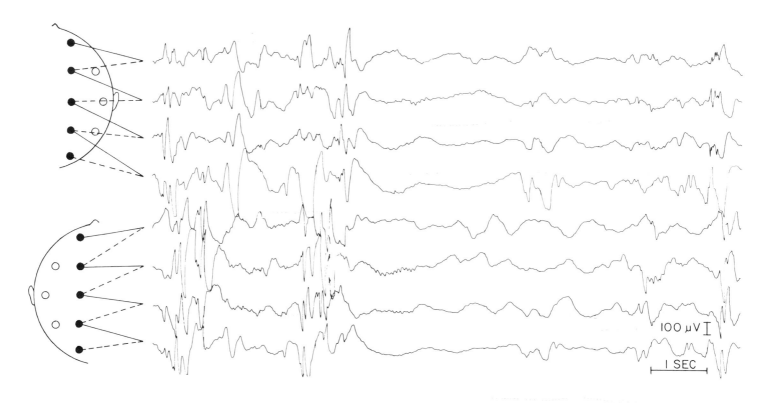

Fig. 19.5. Pattern of hypsarrhythmia interrupted by an electrodecremental seizure in the same patient as in Fig. 19.4. The hypsarrhythmic pattern at the beginning is abruptly replaced by very slow waves of much lower amplitude which were associated with mild spasmodic flexion of the arms.

Hypsarrhythmia is most pronounced during Non-REM sleep and is often greatly attenuated or transiently abolished during REM sleep. Less often, wakefulness or arousal from Non-REM sleep causes a reduction or transient disappearance of the pattern.

Modified hypsarrhythmia is a term used to describe commonly occurring variations of the classical hypsarrhythmia pattern. Generally accepted modified hypsarrhythmic patterns include: (1) predominantly high voltage, generalized, asynchronous, slow wave activity; (2) unilateral or asymmetrical hypsarrhythmia; (3) a discontinuous pattern with frequent epochs of widespread or localized attenuation similar in appearance to the suppression-burst pattern; and (4) hypsarrhythmia with increased interhemispheric synchrony. The suppression-burst variant in particular carries a guarded prognosis with high mortality and little likelihood of normal development. The unilateral or asymmetric pattern is more likely to be non-idiopathic and to be associated with underlying localized structural or functional abnormalities.

The ictal patterns associated with hypsarrhythmia usually include: (1) the *electrodecremental pattern* (Fig. 19.5) characterized by a sudden attenuation of amplitude, often preceded by either a frontal dominant, high amplitude, paroxysmal slow wave or a generalized sharp and slow wave complex, (2) generalized sharp and slow wave complexes or generalized paroxysmal slow waves only, or (3) fast activity appearing during the period of amplitude attenuation. The most common ictal pattern is the electrodecremental pattern.

The clinical seizures consist mainly of infantile spasms (95% of cases) and tonic seizures. Infants and children with hypsarrhythmia and modified hypsarrhythmia often show an arrest of development of perceptual and motor skills. The combination of infantile spasms, mental retardation and hypsarrhythmia is referred to as *West syndrome*. Approximately 60% of children with infantile spasms will demonstrate hypsarrhythmia. Although relative normalization of the EEG may oc-

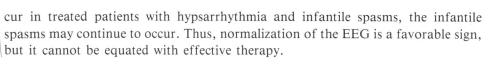

cur in treated patients with hypsarrhythmia and infantile spasms, the infantile spasms may continue to occur. Thus, normalization of the EEG is a favorable sign, but it cannot be equated with effective therapy.

Clinical conditions causing hypsarrhythmia comprise a great variety of disorders of prenatal, perinatal or postnatal onset (Table 19.1, Column 4). Most are due to diffuse or multifocal structural damage, but a few are due to metabolic disorders and are reversible, for instance hypoglycemia, pyridoxine deficiency and phenylketonurea. Rarely, local cerebral lesions such as the choroid plexus papilloma or the lesions seen in Sturge–Weber syndrome may be associated with hypsarrhythmia. In cases where there is a known and irreversible etiology for hypsarrhythmia with infantile spasms the long-term prognosis is poor. Only 5% of such patients develop normally or with only mild impairments. In contrast, the outcome is favorable in approximately 40% of idiopathic cases of hypsarrhythmia with infantile spasms.

19.2.2 *Slow spike-and-wave pattern* (formerly called 'petit mal variant'). *The interictal pattern* consists of spike-and-wave complexes, polyspike-and-wave complexes or sharp-and-slow wave complexes which occur intermittently or repeat at about 1.5–2.5 Hz for up to a few seconds (Fig. 19.6). They may be symmetrical and bisynchronous, or asymmetrical and even asynchronous. They may have a focal onset.

The ictal patterns are generalized and consist of (1) repetition of the interictal discharges for more than a few seconds, often up to 1 minute; (2) low amplitude fast activity of about 20 Hz with increasing amplitude; (3) rhythmical activity of about 10 Hz with increasing amplitude and decreasing frequency, occasionally interrupted by rhythmical slow waves and forming polyspike-and-wave or spike-and-wave complexes (Fig. 19.7); (4) a mixture of rhythmical slow waves and fast waves occasional-

366

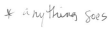

* anything goes

ly forming spike-and-wave patterns; (5) a simple reduction of amplitude leading to apparent flattening of the EEG; (6) generalized slow waves of delta or theta frequency; (7) a biphasic discharge of the type associated with generalized tonic-clonic seizures in adults.

Clinical seizures are of various types. Absence attacks may occur with the ictal patterns (1), (2) or (3). These attacks have been called 'atypical absences' in contrast to 'typical absences' (16.2) associated with bilaterally synchronous and symmetrical 3 Hz spike-and-wave discharges (18.1.2). Tonic, clonic and other generalized motor seizures occur with patterns (2)–(6). Pattern (7) is associated with tonic-clonic seizures similar to those of adults (16.2). Many patients have more than one type of seizure.

The combination of the EEG pattern of slow spike-and-waves, intractable seizures and mental retardation has the name 'Lennox syndrome' or 'Lennox-Gastaut syndrome'.

Clinical conditions causing slow spike-and-wave discharges are the same as those causing hypsarrhythmia in younger patients. Subacute sclerosing panencephalitis may cause slow spike-and-wave patterns in exceptional cases.

19.2.3 *Independent multifocal spikes.* *The interictal pattern* shows spikes arising independently from more than two foci (Fig. 19.8). In contrast to hypsarrhythmia, the foci of the spike discharges are constant, i.e. they do not shift in the same recording; the background shows less abnormal slow wave activity or is normal. Some spike foci may disappear and other, new, foci may appear from one recording to the next to give the appearance of migrating foci.

The ictal patterns vary widely and include both focal and generalized seizure discharges of all types seen in adults (Tables 17.1 and 18.1, Column 2).

Clinical seizures also vary widely and include partial, secondary and primary generalized seizures of most types (Tables 17.1 and 18.1, Column 3). Most patients

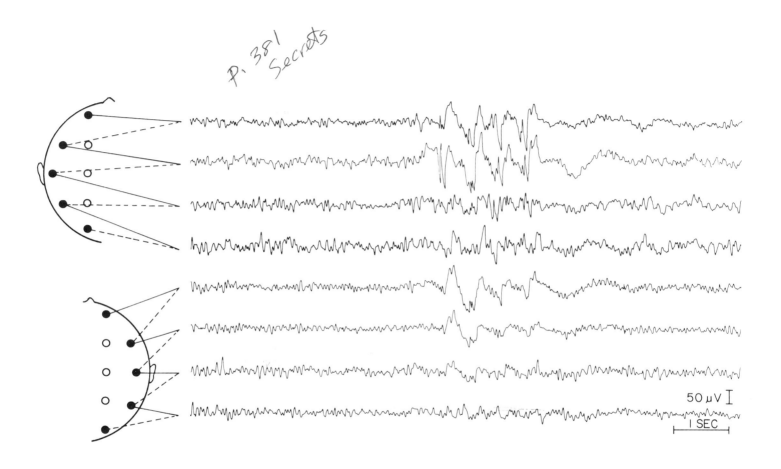

P. 381
Secrets

50 µV

1 SEC

Fig. 19.6. Pattern of slow spike-and-waves at 1.5–2 Hz, maximal over the left anterior head. This 8-year-old girl has a history of generalized seizures of many types since birth; she is slightly retarded but without other neurological abnormalities.

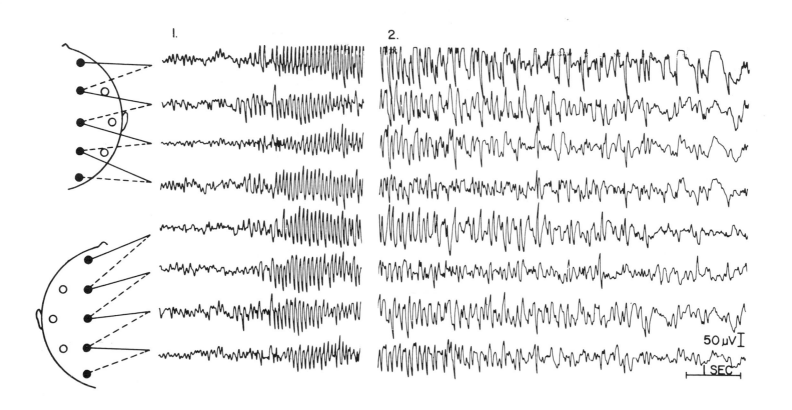

Fig. 19.7. Generalized seizure discharge in the same patient as in Fig. 19.6. 1. Generalized rhythm of high amplitude spikes at 12–14 Hz; 2. Fifteen seconds after the end of Part 1, the frequency of the spikes has slowed and slow waves begin to interrupt the spikes. This episode was associated with a mild generalized tonic seizure.

have generalized motor seizures, and many have more than one type of seizure. As is true for patients with hypsarrhythmia and slow spike-and-waves, the majority of patients with multifocal independent spikes suffer from a combination of seizures and mental retardation indicating severe and widespread cerebral damage.

Clinical conditions causing multiple independent focal spikes are the same as those causing hypsarrhythmia in younger or more severely involved patients.

see Table 19.1

19.3 PERIODIC COMPLEXES

The patterns described in this section (Table 19.2) are similar to each other in that (1) they consist of complexes which recur at fairly regular intervals on a background of slow waves of usually low amplitude; (2) most of them are generalized or widespread in distribution and synchronous in timing over different parts of the head; (3) the complexes are due to acute or subacute structural cerebral damage except in most cases of triphasic waves; (4) longer, ictal EEG discharges and clinical seizure episodes are rare: periodic complexes essentially are interictal activity; (5) some of the complexes caused by structural damage are associated with myoclonic jerks. The jerks may occur before, during or after the complexes or have a variable time relation; jerking may disappear with or without change of the complexes, but rarely do jerks appear without complexes.

19.3.1 *Periodic lateralizing epileptiform discharges (PLEDs).* The EEG pattern shows complexes which consist of a di- or polyphasic spike or sharp wave and may include a slow wave (Fig. 19.9). Complexes usually last for only a fraction of a second. They commonly appear in a wide distribution on one side of the head. In some instances, they have a focal origin and in others they are bilateral but usually with a clear maximum on one side. They may have a different shape in different

Fig 19.9

370

areas and they often vary in the same patient with time. The complexes recur every 1–2 seconds and are separated by low amplitude slow waves or by no detectable activity at regular gain. The background in regions not showing PLEDs is often abnormal. PLEDs may be interrupted by the appearance of a focal seizure discharge which may generalize.

PLEDs usually occur in the setting of an acute or subacute cerebral lesion. Among 170 reported cases etiologies included stroke (38%), neoplasm (20%), epilepsy (17%), and miscellaneous disorders including herpes encephalitis, sickle cell disease, hypoglycemia, electrolyte imbalance, subdural hematoma, tuberculoma, and unspecified infectious diseases (34%). Impaired consciousness was nearly always present, and seizures were evident in 77% of cases. The seizures were either partial or generalized and the partial seizures were always contralateral to the PLEDs.

The individual epileptiform complexes of the PLED pattern are usually not associated with any convulsive activity, but in some cases they occur in synchrony with myoclonic jerks of the opposite side of the body. Focal or generalized electrographic seizure patterns may appear to arise directly from PLEDs or they may occur simultaneously without interrupting the PLED pattern.

Although PLEDs are often considered to be continuous and invariant they may transiently attenuate or disappear during state changes, particularly during periods of arousal. The natural history of PLEDs consists of a gradual simplification of the morphology of complexes with increasingly longer repetition intervals and decreasing amplitude. This may occur over a period of days or weeks. Rarely, PLEDs may persist for years.

PLEDs may also occur independently over both hemispheres, a pattern referred to as bilateral independent periodic lateralized epileptiform discharges (BIPLEDs). In patients exhibiting BIPLEDs, diffuse or bilateral multifocal cerebral diseases, rather than those with single focal lesions, are the rule. Thus, BIPLEDs are most

371

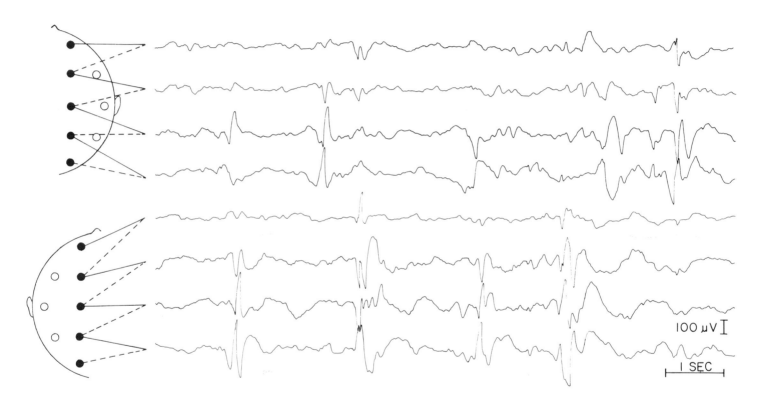

Fig. 19.8. Multifocal independent spikes. This EEG is of the same patient as in Figs. 19.1 and 19.2, now at an age of 13 months.

TABLE 19.2
Periodic and pseudoperiodic complexes

Pattern name	Wave shape	Wave duration	Interval activity	Interval duration	Distribution	Clinical seizure manifestations	Common underlying disorders	Special features
1. Periodic lateralizing epileptiform discharges ('PLEDs')		0.06–0.5 sec	Low amplitude delta, or no activity at regular gain	1–2 sec	Unilateral or bilateral and asymmetric	Epilepsia partialis continua	Recent infarction, epilepsy, encephalitis, tumor, other cortical lesions	Rarely reactive to stimuli or changes in state; usually persist into sleep
2. Periodic generalized sharp waves, often associated with Jakob-Creutzfeldt disease	Mono-, di- or triphasic sharp waves	0.15–0.6 sec	Low amplitude slow	0.5–2 sec 1/sec	Generalized, bisynchronous	Myoclonic jerks	Jakob-Creutzfeldt disease, postanoxic encephalopathy, fat embolism	Triggered by loud noise, flashes
3. Periodic generalized complexes, often associated with SSPE	One or more polyphasic sharp waves, with delta waves	0.5–3 sec	Asynch. and bisynch. theta and delta; focal spikes and slow waves	3–20 sec 4sec	Generalized, symmetrical, synchronous	Myoclonic jerks	SSPE, postanoxic myoclonus, Lennox–Gastaut syndrome, tuborous sclerosis, ketamine	Usually not triggered by stimuli; sleep may enhance or obscure the pattern
4. Suppression-burst	Irregular or regular slow waves, with or without sharp waves	1–3 sec	Low amplitude delta, or no activity at regular gain	2 sec–many minutes	Bilateral, unilateral, regional	None	Anesthesia, CNS depressant drugs, hypothermia, postanoxic encephalopathy, isolated cortex	Unreactive to stimuli
5. Triphasic waves	Major positive sharp wave, preceded and followed by minor negative waves	0.2–0.5 sec	Asynchronous and bisynchronous slow waves	0.5–2 sec	Generalized, maximal frontal or occipital	None	Hepatic, uremic and other metabolic encephalopathies, post-anoxic encephalopathy	Incidence increases with age; rare under 20 years of age; may have longitudinal delay

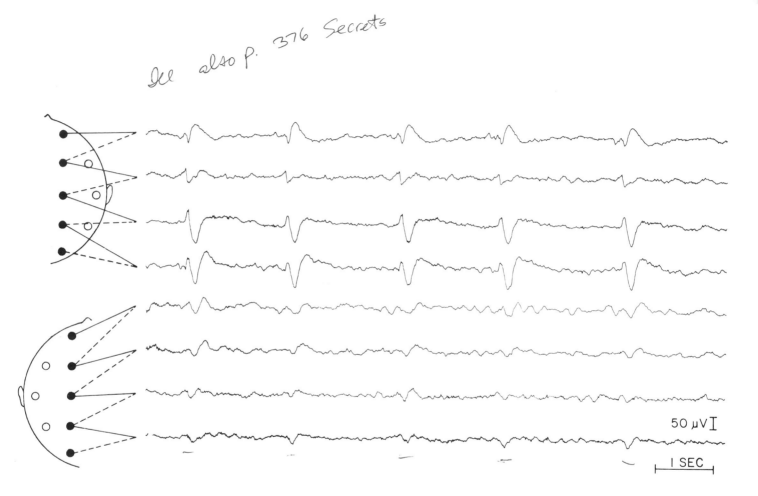

See also p. 376 Secrets

50 μV

1 SEC

Fig. 19.9. Pattern of periodic lateralizing epileptiform discharges (PLEDs) on the right side. This 70-year-old woman suddenly developed weakness and rhythmical twitching of the left arm on the day of the recording; her condition was later diagnosed as a cerebral infarct.

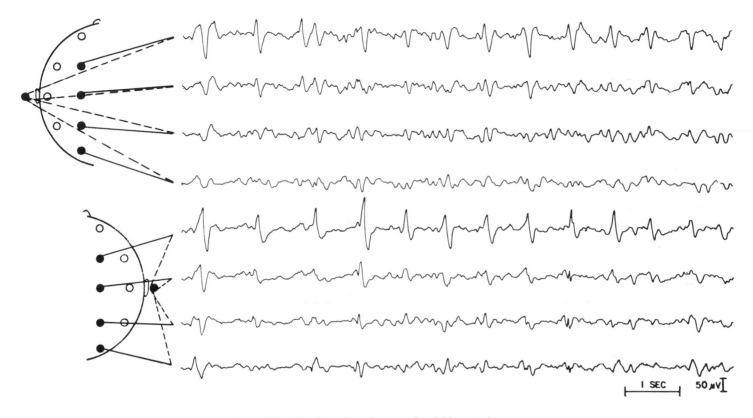

Fig. 19.10. Periodic bilateral sharp waves at about 1 Hz with a frontal maximum and variable posterior extension in a patient with Jakob-Creutzfeldt disease. This 83-year-old woman began to become confused 5 months earlier and then gradually developed dressing apraxia and illusions of a spatial distortion of objects in her left visual field. Startle myoclonus and spontaneous generalized myoclonus began soon after this EEG recording. She died 3 weeks later and her autopsy confirmed the clinical diagnosis of Jakob-Creutzfeldt disease.

often seen with <u>infections</u> (particularly <u>herpes</u> simplex encephalitis and other encephalidities), anoxic encephalopathy, epilepsy, and sickle cell anemia.

19.3.2 *Periodic generalized sharp waves, often associated with Jakob-Creutzfeldt disease. The EEG pattern* is dominated by sharp waves which usually have one, two or three phases and last up to 0.6 seconds (Fig. 19.10). When fully developed, the sharp waves appear <u>synchronously</u> in a wide distribution over both hemispheres, sometimes with a frontal maximum; while they develop, they may be focal or unilateral. The background is usually <u>highly abnormal</u> and consists of generalized asynchronous slow waves of low amplitude. Sharp waves may be triggered by startling stimuli and by light flashes.

Clinical conditions causing these sharp waves include mainly Jakob-Creutzfeldt disease. The sharp waves appear usually within <u>12 weeks</u> of the onset of clinical symptoms and are present during the fully developed disease in over 90% of all patients; they persist through the course of the disease and at the end become slower and <u>disappear</u> in a background of low amplitude. Similar sharp waves are occasionally seen in <u>postanoxic</u> encephalopathy and in <u>cerebral fat</u> embolism.

Seizure manifestations consist of widespread myoclonic jerks associated with the complexes. Startling and flash stimuli which produce sharp waves often also induce myoclonic jerks.

19.3.3 *Periodic generalized complexes, often associated with subacute sclerosing panencephalitis (SSPE).   The EEG pattern* consists of <u>high-voltage</u> (300–1500 µV) complexes containing one or more sharp waves and delta waves. Complexes last 0.5–3 seconds and recur every 3–20 seconds. The background consists of asynchronous and bisynchronous theta and delta waves; <u>bisynchronous slow spike-and-wave</u> discharges, focal spikes and slow waves may also be present. Early in the course of the disease, the background may be fairly normal and the complexes may appear in a limited distribution. Later, however, the complexes usually become

376

generalized, symmetrical and synchronous. Their shape may change with time and become disorganized before death. The complexes are usually not triggered by sensory stimuli. Sleep may enhance or obscure them.

Seizure manifestations consist of myoclonic jerks occurring with the complexes. Tonic seizures may occur with electrodecremental ictal patterns (19.2).

Clinical conditions causing these complexes include mainly subacute sclerosing panencephalitis (SSPE). The complexes may appear at any stage of the disease. Similar complexes may be seen in postanoxic encephalopathy, after head injury, in drug intoxications, lipidoses, herpes simplex encephalitis, and tuberous sclerosis.

19.3.4 *Suppression-burst pattern. The EEG pattern* consists of bursts of irregular or regular slow waves of very low frequency. They are usually widespread and bisynchronous, but they may be limited to one hemisphere or part of it. Bursts last 1–3 seconds and are separated from each other by low amplitude delta waves or by periods of no activity recognizable at regular gain (Fig. 19.11). Successive bursts may vary in shape. The duration of the intervals between the bursts is often fairly regular in a given recording and ranges from 2 to 10 seconds. The duration increases as the patient's condition worsens. Before death, bursts become shorter, simpler and of lower amplitude; periods of suppression become longer until complete electrocerebral silence supervenes. The complexes are not responsive to stimuli.

Seizure manifestations are not associated with this pattern.

Clinical conditions causing burst-suppression patterns include a variety of severe disorders of cerebral structure or function. Structural lesions include acute strokes, postanoxic encephalopathy, head injury, Wernicke's disease and encephalitis. Local burst-suppression patterns can be seen over surgically isolated cerebral cortex. Reversible disorders causing this pattern include deep anesthesia and coma due to barbiturates and other CNS depressant drugs, hypothermia and Reye's syndrome.

*p. 352 K+D
↳ contrary to SSPE

* δ or ō sharp waves –p. 352 K+D, p. 384 Secrets

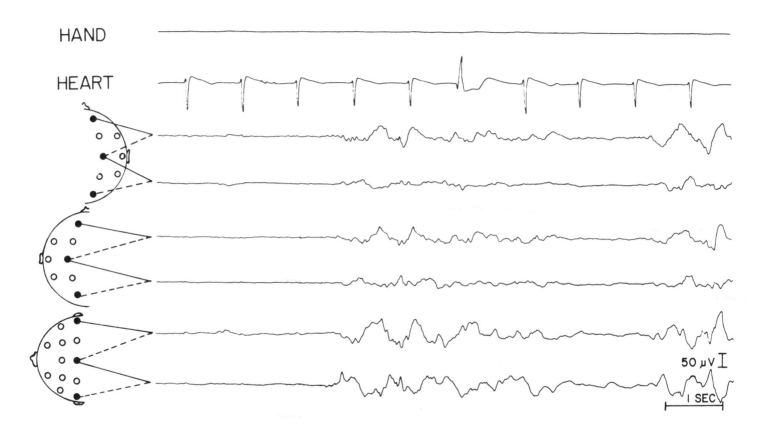

HAND

HEART

Fig. 19.11.Burst-suppression pattern recorded from a 60-year-old man in deep coma from a lethal barbiturate overdose. This recording was made in the intensive care unit with widely spaced electrodes and with monitoring of hand movement and heart beat.

50 µV

I SEC

19.3.5 *Triphasic wave pattern.* Triphasic waves are not directly associated with seizures but are included here because they frequently appear in an approximately periodic pattern. They consist of wave forms with three phases of increasing duration that clearly stand out from the background and other slow waves. The total duration of each triphasic wave complex varies between approximately 1/4 and 1/2 sec. The second phase is relatively positive in polarity and usually has the greatest amplitude of the 3 phases (Fig. 19.12). Occasionally a relatively low amplitude positive phase can be seen consistently preceeding the subsequent 3 phases. Triphasic waves may appear sporadically or periodically at 0.5–1 sec intervals.

Although the amplitude distribution of triphasic waves varies in individual cases between either anterior or posterior dominance (with some individuals showing both simultaneously or at different times in the same record), in most cases triphasic waves are maximal over the anterior head regions. In instances in which maximal amplitudes occur at Fp1 and Fp2, triphasic waves may closely resemble vertical eye movement artifact. In longitudinal bipolar recordings triphasic wave phase reversals may occur over the anterior or posterior head regions. In contrast, waves with 3 phases that have prominent phase reversals over the mid-temporal or central head regions suggest an electrographic disturbance other than the triphasic wave pattern. Triphasic waves that are consistently asymmetric suggest the presence of an additional unilateral abnormality that is often structural and usually, but not always, involves the hemisphere with lower amplitude triphasic waves.

In many cases there is an apparent phase lag (time delay) of the second phase when comparing the anterior and posterior derivations of longitudinal bipolar montages. This delay can occur in either the anterior to posterior or posterior to anterior direction and may last more than 100 msec. The majority of such phase lags are more apparent than real since they are far less common if reference montages (such as ipsilateral or linked ears) are used.

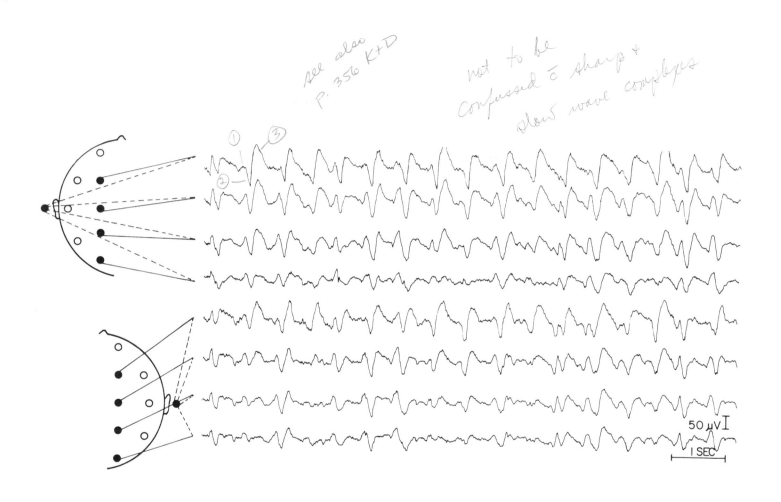

Fig. 19.12. Pattern of triphasic waves at 1–2 Hz with frontal maximum, recorded from a 68-year-old chronic alcoholic in hepatic coma.

The pathophysiology of triphasic waves is poorly understood. As with other bisynchronous patterns, thalamic pacing appears to play an important role. Unilateral lesions that attenuate thalamically generated rhythms such as sleep spindles may also attenuate triphasic waves. It is likely that triphasic wave generation is enhanced by biochemical changes associated with aging: well developed triphasic wave patterns rarely occur in individuals less than 20 years of age, are infrequent before age 30, and increase in incidence thereafter.

Clinical conditions associated with the triphasic wave pattern are mainly metabolic/toxic disturbances with the most common being hepatic failure, renal failure and anoxia. Sporadic triphasic waves are also not uncommon in elderly individuals with clinically advanced dementing disorders. The triphasic wave pattern has also been associated with other disorders including: hypo- or hypernatremia, hypercalcemia, hypoglycemia, stroke, hypertensive encephalopathy, cerebral abcess, encephalitis, congestive heart failure, septic shock, lithium intoxication and the postictal state. In the past a distinction was made between 'typical' and 'atypical' triphasic wave patterns because it was thought that 'typical' triphasic waves were highly characteristic of hepatic encephalopathy. This distinction is no longer considered valid. Indeed, the only feature that may be helpful in narrowing the list of diagnostic possibilities is severe background slowing characterized by mainly smoothly contoured background waveforms with little or no superimposed activity greater than 5 Hz. This finding is almost always seen in the setting of either hepatic, renal or anoxic encephalopathy. The reason for this association may simply be that such severe background slowing is less likely to occur in the other disorders associated with triphasic waves.

19.4 ICTAL PATTERNS WITHOUT SPIKES AND SHARP WAVES

The patterns in this section (Table 19.3) are described in the chapters dealing with local and generalized epileptiform activity. They are joined here because they are

381

TABLE 19.3
Ictal patterns without spikes and sharp waves

Ictal pattern	Distribution	Interictal patterns	Clinical seizure type
1. Three hertz rhythmical slow waves	Generalized	3 Hz spike-and-wave, 3 Hz slow waves, or normal	Absence, absence status, generalized seizures
2. Theta or delta waves	Generalized	Slow spike-and-wave	Tonic seizures
3. Rhythmical 4–6 (2–10) Hz waves	Bilateral or unilateral, temporal or fronto-temporal	Spikes or sharp waves in the temporal area	Complex partial seizures
4. Delta or theta waves in periodic complexes	Generalized	Complexes of SSPE	Myoclonic jerks
5. Periodic or rhythmical slow waves	Localized	None	Epilepsia partialis continua
6. Loss of amplitude ('electro-decremental seizures')	Generalized	Hypsarrhythmia, slow spike-and-wave	Infantile spasms, tonic seizures
7. Paroxysmal low voltage	Temporal, fronto-temporal, bilateral or unilateral	Spikes or sharp waves in the temporal area	Complex partial seizures
8. No change of background	–	Spikes or sharp waves in the temporal area	Complex partial seizures
9. No change of background	–	None	Epilepsia partialis continua
10. Alpha waves	Focal, unilateral	Spikes, sharp waves, abnormal newborn patterns	Neonatal seizures
11. Beta waves	Focal, unilateral	Spikes, sharp waves, abnormal newborn patterns	Neonatal seizures
12. Beta waves	Central	Spikes, polyspikes or normal	Action myoclonus
13. Beta waves (14–20 Hz)	Bilateral or unilateral, maximum temporal or fronto-temporal	Spikes or sharp waves in the temporal area	Complex partial seizures

related to each other in that they represent ictal activity which (1) has no spikes or sharp waves; (2) usually begins and ends abruptly; and (3) is often recognized only by its association with clinical seizure manifestations. Some of these patterns are local, others are generalized; some occur mainly with one type of interictal pattern or seizure, others occur with a variety of interictal patterns and seizure types.

19.4.1   *Generalized ictal slow waves.*   *Rhythmical bisynchronous slow waves at 3 Hz* are occasionally seen instead of 3 Hz spike-and-wave discharges in absence attacks, especially in absence status. Similar slow waves may occur as interictal activity in patients with attacks of absences or of other primary generalized seizures.

Theta or delta waves, often irregular, asynchronous and arrhythmical, may be associated with tonic seizures which occur especially in patients with slow spike-and-wave discharges.

Rhythmical 4–6 Hz waves or, occasionally, 2–10 Hz waves with a maximum in both temporal of fronto-temporal regions are a common ictal pattern of complex partial seizures even in patients who have spike foci in only one temporal lobe.

Slow waves in periodic complexes and hypsarrhythmia may be associated with myoclonic jerks, for instance in subacute sclerosing panencephalitis.

19.4.2   *Local ictal slow waves.*   *Rhythmical 4–6 Hz waves,* or 2–10 Hz waves, with a maximum in the temporal or fronto-temporal regions of one hemisphere occur in complex partial seizures.

Periodic or rhythmical slow waves are seen instead of periodic lateralizing discharges in some patients with epilepsia partialis continua.

19.4.3   *Generalized decrease of amplitude.*   *Electrodecremental seizures* are associated with sudden reduction of high amplitude background activity such as occurs in hypsarrhythmia and in recordings showing slow spike-and-wave activity;

these patterns are replaced by ictal generalized flattening of the tracing or low amplitude fast activity which lasts for several seconds and are often associated with infantile spasms and tonic seizures. Electrodecremental events also occur in some adults during tonic seizures.

The sudden appearance of low voltage activity, replacing a background which usually does not contain epileptiform activity, is one seizure pattern of complex partial seizures.

Sudden loss of amplitude or low voltage fast activity also occurs in non-epileptic attacks of decerebration, often called 'cerebellar fits'.

19.4.4 *No change of background activity* is a rare accompaniment of complex partial seizures and of epilepsia partialis continua.

19.4.5 *Alpha waves,* usually unilateral or focal in distribution, can be seen in newborn and very young infants with partial, unilateral and generalized seizures or status epilepticus; unilateral or bilateral waves of alpha frequency are also the ictal pattern of some patients with complex partial seizures.*

19.4.6 *Beta waves* may appear instead of the ictal alpha activity in some newborn infants. Fast waves of 14–20 Hz may appear with a maximum in the temporal or fronto-temporal regions in complex partial seizures at any age after infancy. Central rhythmic beta activity, with or without spikes, may be associated with movement-activated myoclonus in adults, usually as a result of cerebral anoxia.

see Table 19.3

19.5 EPILEPTIFORM PATTERNS WITHOUT PROVEN RELATION TO SEIZURES ('PSEUDO-EPILEPTOGENIC PATTERNS')

These patterns (Table 19.4) are similar to each other in that they (1) consist of

* PCS et can have almost any ictal pattern

epileptiform activity of usually short duration, (2) have no corresponding ictal patterns, and (3) are not known to be associated with seizures or neurological diseases except that the first of the patterns listed below may be difficult to distinguish from the interictal activity of some patients with seizures and the second pattern is occasionally seen in hepatic encephalopathy. In the past, unsubstantiated claims have been made that the first four patterns below are commonly seen in patients with seizures, in persons with various symptoms referable to the autonomic nervous system (especially dizziness, syncope, nausea, headaches), and in subjects with personality or behavior disorders.

19.5.1 *Six-per-second spike-and-wave discharges* ('phantom spike-wave') consist of a 4–7 Hz repetitive spike-and-wave complex with a relatively low amplitude (less than 40 µV), fast spike (less than 30 msec) followed by a 5–7 Hz wave of equal or greater amplitude. Each burst usually appears in a bisynchronous fashion, lasts less than 1 sec, and occurs during drowsiness or during eye closure at rest.

Two different forms of the 6-per-second spike-and-wave discharge have been described. The classical form is relatively low in amplitude and is maximal over the posterior head regions (Fig. 19.13). Its incidence in normal individuals is increased significantly by intravenous diphenhydramine and it is clearly not associated with seizures. The second form is frontally dominant, often moderate or high in amplitude, but the spikes appear with lower amplitude than intervening waves. This form of 6-per-second spike-and-wave discharge overlaps with abnormal epileptiform patterns with rapid repetition rates. The likelihood that frontally dominant rapid spike-and-wave discharges are associated with seizure disorders increases if the repetition rate is less than 5 Hz or the spikes are clearly much greater in amplitude than the intervening slow waves. The interpretation of anterior dominant spike-and-wave patterns with rapid repetition rates therefore requires careful consideration.

385

TABLE 19.4
Pseudo-epileptiform patterns

[handwritten top margin: "most are temporal"; "all during sleep/drowsiness. ↑ some also alert"]

[handwritten left margin: "Fig page", "387", "388", "389", "390", "p.49 Epstein", "394", "392"]

Pattern name	Wave shape	Duration	Distribution	Age	Vigilance
1. Six hertz spike-and-slow-wave ('wave and spike phantom')	Miniature spike-and-wave at 4–7 Hz	Less than 1 sec *(in trains)*	Generalized, maximum often posterior	Adults, less often adolescents	Drowsy, awake
2. Fourteen and six hertz positive bursts *(spikes)*	Repetitive positive spikes arch-shaped	Less than 1–2 sec	Posterior temporal, parietal, bilaterally independent or synchronous	Adolescents, children; less often adults	Sleep, drowsiness
3. Rhythmical mid-temporal discharge ('RMTD') ('Psycho-motor variant')	6 (4–7) Hz negative sharp waves with notched or flat positive phases	Up to a few seconds	Midtemporal, unilateral, bilateral, independent or bisynchronous	Slightly more in middle-aged females	Sleep
4. Small sharp spikes ('sss'), benign epileptiform transients of sleep ('BETS')	Short spikes, usually small	Less than 50 msec for single phase	Mid- and anterior temporal, often shifting in distribution; unilateral, bilaterally independent or bisynchronous	Adults, adolescents	Sleep
5. Wicket spikes	Often repetitive spikes forming arches *(big)*	Repeating up to a few seconds	Anterior and middle temporal ⊙	Mainly adults *('wicked')*	Awake, asleep
6. Occipital spikes and sharp waves of blind persons	Focal spikes and sharp waves	Up to 200 msec	Occipital, unilateral or bilateral	Often children	Awake, asleep
7. SREDA	Mono- or bi-phasic sharp wave(s) followed by rhythmic 4–7-Hz waves	Less than 10 sec to more than 5 min; usually 40–80 sec	Often symmetrical and posterior temporal and parietal maximal but may be unilateral or asymmetric	Adults	Awake, asleep *[most common]*
8. Paroxysmal hypnogogic hypersynchrony	3–5-Hz moderate to high amplitude rhythmic bursts with intermixed spikes, *notching*	1–6 sec	Generalized, maximum anterior or posterior	Children	Drowsy
9. Midline theta * rhythms (of Cigánek)	4–7 Hz rhythmic trains with sinusoidal, spiky or arciform shape	Typically 4–20 sec	Midline, usually central	Children and adults	Awake, drowsy

386   *[handwritten: * not in text]*   *[handwritten: Δ as RMTD]*

[handwritten: ⊙ unlike me]

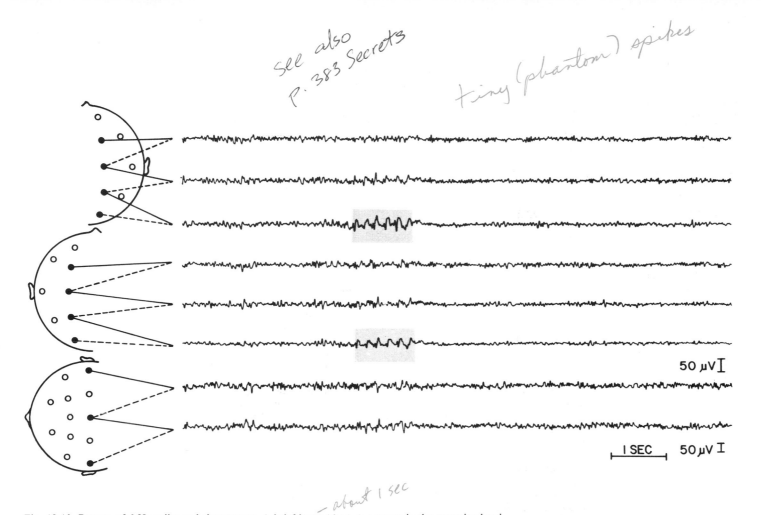

see also
P. 383 Secrets

tiny (phantom) spikes

50 μV

1 SEC   50 μV

about 1 sec

Fig. 19.13. Pattern of 6 Hz spike-and-slow-waves. A brief burst (shaded) appears in the posterior head regions during drowsiness. This 40-year-old woman has a history of headaches, no abnormal findings.

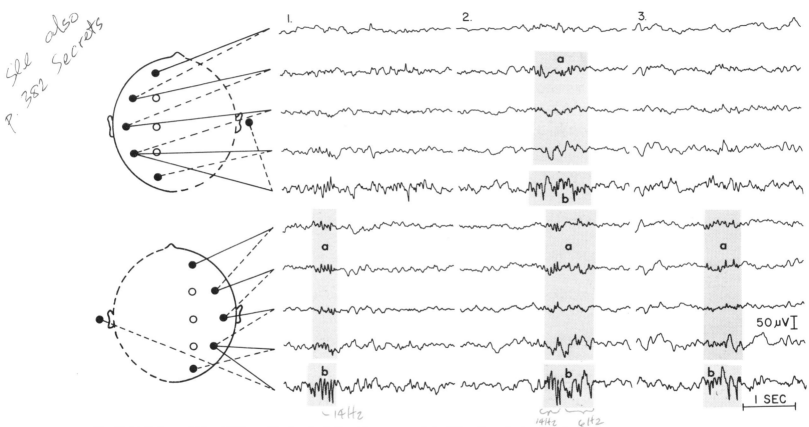

Fig. 19.14. Pattern of 14 and 6 Hz positive bursts. 1, 2 and 3 were recorded within a few minutes of each other during light sleep. Note that the bursts are barely distinguishable in conventional bipolar linkages between adjacent electrodes (a), but are greatly enhanced by the use of long interelectrode distances between posterior temporal electrodes and the opposite ear (b). This 12-year-old girl had a slight concussion 4 days earlier; the neurological examination is normal.

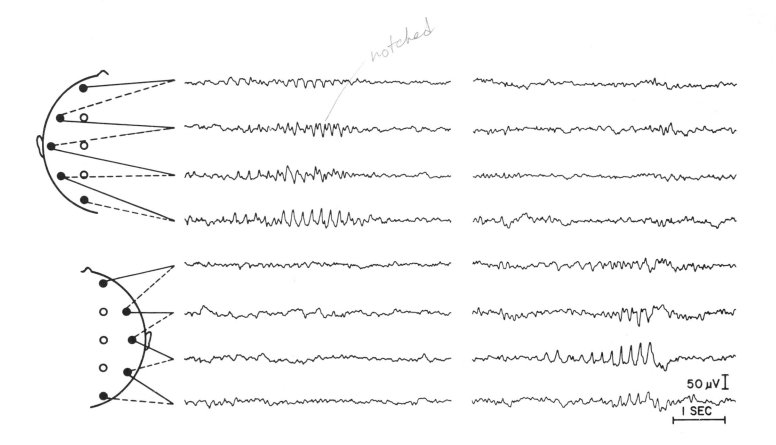

notched

Fig. 19.15. Rhythmical midtemporal discharges (RMTD) at about 6 Hz, occurring independently on either side during light sleep. The patient is a 19-year-old girl with one seizure 5 years earlier, now normal.

389

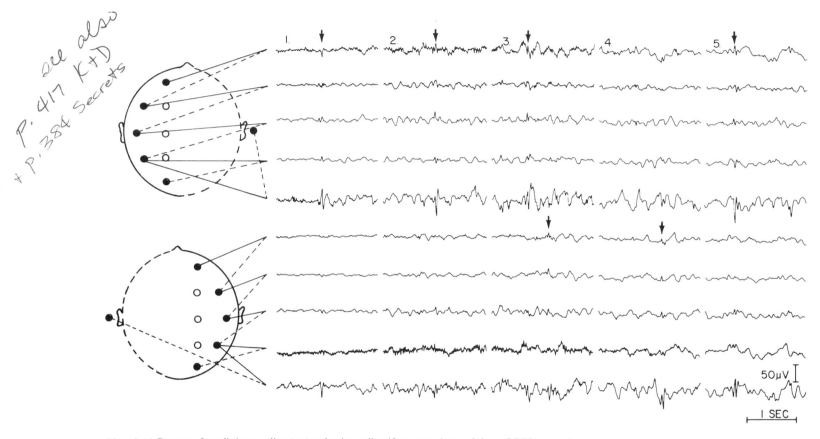

P. 417 K+D *see also* *+ P. 384 Secrets*

Fig. 19.16. Pattern of small sharp spikes (sss) or benign epileptiform transients of sleep (BETS) occurring independently in the temporal regions during light sleep. 1–5. were recorded within five minutes. Note that the amplitude of the spikes (arrows) is greatly increased in interelectrode linkages from the posterior temporal electrodes to the opposite ears. This 15-year-old girl complains of dizziness which is probably due to hyperventilation.

390

19.5.2 *Fourteen- and six-per-second positive spikes* ('ctenoids') consist of brief runs (usually less than 1 sec) of positive spikes repeating at approximately 14 or 6 Hz. This pattern occurs either bisynchronously or unilaterally (usually involving both hemispheres at different times). It may be difficult to recognize in bipolar montages and is best seen in ear reference montages or those with long interelectrode distances. The 14-Hz pattern is far more common than the 6-Hz pattern, but both may occur simultaneously (Fig. 19.14). The 14-Hz pattern often looks like a sleep spindle with a sharp positive phase, although its location is quite different; it is greatest in amplitude over the posterior temporal head regions. The sharp components often have a negative polarity in nasopharyngeal recordings.

Fourteen- and six-per-second positive spikes are most likely to occur during sleep in adolescents. Their peak incidence (over 25% of normal subjects) occurs between ages 12 and 13. An unexplained finding is 14- and 6-per-second positive spikes in comatose patients with acute Reye's syndrome, in severe toxic liver disease, or other metabolic and postanoxic encephalopathies. In such cases the pattern may differ from that seen in normal individuals in that the frequency is often more variable and the bursts can be elicited by alerting stimuli.

19.5.3 *Rhythmical midtemporal discharges* (formerly also called 'psychomotor variant') are bursts of rhythmical sharp waves at about 6 Hz (range of 4–7 Hz) which often have a top which is flat or notched by a small 12 Hz component (Fig. 19.15). These bursts may last for up to a few seconds. They often begin and end with a gradual increase and decrease of amplitude. They occur in the midtemporal regions, either on one side or on both and then either independently or simultaneously. They are mostly seen in young adults during light sleep. These bursts are distinguished from ictal discharges in patients with interictal temporal lobe spikes in that they do not vary much in duration and wave shape and thus resemble neither the

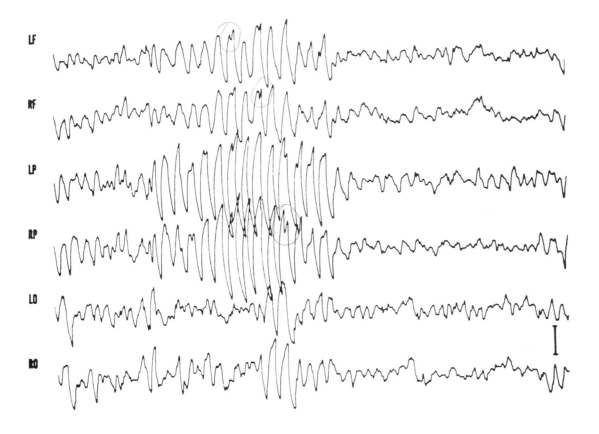

LF

Rf

LP

RP

LO

RO

Fig. 19.17. Paroxysmal hypnogogic hypersynchrony. Notched pattern. Courtesy P. Kellaway, Current
Practice of Clinical Electroencephalography, 1979.

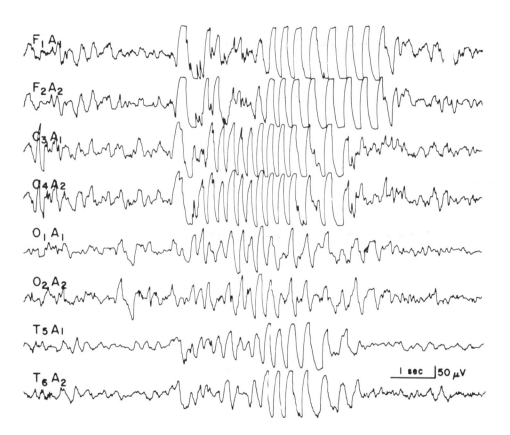

Fig. 19.18. Paroxysmal hypnogogic hypersynchrony. Irregular intermixed spike patterns. Courtesy P. Kellaway, Current Practice of Clinical Electroencephalography, 1979.

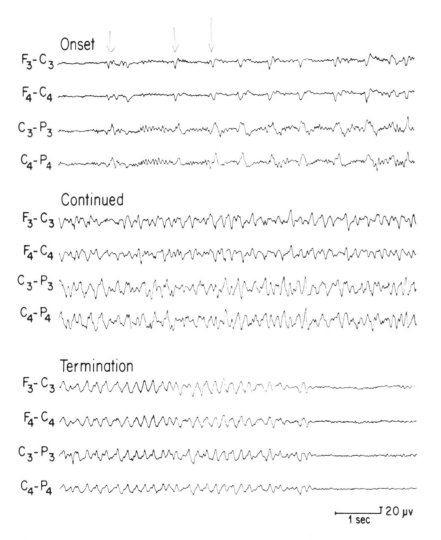

Fig. 19.19. Subclinical rhythmic EEG discharge of adults (SREDA) in a 60-year-old woman during wakefulness with abrupt onset and gradual evolution to 5-Hz rhythmic activity. Courtesy, B.F. Westmoreland, EEG clin. Neurophysiol. 51: 186–191, 1981.

interictal single spikes nor the ictal, sustained and changing discharges of temporal lobe foci.

19.5.4 *Small sharp spikes.*

Small sharp spikes, or *benign epileptiform transients of sleep* ('BETS'), are sharply contoured mono- or bi-phasic (rarely tri- or quadri-phasic) low amplitude, very brief duration (less than 65 msec) waveforms (Fig. 19.16). Identifying features of small sharp spikes include their typically widespread distribution and horizontal dipole configuration. Although they are often greatest in amplitude over the temporal head regions (as shown in depth electrode recordings), they are characteristically difficult to localize precisely and often appear in both hemispheres either independently or bisynchronously. They frequently demonstrate an opposite polarity in the anterior to posterior direction in a single hemisphere or transversely between hemispheres when they occur bisynchronously (i.e., a horizontal dipole configuration; true phase reversals). Another distinguishing feature of small sharp spikes is that they rarely repeat with the same distribution and morphology more than once per second. Although the name 'small' suggests they are always very low in amplitude, this may not be the case, particularly in montages with long interelectrode distances or in nasopharyngeal electrode recordings.

19.5.5 *Wicket spikes*

occur in the anterior or middle temporal areas with a negative polarity and an amplitude of up to more than 200 μV. They differ from other, abnormal, spikes in that they appear not only intermittently but also repetitively in trains of arch-shaped rhythms resembling mu rhythm.
They therefore represent a sudden accentuation of individual waveforms arising from a sharply contoured background. Although wicket spikes were originally described as temporal in location and mainly occurring in older individuals, it is important to be aware that similar isolated sharply contoured waveforms may occur over *any* head region where there is sharply contoured background activity.

395

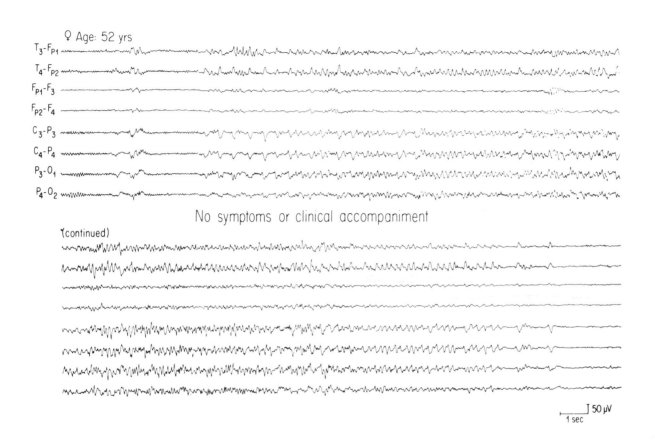

Fig. 19.20. Subclinical rhythmic EEG discharge of adults (SREDA) in a 52-year-old woman with headaches preceded by a widespread, moderate to high amplitude, biphasic waveform. Courtesy, B.F. Westmoreland, EEG clin. Neurophysiol. 51: 186–191, 1981.

19.5.6 *Occipital spikes of blind persons* may occur after lesions of the visual path anterior to the occipital cortex, usually in congenital or long-standing acquired blindness. Associated abnormalities are disorganization of alpha rhythm, loss of photic responses and absence of lambda waves and POSTs. This condition differs from cerebral blindness due to bilateral occipital lesions which may be associated with epileptiform activity and seizures. *see Table 19.4*

19.5.7 *Paroxysmal hypnogogic hypersynchrony* is a variant of hypnogogic hypersynchrony and therefore occurs in normal children during drowsiness or arousal from sleep. It consists of low amplitude spikes intermixed with rhythmical moderate to high amplitude 3–5 Hz bisynchronous bursts. The spike-like components most often take the form of a simple notching of the slow waves (Fig. 19.17). In other cases they are irregularly intermixed with the slow waves or may form brief runs with the appearance of multiple spike complexes (Fig. 19.18). A distinguishing feature of the irregularly intermixed spike components is their superimposed appearance; there is an inconsistent time relationship between the spikes and the slow waves.

19.5.8 *Subclinical rhythmic EEG discharge of adults (SREDA).* Like rhythmical midtemporal discharges (RMTD), SREDA is likely to be misinterpreted as an ictal epileptiform pattern. Unlike RMTD, SREDA occurs mainly in elderly* individuals during wakefulness (in nearly all cases), during or shortly after hyperventilation (in some individuals only during hyperventilation), and occasionally during sleep. It also differs from RMTD in its topographic distribution and it does not contain prominent harmonically related waveforms. Since SREDA invariably occurs while the patient is awake, response testing can be performed to demonstrate that, in contrast to many epileptic events, consciousness and mentation are preserved. Other distinctive characteristics of this pattern are: (1) its tendency to occur several times in a

397

*... of adults

single routine recording (over 15 times in some reported cases); and (2) its tendency to be present in subsequent EEGs, even when more than 12 years have elapsed between recordings.

SREDA typically begins abruptly (Fig. 19.19) or is delayed 1 to several seconds after a single high amplitude mono- or bi-phasic sharp or slow wave component (Fig. 19.20). Once established, the pattern consists of repetitive monophasic sharp waveforms (approximately 150–300 msec in duration) that repeat every 1–2 sec and gradually evolve into a sustained sinusoidal 4–7 Hz pattern (usually 5–6 Hz). The pattern may either end abruptly or gradually diminish and merge with the background.

In approximately two-thirds of cases the discharges are bisynchronous and symmetrically distributed and are maximal over the parietal and posterior temporal regions. In other cases it is either asymmetric or unilateral. The average duration of the discharge is typically 40–80 sec, but it may be less than 10 sec or more than 5 min. In most cases it replaces the ongoing background activity. In other cases the background may persist. For example, during wakefulness reactivity of the alpha rhythm may be discernable and during sleep vertex waves and sleep spindles may be seen.

REFERENCES

Aicardi, J. (1986) Epilepsy in Children. Raven, New York.

Aicardi, J. and Gomes, A.L. (1989) The myoclonic epilepsies of childhood. Cleveland Clin. J. Med. 56 (Suppl. 1): S34–39.

Blume W.T. (1978) Clinical and electroencephalographic correlates of the multiple independent spike foci pattern in children. Ann. Neurol. 4: 541–547.

Blume, W.T. (1987) Lennox-Gastaut Syndrome. In: Luders, H. and Lesser, R.P. (Eds.), Epilepsy: Electroclinical Syndromes. Springer, New York, pp. 73–92.

Catani, P., Salzarulo, P. and Findji, F. (1978) Occipital spikes and eye movement activity during paradoxical sleep in visually defective children. Electroenceph. clin. Neurophysiol. 44: 782–784.

Celesia, G.G. (1973) Pathophysiology of periodic EEG complexes in subacute sclerosing panencephalitis (SSPE). Electroenceph. clin. Neurophysiol. 35: 293–300.

Charlton, M.H. (1975) Myoclonic Seizures. Excerpta Medica, Amsterdam.

Chatrian, G.E., Shaw, C.M. and Leffman, H. (1964) The significance of periodic lateralized epileptiform discharges in EEG: An electrographic, clinical and pathological study. Electroenceph. clin. Neurophysiol. 17: 177–193.

Ch'ien, L.T., Boehm, R.M., Robinson, H., Liu, C. and Frenkel, L.D. (1977) Characteristic early electroencephalographic changes in herpes simplex encephalitis. Clinical and virologic studies. Arch. Neurol. 34: 361–364.

Chiofalo, N., Fuentes, A. and Gálves, C. (1980) Serial EEG findings in 27 cases of Creutzfeldt-Jakob disease. Arch. Neurol. 37: 143–145.

Clancy, R.R. and Legido, A. (1987) The exact ictal and interictal duration of electroencephalographic neonatal seizures. Epilepsia 28: 537–541.

Clancy, R.R., Legido, A. and Lewis, D. (1988) Occult neonatal seizures. Epilepsia 29: 256–261.

Cobb, W.A. (1979) Evidence on the periodic mechanism in herpes simplex encephalitis. Electroenceph. clin. Neurophysiol. 46: 345–350.

De la Paz, D. and Brenner, R.P. (1981) Bilateral independent periodic lateralized epileptiform discharges. Arch. Neurol. 38: 713–715.

Drury, I. (1989) Epileptiform patterns of children. J. Clin. Neurophysiol. 6: 1–39.

Drury, I., Klass, D.W., Westmoreland, B.F. and Sharbrough, F.W. (1985) An acute syndrome with psychiatric symptoms and EEG abnormalities. Arch. Neurol. 35: 911–914.

Eeg-Olofsson, O. (1971) The development of the electroencephalogram in normal children from the age of 1 through 15 years. 14 and 6 Hz positive spike phenomenon. Neuropaediatrie 2: 405–427.

Fisch, B.J. and Klass, D.W. (1988) The diagnostic specificity of triphasic wave patterns. Electroenceph. clin. Neurophysiol. 70: 1–8.

Fisch, B.J. and Pedley, T.A. (1985) Evaluation of focal cerebral lesions. Role of electroencephalography in the era of computerized tomography. In: Aminoff, M.J. (Ed.), Electrodiagnosis, Neurologic Clinics. Saunders, Philadelphia, pp. 649–662.

Gabor, A.J. and Seyal, M. (1986) Effect of sleep on the electroencephalographic manifestations of epilepsy. J. clin. Neurophysiol. 3: 23–38.

Gibbs, F.A. and Gibbs, E.L. (1952) Atlas of Electroencephalography, Vol. 2, Epilepsy, Addison-Wesley, Cambridge, MA.

Gurvitch, A.M., Zarzhetsky, Y.V., Trush, V.D. and Zonov, V.M. (1984) Experimental data on the nature of post-resusitation alpha frequency activity. Electroenceph. clin. Neurophysiol. 58: 426–437.

Harrison, A., Lairy, G.C. and Leger, E.M. (1970) EEG et privation visuelle. Electroenceph clin. Neurophysiol. 29: 20–37.

Hrachovy, R.A. and Frost Jr., J.D. (1989) Infantile spasms. Cleveland Clin. J. Med. 56 (Suppl.1): S10–16.

Hrachovy, R.A., Frost Jr., F.D. and Kellaway, P. (1984) Hypsarrhythmia: variations on the theme. Epilepsia 25: 317–325.

Kellaway, P., Hrachovy, R.A., Frost Jr., J.D. and Zion, R. (1979) Precise characterization and quantification of infantile spasms. Ann. Neurol. 6: 214–218.

Kellaway, P. and Mizrahi, E.M. (1987) Neonatal seizures. In: Luders, H. and Lesser, R.P. (Eds.), Epilepsy: Electroclinical Syndromes. Springer, New York, pp. 151–187.

Klass, D.W. and Westmoreland, B.F. (1985) Nonepileptogenic epileptiform electroencephalographic activity. Ann. Neurol. 18: 627–635.

Kuroiwa, Y. and Celesia, G.G. (1980) Clinical significance of periodic EEG patterns. Arch. Neurol. 37: 15–20.

Lai, C.-W. and Gragasin, M.E. (1988) Electroencephalography in Herpes Simplex encephalitis. J. clin. Neurophysiol. 5: 87–103.

Lee, S.I. (1983) Electroencephalography in infantile and childhood epilepsy. In: Dreifuss, F.E. (Ed.), Pediatric Epileptology. John Wright, Boston, pp. 33–64.

Lee, S.I. and Kirby, D. (1988) Absence seizure with generalized rhythmic delta activity. Epilepsia 29: 262–267.

Lee, B.I. and Schauwecker, D.S. (1988) Regional cerebral perfusion in PLEDs: A case report. Epilepsia 29: 607–611.

Levy, S.R., Chiappa, K.H., Burke, C.J. and Young, R.R. (1986) Early evolution and incidence of electroencephalographic abnormalities in Creutzfeldt–Jacob disease. J. clin. Neurophysiol. 3: 1–21.

Lipman, I.J. and Hughes, J.R. (1969) Rhythmic mid-temporal discharges. An electroclinical study. Electroenceph. clin. Neurophysiol. 27: 43–47.

Lombroso, C.T., Schwartz, I.H., Clark, D.M., Muench, H. and Barry, J. (1966) Ctenoids in healthy youths. Controlled study of 14- and 6-per second positive spiking. Neurology 16: 1152–1158.

Lombroso, C.T. (1987) Neonatal Electroencephalography. In: Niedermeyer, E. and Lopes da Silva, F. (Eds.), Electroencephalography: Basic Principles, Clinical Applications and Related Fields. Urban and Schwarzenberg, Baltimore, pp. 725–762.

McCutchen, C.B., Coen, R. and Iragui, V.J. (1984) Periodic lateralized epileptiform discharges in asphyxiated neonates. Electroenceph. clin. Neurophysiol. 61: 210–217.

MacGillivray, B.B. (1976) Section III. The EEG in liver disease. In: Rémond, A. (Ed.), Handbook of Electroenceph. clin. Neurophysiol., Vol. 15C. Elsevier, Amsterdam, pp. 26–50.

Markand, O.N. and Panszi, J.G. (1975) The electroencephalogram in subacute sclerosing panencephalitis. Arch. Neurol. 32: 719–726.

Maulsby, R.L. (1979) EEG patterns of uncertain diagnostic significance. In: Klass, D.W. and Daly, D.D. (Eds.), Current Practice of Clinical Electroencephalography. Raven, New York, pp. 411–419.

Miller, C.R., Westmoreland, B.F. and Klass, D.W. (1985) Subclinical rhythmic EEG discharge of adults (SREDA): Further observations. Am. J. EEG Technol. 25: 217–224.

Mizrahi, E.M. and Kellaway, P. (1987) Characterization and classification of neonatal seizures. Neurology 37: 1837–1844.

Mizrahi, E.M. and Tharp, B.A. (1982) A characteristic EEG pattern in neonatal herpes simplex encephalitis. Neurology 32: 1215–1220.

Mokrán, V., Cigánek, L. and Kabátnik, Z. (1971) Electroencephalographic theta discharges in the midline. Eur. Neurol. 5: 288–293.

Noriega-Sanchez, A. and Markand, O.N. (1976) Clinical and electroencephalographic correlation of independent multifocal spike discharges. Neurology 26: 667–672.

PeBenito, R. and Cracco, J. (1979) Periodic lateralized epileptiform discharges in infants and children. Ann. Neurol. 6: 47–50.

Pedley, T.A. (1981) EEG patterns that mimic epileptiform discharges but have no association with seizures. In: Henry, C. (Ed.), Current clinical Neurophysiology. Elsevier, Amsterdam, pp. 307–336.

Pettit, R.E. (1987) Pyridoxine dependency seizures: Report of a case with unusual features. J. Child Neurol. 2: 38–40.

Reiher, J. and Lebel, M. (1977) Wicket spikes: Clinical correlates of a previously undescribed EEG pattern. Can. J. Neurol. Sci. 4: 39–47.

Rose, A.L. and Lombroso, C.T. (1970) Neonatal seizure states. A study of clinical, pathological, and electroencephalographic features in 137 full-term babies with long-term follow-up. Pediatrics 45: 404–425.

Schraeder, P.L. and Singh, N. (1980) Seizure disorders following periodic lateralized epileptiform discharges. Epilepsia 21: 647–653.

Schwartz, M.S., Prior, P.F. and Scott, D.F. (1973) The occurrence and evolution in the EEG of a lateralized periodic phenomenon. Brain 96: 613–622.

Shibasaki, H., Yamashita, Y. and Kuroiwa, Y. (1978) Electroencephalographic studies of myoclonus. Myoclonus-related cortical spikes and high amplitude somatosensory evoked potentials. Brain 101: 447–460.

Smith, J.B., Westmoreland, B.F., Reagan, T.J. and Sandok, B.A. (1975) A distinctive clinical EEG profile in herpes simplex encephalitis. Mayo Clin. Proc. 50: 469–474.

Snodgrass, S.M., Tsuburaya, K. and Ajmone-Marsan, C. (1989) Clinical significance of periodic lateralized epileptiform discharges: Relationship with status epilepticus. J. clin. Neurophysiol. 6: 159–172.

Tharp, B.R. (1986) Neonatal and pediatric electroencephalography. In: Aminoff, M.J. (Ed.), Electrodiagnosis in Clinical Neurology. Churchill/Livingstone, New York, pp. 77–124.

Thomas, J.E., Reagan, T.J. and Klass, D.W. (1977) Epilepsia partialis continua. Arch. Neurol. 34: 266–275.

Thomas, J.E. and Klass, D.W. (1968) Six-per-second spike-and-wave pattern in the electroencephalogram: A reappraisal of its clinical significance. Neurology 18: 587–593.

Walsh, J.M. and Brenner, R.P. (1987) Periodic lateralized epileptiform discharges: Long term outcome in adults. Epilepsia 28: 533–536.

Werner, S.S., Stockard, J.E. and Bickford, R.G. (1977) Atlas of Neonatal EEG. Raven, New York.

Westmoreland, B.F., Groover, R.V. and Sharbrough, F.W. (1979) Electrographic findings in three types of cerebromacular degeneration. Mayo Clin. Proc. 54: 12–21.

Westmoreland, B.F., Sharbrough, F.W. and Donat, J.R. (1979) Stimulus-induced EEG complexes and motor spasms in subacute sclerosing pancencephalitis. Neurology 29: 1154–1157.

Westmoreland, B.F. and Gomez, M.R. (1987) Infantile Spasms (West Syndrome). In: Luders, H. and Lesser, R.P. (Eds.), Epilepsy: Electroclinical Syndromes. Springer, New York, pp. 49–72.

Westmoreland, B.F. and Klass, D.W. (1981) A distinctive rhythmic EEG discharge of adults. Electroenceph. clin. Neurophysiol. 51: 186–191.

Westmoreland, B.F. and Klass, D.W. (1986) Midline theta rhythm. Arch. Neurol. 43: 139–141.

Westmoreland, B.F., Reiher, J. and Klass, D.W. (1979) Recording small sharp spikes with depth electroencephalography. Epilepsia 20: 599–606.

White, J.C., Langston, J.W. and Pedley, T.A. (1977) Benign epileptiform transients of sleep. Neurology 27: 1061–1068.

Yamada, T., Young, S. and Kimura, J. (1977) Significance of positive spike bursts in Reye syndrome. Arch. Neurol. 34: 376–380.

Local slow waves

20

SUMMARY

(20.1) *The pattern* of local slow waves consists of waves which have a frequency under 8 Hz and a limited distribution; they are usually restricted to one or a few neighboring electrodes, i.e., to a focus of slow waves; less often, they occupy an entire hemisphere.

(20.2) *The cause* of local slow waves is a circumscribed abnormality located superficially or deeply in a hemisphere. Commonly the abnormality is a structural lesion which has an acute onset or a progressive course. In the case of acute lesions, the slow waves develop at the time of the damage and persist for weeks or months. Slow waves may also occur as a result of transient local abnormalities such as epileptiform activity and ischemia and then outlast the transient event by several hours or a few days.

(20.3) *Other EEG abnormalities* are often associated with focal slow waves and may further clarify the location and type of the underlying lesion.

(20.4) *Mechanisms* generating focal slow waves include functional or structural interruption of corticocortical and corticosubcortical fiber connections.

(20.5) *Specific disorders* associated with focal slow waves include a variety of structural lesions such as tumors, infarcts, hemorrhages, abscesses and several kinds of transient abnormalities such as transient ischemic attacks, migraine, partial seizures and hypertensive encephalopathy.

20.1 DESCRIPTION OF PATTERN

Local slow waves consist of waves of less than 8 Hz which commonly appear at only one or a few electrodes, i.e. in a focal distribution (Figs. 20.1; 20.3; 20.4); less common are slow waves which are distributed over an entire hemisphere, i.e. unilateral slow waves (Fig. 20.2). Individual slow waves are often irregular and successive slow waves often are arrhythmical, i.e. composed of different fre-

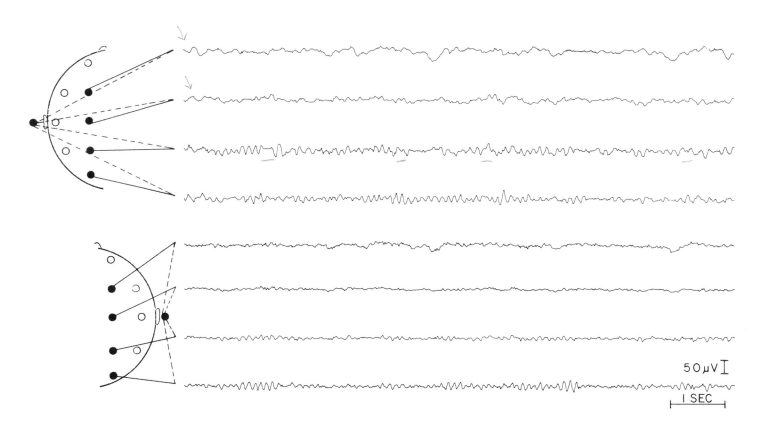

Fig. 20.1. Left fronto-central slow wave focus; the right frontal slow waves are largely due to eye movements. The patient is a 53-year-old man with a 3 year history of partial complex seizures which begin with olfactory hallucinations. A left frontal oligodendroglioma was removed surgically a few days after this EEG recording.

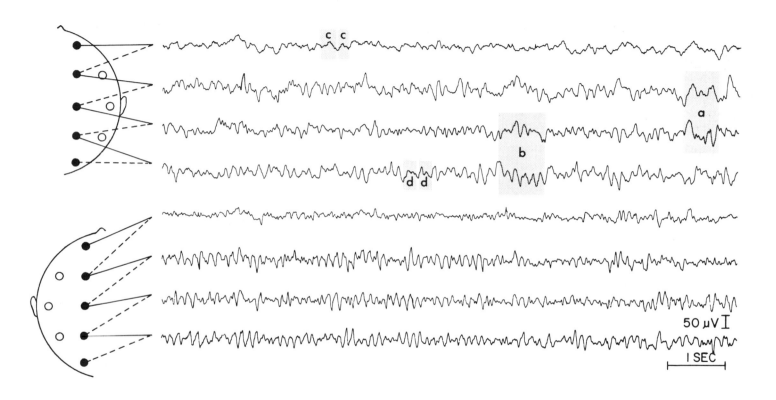

Fig. 20.2. Right centro-parietal slow wave focus. Delta waves have a maximum in the right central (a) and parietal (b) areas; theta waves appear in the right frontal (c) and occipital (d) areas. Occipital alpha rhythm on the right is slower than that on the left. This 76-year-old man had a large cerebral infarct in the distribution of the right middle cerebral artery two days before the EEG.

quencies. Focal irregular delta activity is also referred to as focal polymorphic delta activity.

The slow waves at the center of a focus are usually more persistent and usually of lower frequency than slow waves at the periphery; foci of delta waves are often surrounded by theta waves. The amplitude of slow waves does not always have a maximum at the center; the surrounding slow waves may be larger. Focal slow waves often do not entirely replace the background activity (Figs. 20.1–4). Focal slow waves of low amplitude may be difficult to distinguish from normal background activity. Arrhythmical focal delta waves generally are not much attenuated by eye opening and alerting nor facilitated by hyperventilation, but surrounding slow waves of theta frequency may show such reactions. Local slow waves are most conspicuous during wakefulness, but may persist into sleep.

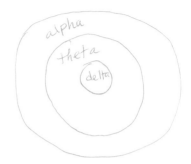

20.2 CLINICAL SIGNIFICANCE OF FOCAL SLOW WAVES

20.2.1 *Types of underlying lesions.* *Focal slow waves* indicate a circumscribed lesions which may be due to either lasting structural damage or a transient disturbance in an area of the subcortical white matter or in the thalamic nuclei; however, lesions of the meninges or the subdural space that invade or compress the underlying hemisphere can also cause focal slow waves. Beyond these general characteristics, focal slow waves do not indicate the specific nature of the local lesion and may thus be due to a variety of conditions.

The classic electrographic sign of a focal disturbance in cerebral function is focal delta activity. A structural lesion is most likely if the delta activity is continuously present, shows variability in waveform, amplitude, duration, and morphology (so-called *polymorphic delta activity*), and persists during changes in physiologic state. Delta waves that are suppressed with eye opening (or other alerting maneuvers), or fail to persist into sleep, are less indicative of structural pathology.

Transient cerebral disorders which can cause episodic focal slow waves are transient ischemic attacks, migraine attacks associated with focal neurological signs, hypertensive and metabolic encephalopathies, some partial seizures, postictal depression, and mild local head injuries. The slow waves should disappear within hours or a few days of the acute disorder; slow waves which persist longer suggest that lasting damage has occurred.

20.2.2 *The temporal relation between slow waves and underlying damage* is not perfect. The correlation is best at the beginning: Focal slow waves appear at the onset of sudden structural damage. For instance, focal slow waves are present from the beginning of cerebral infarcts and develop soon after head injuries, giving the EEG a distinct advantage over isotopic and computerized brain scans in the early recognition of these lesions. The correlation between slow waves and the clinical signs of cerebral damage deteriorates with time in that focal slow waves may disappear weeks or months after acute damage even though the clinical signs persist; this discrepancy suggests that further clinical improvement is unlikely. Rarely do slow waves persist after neurological signs have cleared; a persistence of slow waves indicates persistent cerebral damage.

In many slowly progressive structural lesions, slow waves appear only at or after the onset of clinical signs; however in some cases focal slow waves associated with tumors may be seen at a time when the patient has only vague symptoms.

20.2.3 *The spatial relationship between focal slow waves and the underlying cerebral lesion varies.* Slow waves in superficial lesions generally are fairly precise indicators of the site of the abnormality. However, in some cases, the slow wave focus may appear in a more lateral and anterior location than that of the cerebral lesion. Rarely do slow wave foci appear far away from the lesion. Lesions which are small and deep, for instance infarcts of the internal capsule, do not produce continuous irregular focal delta activity in the EEG even though the patient may show considerable neurological abnormalities.

The localizing value of focal delta is increased when it is topographically discrete or associated with a depression of intermixed faster background frequencies. Superficial lesions tend to produce more restricted EEG changes, whereas deep cerebral lesions may result in hemispheric, or even bilateral, delta. Lesions involving the central and parietal areas are less likely to present with a circumscribed delta focus, and are also more apt to produce delta activity falsely localized to the temporal areas.

Focal delta is usually, but by no means always, maximal over the lesion. If sufficient destruction of the cortex has occurred, the amplitude of delta activity may actually be reduced over the area of maximal cortical involvement and thus be higher in the areas bordering the lesion. If two or more delta foci are present, the one that is most persistant, least rhythmic, and contains less activity above 4 Hz indicates the site of the major lesion, regardless of voltage.

Focal slow waves over an abnormality in one hemisphere may be associated with similar slow waves, usually of lower amplitude, in the opposite hemisphere, particularly in cases of frontal (Fig. 20.1) and occipital lesions. This phenomenon has several possible explanations: (a) an acute infarct or a tumor may produce compression, edema or ischemia in neighboring parts of the opposite hemisphere; (b) impulses from slow wave foci in one hemisphere may travel via commissural fibers to the corresponding area of the other hemisphere to produce slow waves there; (c) the electrical field of a slow wave focus may be conducted through the volume of the interposed tissue to the electrodes over the opposite hemisphere. In the first two instances, bilateral asynchronous frontal or occipital slow wave foci may make it difficult to distinguish between unilateral and bilateral cerebral lesions. In such cases, slight differences in the distribution and timing of slow waves may indicate the area of the primary abnormality. In the case of volume conduction, slow waves

408   ⁎ FIRDA

in the opposite hemisphere are synchronized, although attenuated, copies of the slow waves of the major focus.

Lesions in the posterior fossa cause focal slow waves only very rarely. Infratentorial lesions may produce arrhythmical slow waves in the occipital regions; these waves are usually bilateral, sometimes asymmetrical and rarely focal. They may be due to pressure on, or ischemia of, the occipital lobes, caused by the infratentorial lesion.

20.3 OTHER EEG ABNORMALITIES ASSOCIATED WITH FOCAL SLOW WAVES

In many cases of focal slow waves, the EEG shows other abnormalities which may be helpful in making the clinical diagnosis. In a few instances such abnormalities precede the appearance of focal slow waves and thus become the earliest indication of a local lesion; this is particularly true in cases of cerebral tumors.

20.3.1 *Widespread asynchronous slow waves* are commonly seen in a hemisphere having a delta focus, or in both hemispheres (Fig. 20.2). They are more common in acute than in chronic lesions and suggest cerebral disturbances due to such possible mechanisms as local distortion of brain tissue, edema, vascular, metabolic or other changes. Widespread slow waves can accompany the reduction of alertness which occurs in some deeply located hemispheric strokes and tumors. The generalized slow waves may become so prominent as to obscure the focal slow waves.

20.3.2 *Bilaterally synchronous slow waves* usually appear intermittently and in a wider distribution than the more persistent focal slow waves (Fig. 20.3). The bisynchronous slow waves may be larger or more persistent on the side of the focal slow waves but often have a frontal maximum independent of the distribution of the focal slow waves. Bisynchronous slow waves often suggest that the lesion causing

409

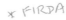 * FIRDA

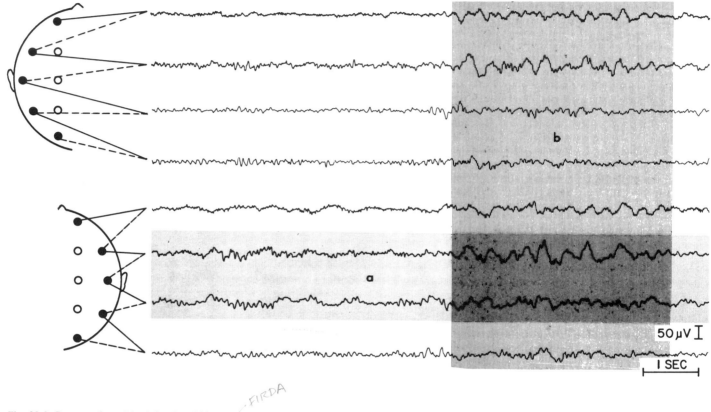

FIRDA

Fig. 20.3. Pattern of combined focal and bisynchronous slow waves. Focal slow waves of 0.5–2 Hz (a) occur continuously in the right temporal area; a burst of bisynchronous slow waves of 2–3 Hz (b) appears with a maximum in the anterior head regions, slightly greater on the right. The patient is a 62-year-old woman with a history of syncope and a decreased left nasolabial fold. Further workup was prompted by the EEG findings and revealed a right sphenoid wing meningioma.

focal slow waves has involved deep midline structures in the anterior, middle or
posterior fossa, especially the mesencephalon or diencephalon, by directly invading
these structures, by compressing or distorting them, or by rendering them ischemic.
Indeed, *the combination of frontal or occipital dominant intermittent rhythmic
delta activity (FIRDA or OIRDA) and continuous focal irregular delta activity is the
classic electrographic sign of impending cerebral herniation* from a focal structural
lesion. The referring physician should, therefore, be informed immediately if this
combination of patterns is present. However, the same combination of patterns may
also be seen in patients with focal structural lesions and co-existant toxic or
metabolic encephalopathies.

20.3.3 *Focal spikes and sharp waves* may be caused by the same lesion which
causes the focal slow waves (Fig. 20.4). On the other hand, slow waves associated
with focal spikes or sharp waves may be entirely the result of ongoing epileptiform
activity (20.6.6).

20.3.4 *Asymmetry of the alpha rhythm* may result from a reduction of the amplitude and frequency (Fig. 20.2) of the alpha rhythm in the hemisphere showing focal
slow waves. This happens more often with lesions in the posterior parts of the
hemisphere than with anterior lesions, possibly as a result of compression of the
posterior structures involved in the production of the alpha rhythm. Occasionally,
the alpha rhythm is reduced on the side opposite to a slow wave focus, perhaps due
to compression, or interference with blood supply, of that hemisphere.

20.3.5 *Asymmetries of the beta rhythm, mu rhythm, vertex waves, K complexes,
sleep spindles, FIRDA, OIRDA, and triphasic waves* may be due to a reduction of
all EEG activity in the vicinity of a lesion producing a slow wave focus, especially
a lesion near the central regions. An isolated depression of beta activity, however,

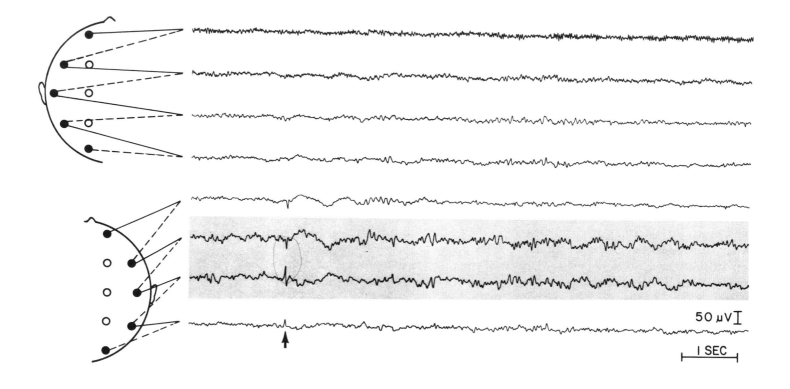

Fig. 20.4. Pattern of combined focal slow waves and focal spikes. Focal slow waves of 1–3 Hz (shaded) appear continuously in the right temporal region; a spike (arrow) appears in the same distribution. The recording was made during drowsiness. The patient is the same as in Fig. 20.3, one year after surgical removal of the meningioma; she had one generalized seizure 10 days before this EEG recording.

* phase reversing at T4

is not always a reliable localizing sign because beta activity may be (rarely) increased on the side of a tumor and is often increased by an underlying skull defect.

20.4 MECHANISMS CAUSING FOCAL SLOW WAVES

Clinical and experimental observations indicate that continuous, irregular, delta activity results primarily from lesions affecting cerebral white matter. Involvement of superficial cortex is not essential, and indeed, lesions restricted to the cortical mantle do not generally produce significant focal delta activity. It is likely that functional deafferentation of cortex, rather than a change in cortical metabolic rate, is critical. Cerebral edema does not appear to make a substantial contribution to the production of delta waves. Lesser degrees of focal slowing probably have a similar pathogenesis, although the mechanism of cortical deafferentation will be more likely due to transient disturbances or relatively small lesions.

20.5 SPECIFIC DISORDERS CAUSING FOCAL SLOW WAVES

20.5.1 *Degenerative, developmental and demyelinating diseases.* Degenerative diseases produce focal slow waves so rarely that the EEG is often used to rule out structural lesions in patients suspected of having degenerative diseases. Exceptions are the temporal slow wave foci which may appear in senile dementia and local slow waves which occur at the beginning of Jakob-Creutzfeldt disease. Developmental diseases cause focal slow waves infrequently even if there is focal cerebral damage. This may be due to the fact that these lesions begin early in life, at a time when local damage produces distortions of background and specific epileptiform patterns (19.1). Later in life, the residual cerebral damage is rarely reflected by discrete focal slow waves.

Senile and presenile dementia (Alzheimer's disease) may be associated with an

413

exaggeration of the intermittent focal slow waves which appear in the temporal areas, particularly on the left side, with advancing age (13.4). However, these focal slow waves are a less reliable indicator of dementia than are generalized asynchronous slow waves.

Jakob-Creutzfeldt disease may show slow waves locally for a short period before they become generalized, and before periodic complexes appear (19.3).

Normal pressure hydrocephalus occasionally produces local or generalized asynchronous slow waves.

Hydrocephalus in children may be associated with focal slow waves in addition to other abnormalities; focal slow waves are more common at the site of shunt insertions.

Porencephaly, tuberous sclerosis, and perinatal cerebral damage may cause residual local slow waves in the EEG after causing generalized abnormalities in infancy.

Holoprosencephaly may cause focal slow waves and focal spikes, emanating from islands of preserved brain tissue.

Multiple sclerosis and Schilder's disease cause focal slow waves much less often than they cause widespread slow waves and other abnormalities.

Bilateral retrobulbar neuritis in children, causing significant visual loss may lead to occipital slow waves in addition to spikes (17.5).

20.5.2 *Metabolic and toxic encephalopathies.* Focal slow waves are seen in these disorders much less often than are generalized slow waves. Focal slow waves may appear on a background of generalized slow waves during metabolic coma or emerge from generalized slow waves after metabolic coma as a result of local vascular complications, namely transient cerebral ischemia or infarction. Very few metabolic disorders cause focal slow waves without causing generalized slow waves and coma. Focal slow waves may occur in: hypoglycemia, hypoxia and CO

414

poisoning, hyperosmolar coma, for instance in nonketotic hyperglycemia, hyper-parathyroidism, porphyria, vitamin B12 deficiency and Wilson's disease. Focal slow waves may occur after myelography with metrizamide.

20.5.3 *Cerebrovascular diseases.* *Strokes* of the cerebral hemispheres caused by ischemia, embolism or hemorrhage are common causes of focal slow waves. Infarcts in the distribution of the middle cerebral artery often cause local slow waves in the temporal, frontal, central and parietal areas (Fig. 20.2). Occlusion of the anterior cerebral artery, especially at the origin of the artery at the base of the brain, may cause frontal intermittent delta activity (22.2), even though this activity is more often due to frontal tumors than to infarctions. A cerebral infarct in the distribution of the posterior cerebral arteries is likely to cause focal slow waves in the occipital and posterior temporal areas. Infarcts of the brainstem rarely produce focal slow waves over the posterior head and are often associated with a normal EEG; they may produce generalized bisynchronous and asynchronous slow waves if they involve the reticular formation in the core of the midbrain or alpha coma patterns if they involve the pontine reticular formation (25.3.2).

Multiple infarcts may be the cause of more than one slow wave focus. Slow wave foci are often acquired in sequence by patients who have successive strokes. The small infarcts responsible for the lacunar state in hypertensive patients often cause no sharply defined slow wave foci but rather result in generalized slow waves. Cerebral air and fat emboli also usually cause generalized rather than focal slow waves.

Transient ischemic attacks of the cerebral hemispheres may cause local slow waves or reductions of amplitude (23.6.3). An EEG is rarely recorded during the attack, but slow waves may persist for many hours after the attack, or longer if an infarct has occurred.

Occlusion of the carotid artery is produced intentionally during surgical repair of a partially occluded artery (carotid endarterectomy). Sudden clamping of the artery may reduce the cerebral blood flow to a level below that needed to prevent infarction. Imminent infarction can be recognized by the appearance of focal or unilateral slow waves within a few minutes after clamping; the slow waves are often followed by loss of amplitude. Lasting cerebral damage can be avoided if a shunt is placed so that blood can bypass the clamped segment of the artery until surgery is completed. Monitoring of the EEG during carotid endarterectomy can thus help to determine the need for shunting and detect the occurrence of intraoperative stroke.

Migraine attacks can produce local slow waves, especially if the attacks are associated with unilateral neurological abnormalities other than visual symptoms. The slow waves are presumably due to local cerebral ischemia occurring during the attack. If they persist for hours or a few days after the attack, the slow waves may be due to local cerebral ischemia; if they persist longer, they can be presumed to be due to infarction. Attacks of basilar artery migraine may be associated with focal slow waves in the posterior head regions on one or both sides, or with generalized slow waves; this form of migraine may also produce epileptiform activity in the same distribution. Slow wave foci in patients with headaches unexplained by a recent attack of migraine are sufficiently rare to warrant a workup for mass lesions or vascular malformations.

Chronic subdural hematoma commonly causes focal slow waves even though a regional reduction of amplitude is more characteristic. Bilateral subdural hematomas may be associated with any combination of unilateral and bilateral slow waves and asymmetries, including slow waves on one side and amplitude reductions on the other.

Subarachnoid hemorrhage produces focal slow waves only occasionally and by one of several possible mechanisms. The hemorrhage may damage the brain locally. Spasm of the bleeding vessel may cause local ischemia or infarction. Bleeding may

416

come from an aneurysm or a vascular malformation which locally compresses the brain. Slow wave foci in the central region suggest bleeding from an aneurysm of the middle cerebral artery; foci in the posterior temporal region have no localizing value. Subarachnoid hemorrhage may cause ipsilateral decrease of amplitude and decrease of alpha frequency; when associated with a lowered level of consciousness, generalized slow waves are practically always present.

20.5.4 *Cerebral trauma.*   *Head injuries* may lead to focal slow waves in addition to the more common initial decrease of amplitude and subsequent wide-spread slow waves. In many cases, focal slow waves after head injury are transient, variable in distribution and unassociated with focal neurological signs. They therefore probably do not represent local structural damage but may be explained by temporary local changes of cerebral cirulation or edema. In other instances, they last longer and are due to contusions, intracerebral hemorrhages, acute traumatic subdural or epidural hematoma.

Progressive traumatic encephalopathy may produce one or more slow wave foci initially before leading to generalized slow waves.

Brain surgery involving the cerebral hemispheres is often followed by focal slow waves. They suggest local brain damage. However, this must be distinguished from the effects of a skull defect which can locally increase the amplitude of generalized slow waves (23.4).

Hemispherectomy may cause unilateral slow waves in addition to amplitude reductions.

20.5.5 *Brain tumors.*   *Supratentorial brain tumors* are among the most important causes of focal slow waves, and focal slow waves are the most characteristic sign of a supratentorial tumor (Fig. 20.1,3). Focal slow waves of tumors may be associated with other EEG abnormalities such as focal epileptiform activity (Fig. 20.4) and gen-

417

eralized slow waves (Fig. 20.3) which have the implications described earlier (20.3).

Studies of the EEG in patients with brain tumors have revealed several important pieces of clinical information. Frontal tumors tend to produce a considerable amount of focal slow wave activity not only on the side of the tumor but also on the opposite side (Fig. 20.1). Tumors deep in the parietal lobe may cause focal parietal theta rhythm. Multiple metastases occasionally cause more than one slow wave focus. Tumors in older persons are more likely to produce bisynchronous slow waves than are tumors in persons of other ages. Infratentorial tumors, while often causing bisynchronous slow waves, produce local slow waves in the posterior head regions only rarely in adults and slightly more commonly in children. Slow wave foci in the temporal region do not have localizing value.

20.5.6 *Seizure disorders. Postictal* continuous irregular focal delta waves often appear after a single isolated seizure of focal onset, but rarely persist more than 20 minutes unless an underlying structural abnormality is present. In a patient who is known to have had a recent seizure but who shows no epileptiform activity in the EEG, focal slow waves can suggest a focal origin of the seizure.

Interictal focal slow waves raise the suspicion of a local lesion such as a tumor, stroke, injury or malformation which can both damage subcortical tissue, giving rise to the slow waves, and irritate cortical tissue, producing epileptiform activity. However, focal slow waves, mixed with focal spikes or sharp waves, can be seen in stationary epileptogenic lesions as part of the ongoing epileptiform activity.

Ictal focal slow waves are rarely the only EEG manifestation of an ongoing seizure; this may be seen in seizures and status epilepticus of partial seizures and in epilepsia partialis continua (19.3.2).

20.5.7 *Infectious diseases.* *Abscesses* of the cerebral hemispheres are more commonly associated with focal slow waves than with other EEG abnormalities such as unilateral slow waves, focal spikes and sharp waves, periodic lateralizing epileptiform discharges, or local reductions of amplitude. Bisynchronous slow waves are more common with deeply located abscesses. Asynchronous generalized slow waves invariably appear when the level of alertness decreases.

Meningitis and encephalitis produce focal slow waves only rarely and when the infection involves one part of the hemispheres more than others. This is usually the case in the acute necrotizing encephalitis of herpes simplex which produces focal slow waves in one or both temporal areas early in the disease (19.3.1).

Progressive multifocal leukoencephalopathy may begin locally and be associated with focal slow waves for a while before generalized asynchronous slow waves supervene.

20.5.8 *Psychiatric diseases.* *Focal slow waves* have been reported in a great variety of psychiatric disorders. However, this occurrence is so rare and without clear relation to specific diseases that focal slow waves cannot be accepted as manifestation of psychiatric disease and a local cerebral lesion must be excluded by other examinations. This is especially true for patients whose symptoms include dementia where the finding of a slow wave focus in any part of the brain would be strong presumptive evidence for a structural cerebral lesion.

REFERENCES

Fisch, B.J. and Pedley, T.A. (1985) Evaluation of focal cerebral lesions. Role of electroencephalography in the era of computerized tomography. In: Aminoff, M.J. (Ed.), Electrodiagnosis, Neurologic Clinics. Saunders, Philadelphia, pp. 649–662.

Fischer-Williams, M. (1987) Brain tumors and other space occupying lesions (with a section on oncological CNS complications). In: Niedermeyer, E. and Lopes da Silva, F. (Eds.), Electroencephalography: Basic Principles, Clinical Applications and Related Fields. Urban and Schwarzenberg, Baltimore, pp. 163–182.

Gilmore, P.C. and Brenner, R.P. (1981) Correlation of EEG, computerized tomography, and clinical findings: Study of 100 patients with focal delta activity. Arch. Neurol. 38: 371–372.

Gloor, P., Ball, G. and Schaul, N. (1977) Brain lesions that produce delta waves in the EEG. Neurology 27: 326–333.

Goldensohn, E.S. (1979) Use of the EEG for evaluation of focal intracranial lesions. In: Klass, D.W. and Daly, D. (Eds.), Current Practice of Clinical Electroencephalography. Raven, New York, pp. 307–342.

MacDonnell, R.A.L., Donnan, G.A., Bladin, P.F., Berkovic, S.F. and Wriedt, C.H.R. (1988) The electroencephalogram and acute ischemic stroke. Distinguishing cortical from lacunar infarction. Arch. Neurol. 45: 520–524.

Marshall, D., Brey, R.L. and Morse, M.W. (1988) Focal and/or lateralized polymorphic delta activity. Arch. Neurol. 45: 33–35.

Michel, B., Gastaut, J.L. and Bianchi, L. (1979) Electroencephalographic cranial computerized tomographic correlations in brain abscess. Electroenceph. clin. Neurophysiol. 46: 256–273.

Newmark, M.E., Theodore, W.H., Sato, S., de la Paz, R., Patronas, N., Brooks, R., Jabbari, B. and Di Chiro, G. (1983) EEG, transmission computed tomography, and positron emission tomography with fluorodeoxyglucose [18]F: Their use in adults with gliomas. Arch. Neurol. 40: 607–610.

Petty, G.W., Labar, D.R., Fisch, B.J., Pedley, T.A., Mohr, J.P. and Khandji, A. (1988) EEG in lacunar strokes. Ann. Neurol. 24: 129A.

Schaul, N., Green, L., Peyster, R. and Gotman, J. (1986) Structural determinants of electroencephalographic findings in acute hemispheric lesions. Arch. Neurol. 20: 703–711.

Sharbrough, F.W., Messick, J.M. and Sundt, T.M. (1973) Correlation of continuous electroencephalograms with cerebral blood flow measurements during carotid endarterectomy. Stroke 4: 674–683.

Sharbrough, F.W. (1987) Nonspecific abnormal EEG patterns. In: Niedermeyer, E. and Lopes da Silva, F. (Eds.), Electroencephalography: Basic Principles, Clinical Applications and Related Fields. Urban and Schwarzenberg, Baltimore, pp. 163–182.

Van der Drift, J.H.A. and Kok, N.K.D. (1972) Section II. The EEG in cerebrovascular disorders in relation to pathology. In: Rémond, A. (Ed.), Handbook of Electroenceph. clin. Neurophysiol., Vol. 14A, Elsevier, Amsterdam, pp. 12–64.

Vignaendra, V., Ghee, L.T. and Chawla, J. (1975) EEG in brain abscess: Its value in localization compared to other diagnostic tests. Electroenceph. clin. Neurophysiol. 38: 611–622.

SUMMARY

(21.1) *The pattern* of generalized asynchronous slow waves consists of waves of less than 8 Hz which occur over both hemispheres in such a way that the waves on one side have no constant time relationship with the waves on the other side. Asynchronous slow waves usually vary in frequency and often have irregular shapes. They may be reduced by eye opening and alerting and increased by hyperventilation. They may have a local maximum, i.e. an area of higher amplitude and incidence, in some part of the brain; this pattern differs from a slow wave focus surrounded by generalized slow waves in that focal slow waves have usually a lower frequency and sometimes a lower amplitude than the surrounding slow waves and react less to eye opening, alerting and hyperventilation.

(21.2) *Causes* of generalized asynchronous slow waves include many normal and abnormal conditions. In general, these slow waves are present in all normal subjects during drowsiness and sleep. During wakefulness, slow waves are part of the normal background in subjects of all ages except adults. In adults, a mild to moderate excess of generalized slow waves during wakefulness, although an electrographic abnormality, is found in 10–15% of otherwise normal subjects. A mild or moderate amount of asynchronous generalized slow waves in a wakeful adult can therefore only suggest that a person is somewhat more likely to have a cerebral abnormality. However, a marked amount of these slow waves always indicates a cerebral abnormality. The type of abnormality remains unspecified: Generalized asynchronous slow waves occur in such a great variety of widespread cerebral disorders that they are the most common and least specific EEG abnormality.

(21.3) *Other EEG abnormalities* associated with generalized asynchronous slow waves are usually of greater diagnostic significance.

(21.4) *Mechanisms* causing generalized asynchronous slow waves generally interfere with the structure or function of both hemispheres and involve subcortical white matter.

(21.5) *Specific disorders* include a wide variety of cerebral abnormalities.

21.1 DESCRIPTION OF PATTERN

Generalized asynchronous slow waves have a frequency under 8 Hz and occur over

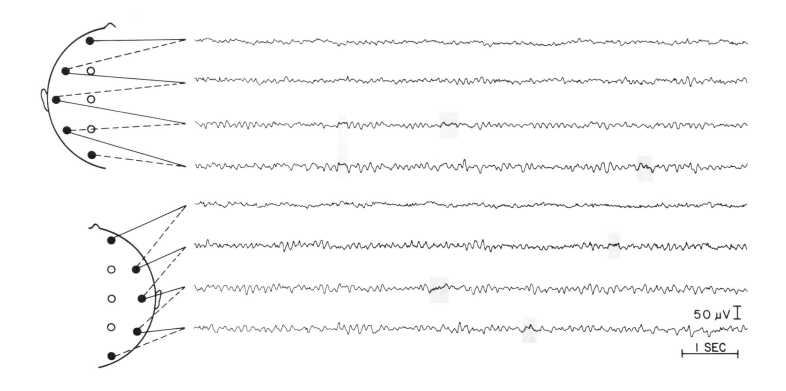

Fig. 21.1. Pattern of generalized asynchronous slow waves with a maximum in the posterior head regions. The slow waves are mainly in the theta range and of low or medium amplitude; a few slow waves are indicated by shading. The slow waves of much lower frequency in the prefrontal regions are eye movement artifacts. The patient is a 53-year-old woman with a schizoid personality disorder and several psychotic episodes, currently treated with 100 mg chlorpromazine every 4 hours.

most or all parts of both hemispheres (Figs. 21.1; 21.2; 21.3). The slow waves in one area have no constant time relationship with slow waves in the corresponding area on the other side. For example, slow waves may appear in some areas when there are no slow waves in other areas; slow waves appearing in different areas at the same time may have different frequency; waves of similar frequency appearing simultaneously in different areas may have varying phase relationship. Even though individual slow waves may often have a fairly regular shape, their rate of repetition usually varies by at least $2-3$ Hz, i.e. they are often arrhythmical. The slow waves are reduced by eye opening and alerting, and increased by relaxation and hyperventilation; in some comatose patients, alerting stimuli may paradoxically increase the slow waves (Fig. 25.4). In general, the reactivity of generalized asynchronous slow waves is greater than that of focal slow waves and less pronounced than that of bisynchronous generalized slow waves. Generalized asynchronous slow waves are best recognized during wakefulness because during sleep they are usually obscured by the generalized slow waves of normal sleep patterns.

Although distributed widely, generalized asynchronous slow waves may be more prominent in some areas than in others (Fig. 21.1). They may have a maximum of amplitude and incidence in corresponding parts of both hemispheres or in one area. This local prominence can usually be distinguished from focal slow waves which appear on a background of generalized slow waves since focal waves arising from a focal structural abnormality usually have a lower frequency, and sometimes lower amplitude, than the surrounding slow waves and they are less reactive to eye opening, alerting and hyperventilation than are generalized asynchronous slow waves.

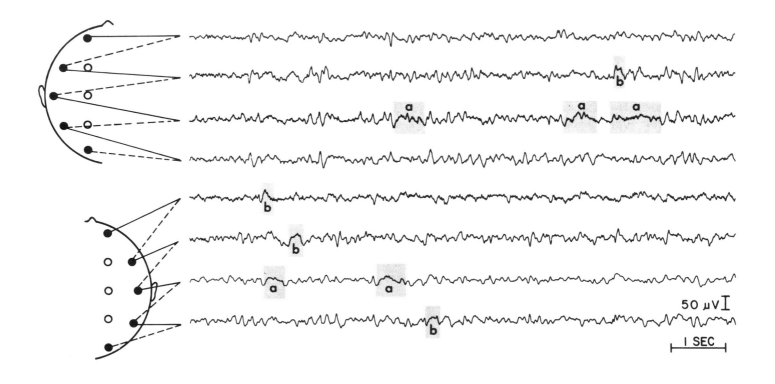

Fig. 21.2. Pattern of generalized asynchronous slow waves of delta (a) and theta (b) frequency and of moderate amplitude. Intermittent rhythmical occipital background activity has a frequency of 5–6 Hz. This 73-year-old man has fairly severe senile dementia.

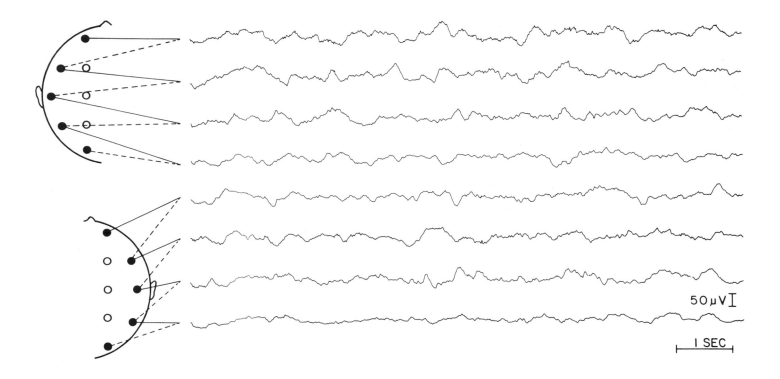

50µV

1 SEC

Fig. 21.3. Pattern of generalized asynchronous slow waves of predominantly delta frequency and moderate to high amplitude. This 69-year-old man had a cardiorespiratory arrest, was resuscitated but remained in postanoxic coma for the 2 days before this recording.

21.2.1 *Normal generalized asynchronous slow waves* occur in drowsiness and sleep at all ages. During wakefulness, they are prominent in infants, gradually diminish in children and adolescents, and reach a minimum in adults; slightly greater amounts appear in older persons. The slow waves are therefore abnormal only if they exceed the normal range for the age of the patient.

21.2.2 *Abnormal amounts of generalized asynchronous slow waves in normal subjects* occur in the waking record of 10–15% of adults and in perhaps even a greater percentage of subjects of other ages; a mild excess is more common than a moderate one. Generalized asynchronous slow waves thus distinguish less sharply between normal and abnormal subjects than do other EEG patterns. This overlap reduces the ability of mild and moderate asynchronous slow wave abnormalities to indicate cerebral abnormalities. Therefore, the finding of this abnormality can only suggest that a patient is more likely to have a cerebral abnormality than a patient with a normal EEG. However, this does not affect the significance of a marked excess of generalized asynchronous slow waves in the waking EEG which indicates a cerebral abnormality in every adult, teenager and child.

21.2.3 *Abnormal generalized asynchronous slow waves* are due to a wide variety of conditions and are the most common and least specific abnormal EEG pattern. However, an EEG showing only an excess of generalized asynchronous slow waves has a certain negative diagnostic value: The absence of other abnormalities reduces the likelihood of a recent focal brain lesion of the hemispheres considerably, and it reduces the probability of a convulsive disorder slightly.

426

21.3.1 *Attenuation, slowing and disorganization of alpha rhythm* often occurs
with mild and moderate generalized slow waves (Fig. 20.1). Marked generalized
slow waves replace alpha rhythm completely (Fig. 20.3).

21.3.2 *Bisynchronous slow waves* often appear intermittently in bursts which
usually have higher amplitude and restricted distribution and therefore stand out
against a background of asynchronous generalized slow waves. Many cerebral
abnormalities which eventually lead to bisynchronous slow waves initially cause disorganization of alpha rhythm and mild or moderate asynchronous slow waves, and
later produce mixtures of bisynchronous and asynchronous slow waves. The bisynchronous slow waves usually are of greater diagnostic importance than the
asynchronous slow waves.

21.3.3 *Focal slow waves, generalized epileptiform activity, periodic complexes and
other abnormal patterns* of greater diagnostic significance than asynchronous
generalized slow waves often appear on a background of these slow waves.

21.4 MECHANISMS CAUSING GENERALIZED ASYNCHRONOUS SLOW WAVES

Generalized asynchronous slow waves may be produced by various mechanisms.
Most of them probably interfere with structure or function of both hemispheres and
involve subcortical white matter in a wide distribution; rarely are the generalized
slow waves an extension of focal slow waves. Widespread interruption or disorganization of cortical input from the brainstem reticular formation may be an

important factor in many cases; brainstem lesions cause widespread asynchronous slow waves in some cases although they seem more likely to produce bisynchronous slow waves.

21.5.1 *Degenerative, developmental and demyelinating diseases.* Most of the degenerative diseases which produce generalized asynchronous slow waves are those which involve the cerebral hemispheres and cause dementia. Degenerative diseases involving the cerebellum, brainstem and spinal cord do not produce EEG abnormalities.

(1) *Senile and presenile dementia (Alzheimer's disease)* is often associated with an exaggeration of age-related EEG changes (13) and thus leads to: (a) excessive generalized asynchronous slow waves; (b) marked slowing, reduction of amplitude and disorganization of alpha rhythm (Fig. 21.2); (c) fairly frequent bursts of focal slow waves, often with sharp contours, appearing in the temporal regions, most often on the left side; (d) the appearance of bilaterally synchronous slow waves. While excessive generalized asynchronous slow waves correlate better with dementia than do the other EEG abnormalities, Alzheimer's dementia usually becomes quite obvious before the EEG becomes definitely abnormal.

(2) *Pick's disease* which can usually not be distinguished from Alzheimer's disease on clinical grounds often produces few or no EEG abnormalities even in the presence of rather severe dementia.

(3) *Parkinson's disease* is associated with a mild or moderate amount of generalized asynchronous slow wave activity in less than half of all patients. This is not of great clinical importance because the diagnosis is not based on the EEG; however, it is worth noting that the finding of generalized asynchronous slow waves

428

in a patient with Parkinson's disease should cause no alarm. Cerebral slow waves in the EEG of a patient with Parkinson's disease must be distinguished from artifacts consisting of intermittent or continuous rhythmical 4–6 Hz waves produced by tremor of the head or neck. These slow waves may fall in phase with motor unit action potentials from nearby scalp muscles and generate patterns resembling spike-and-wave discharges.

(4) *Progressive supranuclear palsy* may lead to generalized slow waves in advanced cases, but the initial abnormalities of sleep patterns and bisynchronous slow waves in the waking record are diagnostically more important.

(5) *Huntington's chorea* may be associated with generalized asynchronous slow waves, but the generalized reduction of amplitude is a more important diagnostic feature.

(6) *Jakob-Creutzfeldt disease* is characterized by progressive and widespread slowing of the EEG and by disintegration of alpha rhythm. Moderate or marked slow waves replace all normal background activity in advanced cases. In the end-stage of the disease, the amplitude of all activity may decrease and the EEG may become nearly flat and featureless. Periodic sharp waves, appearing in the early or middle stages of the disease, are the most characteristic abnormal pattern in this disease (19.3).

(7) *Normal pressure hydrocephalus* often produces no EEG abnormality but may be associated with mild or moderate generalized slow waves or with focal slow waves. The generalized slow waves are asynchronous in most cases, in contrast to bisynchronous slow waves which may appear in obstructive hydrocephalus.

(8) *Hydrocephalus in children,* regardless of its cause, may be associated with asynchronous generalized slow waves and other abnormalities including bi-synchronous slow waves, focal slow waves, and spike foci.

429

OIRDA

FIRDA

(9) *Tuberous sclerosis* in adults can cause asynchronous generalized slow waves in addition to bisynchronous slow waves and focal spikes; infants and young children show different abnormalities.

(10) *Other degenerative and developmental diseases* may produce generalized asynchronous slow waves as the only abnormality or as one of several abnormalities in some patients; other patients with the same diseases may have normal EEGs. These diseases include: Leber's hereditary optic atrophy, Riley-Day syndrome, Seitelberger's disease, Leigh's disease, microcephaly with or without microgyria, macrogyria or agyria, holoprosencephaly, cerebral palsy, infantile hemiplegia, myotonic dystrophy, Mongolian idiocy.

(11) *Multiple sclerosis* produces generalized asynchronous slow waves, reduction of amplitude and other abnormalities in approximately one-half of all cases. The incidence of abnormalities varies widely in different groups of patients, probably depending on acuteness, duration and rate of progression of the disease. Longer duration of the disease may account for higher incidences of abnormalities in some studies of benign multiple sclerosis.

21.5.2 *Metabolic and toxic encephalopathies.* Generalized asynchronous slow waves may occur in any of these conditions when they cause significant encephalopathy and therefore do not distinguish these conditions from each other or from other conditions. Mild or moderate slow waves, often associated with a disorganization of the background, are usually the first abnormality in the EEG and marked slow waves may be the only abnormality found in the severest stages. Asynchronous slow waves in these encephalopathies may combine with bisynchronous slow waves and other abnormalities in adults and children, and with special patterns in infants (19.1.2).

(1) *Congenital encephalopathies such as phenylketonuria, amaurotic familial idiocy, metachromatic and other leukodystrophies (Krabbe's and Pelizaeus-*

Merzbacher's diseases often cause hypsarrhythmia, slow spike-and-waves or multi-focal independent spikes (19.2) in infancy and early childhood, but only excessive slow waves at later ages. Thus, the three infantile epileptiform patterns are often found in the infantile (Tay-Sachs) and late infantile (Bielschowski-Jansky) forms of amaurotic familial idiocy but not in the juvenile (Spielmeyer-Vogt) and adult (Kufs) forms which show only asynchronous generalized slow waves and occasional bi-synchronous slow waves.

(2) *Wilson's disease* produces generalized asynchronous or focal slow waves in about one-half of all patients, especially those with significant liver disease.

(3) *Acquired metabolic encephalopathies* such as those due to hepatic and renal failure, hypoglycemia, hypoxia and electrolyte imbalances often have an initial phase of generalized asynchronous slow waves and disorganized background followed by combinations of these slow waves with prominent bilaterally synchronous slow waves and other abnormalities. Asynchronous slow waves in these encephalopathies are usually present when the patient begins to become confused and somnolent. Residual slow waves may persist after the end of acute encephalopathies suggesting widespread residual cerebral damage. Metabolic encephalopathies and the corresponding EEG abnormalities are listed in Table 22.1. A few other metabolic encephalopathies produce mainly other EEG abnormalities to which generalized asynchronous slow waves may be added in some cases. Hypothyroidism leads to a decrease of the frequency of alpha rhythm and a generalized reduction of overall amplitude, hyperthyroidism causes an increase of alpha rhythm frequency (25.6) and an excess of fast activity.

(4) *Toxic encephalopathies* commonly produce generalized asynchronous slow waves in acute intoxications, especially those associated with reduced levels of alertness. Common examples are intoxications by alcohol, barbiturates, and other drugs depressing the central nervous system. However, slow waves induced by drugs are not always accompanied by clinical manifestations of encephalopathy: intravenous

431

administration of atropine, chronic intake of sedatives and psychotropic drugs, or myelography with metrizamide can induce generalized slow waves without producing overt mental changes.

Alcohol.   *Acute alcohol intoxication* may cause generalized asynchronous slow waves, decrease of alpha frequency and increase of central beta activity.

Chronic alcoholism itself produces no EEG abnormalities, but asynchronous generalized slow waves may be found when chronic alcoholism is associated with cerebral atrophy in patients over 60 years of age.

Acute withdrawal syndrome, delirium tremens, and Korsakoff's psychosis usually induce no more than mild or moderate generalized slow waves; only a few cases of Korsakoff's psychosis show more prominent generalized slow waves similar to those of Wernicke's disease. Beta activity is often prominent and replaces the alpha rhythm or is superimposed on it in a harmonic relation to give it a notched appearance.

Wernicke's encephalopathy usually produces prominent generalized asynchronous slow waves, and often also causes bisynchronous slow waves and a decrease of the alpha rhythm.

Hepatic encephalopathy and subdural hematoma are indirect results of alcoholism which usually are associated with asynchronous slow waves but often with more characteristic abnormalities: hepatic encephalopathy with bisynchronous slow waves, or triphasic waves (19.3); subdural hematoma with focal slow waves and asymmetries of amplitude.

Barbiturates acutely produce prominent central or generalized beta activity and a decrease of alpha rhythm at low or medium blood levels. At higher levels, beta waves and frontal 10–12 Hz waves may persist as generalized asynchronous theta and delta waves emerge and become more prominent until nonreactive delta waves predominate. Then periods of low amplitude activity or of complete electrical silence of a few seconds in duration begin to interrupt the delta waves at short intervals, creating burst-suppression patterns (19.3). With deepening coma, the quiet periods increase in duration and the delta waves in the bursts decrease in amplitude and eventually disappear completely. Electrocerebral silence may persist and ultimately indicate cerebral death although the patient and the EEG may recover even after more than 24 hours without recordable EEG.

Chronic intake of barbiturates may either cause fast waves or produce no effect on the EEG.

Barbiturate withdrawal can produce asynchronous slow waves along with bursts of high amplitude bisynchronous theta waves; photo-convulsive responses and spontaneous generalized epileptiform activity may also occur.

Phenothiazines, haloperidol, rauwolfia derivatives may produce generalized asynchronous slow waves and slowing of alpha rhythm at moderate doses. Large doses can induce bisynchronous slow waves, prominent beta activity, and bilateral spike-and-wave or polyspike-and-wave patterns.

Tricyclic antidepressants may produce generalized asynchronous or bisynchronous slow waves, and bilateral spikes or spike-and-wave discharges.

Carbon monoxide and other poisons causing widespread structural brain damage may produce generalized asynchronous slow waves.

Other toxic agents of many different types can produce generalized asynchronous slow waves. These include: carbon disulfide, methyl chloride and bromide, organic solvents, manganese, mercury, tin, strontium, lead, arsenic, bismuth, lithium, monoamine oxidase inhibitors, opiates, chloralose. Some of these are associated with a slowing of alpha frequency and bisynchronous slow waves, others with epileptiform activity. Most vitamin deficiencies causing asynchronous slow waves also cause bisynchronous slow waves.

21.5.3 *Cerebrovascular diseases:*
(1) *Syncope of various causes including Stokes-Adams attacks, transient ischemic*

433

attacks of the brainstem, and other conditions causing transitory reductions of blood flow to the entire brain or to the brainstem produce generalized slow waves only when consciousness fades; bisynchronous slow waves may be added. The slow waves disappear within minutes or hours after recovery from these conditions; persistence of slow waves suggests that structural damage has occurred.

(2) *Postanoxic encephalopathy* is often the direct result of cardiac and respiratory arrest, or the indirect result of metabolic encephalopathy, intracerebral or subarachnoid hemorrhage, or of severe cerebral injury which causes widespread structural cerebral damage and generalized asynchronous slow waves. Depending on the severity of the underlying damage, asynchronous slow waves show higher amplitude and lower frequency (Fig. 21.3) and may be associated with, or replaced by: (a) bursts of bisynchronous slow waves; (b) rhythmical, widespread and unreactive alpha or theta activity; (c) reduced amplitude; (d) spikes or sharp waves; (e) burst-suppression patterns; or, (f) electrocerebral silence.
cerebral silence (24.6.3).

The prognostic value of the EEG in postanoxic encephalopathy is very limited. During the first six hours after the anoxic insult, the EEG has no relation to outcome. Later, the persistence of electrocerebral silence indicates cerebral death whereas the return of a normal EEG has a good prognosis. Between these extremes, the EEG does not clearly predict the outcome. The presence of elements of normal sleep activity and of any EEG response to alerting stimuli suggests less severe damage and a better prognosis.

(3) *Midbrain strokes* due to thrombosis, embolism or hemorrhage which damage the reticular formation in the central parts of the midbrain reduce the patient's alertness and produce generalized asynchronous slow waves with or without superimposed bisynchronous slow waves. Infarcts in the central parts of the pons may produce coma associated with alpha or theta activity, while infarcts involving the lateral parts of the midbrain or pons usually do not produce alterations of consciousness or EEG abnormalities.

434

(4) *Multiple cerebral infarcts, lacunar state, fat and air embolism* commonly produce generalized asynchronous slow waves.

(5) *Chronic subdural hematoma* commonly produces generalized asynchronous slow waves, but focal slow waves and asymmetries (23.2) often overshadow this abnormality and always are of greater diagnostic significance.

(6) *Migraine and other headaches* are associated with an abnormally high incidence of generalized asynchronous slow waves and other abnormalities between attacks.* Additional abnormalities may appear during migrainous attacks.

21.5.4 *Cerebral trauma:*

(1) *Mild head injuries* that cause only a brief loss of consciousness or no unconsciousness at all may produce diffuse asynchronous theta and delta waves and a decrease of alpha amplitude and frequency; the abnormalities usually disappear within hours or days but may persist for weeks even in patients who recover without complications. The abnormalities are generally more severe in children than in adults.

(2) *Severe head injuries* that cause longer periods of unconsciousness are associated with marked generalized asynchronous slow waves and may also be associated with (a) generalized decrease of amplitude, (b) focal decrease of amplitude, (c) focal slow waves, (d) bisynchronous generalized slow waves, (e) early or late focal epileptiform activity, (f) absence of sleep patterns.

(3) *Progressive traumatic encephalopathy* of boxers and other persons exposed to repeated head injuries is often associated with generalized asynchronous and bisynchronous slow waves; these abnormalities are usually preceded by slowing of alpha rhythm and the appearance of focal slow waves.

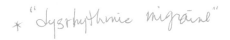

* "dysrhythmic migraine"

435

21.5.5 *Brain tumors:*

(1) *Solitary brain tumors* produce asynchronous generalized slow waves only indirectly, namely when they invade or compress midbrain and diencephalic structures so that alertness is reduced. Focal slow waves or bisynchronous slow waves may precede this development.

(2) *Multiple metastases* cause asynchronous generalized slow waves as the result of initially discrete slow wave foci or as the result of diencephalic or mesencephalic lesions that reduce alertness.

21.5.6 *Seizure disorders:*

(1) *Postictal generalized asynchronous slow waves* may persist for up to several days after a generalized seizure; they may remain for a few weeks after electro-convulsive treatment.

(2) *Interictal generalized asynchronous slow waves* are found in a higher percentage of subjects with epilepsy than in the asymptomatic population; the incidence of interictal slow waves is especially high in patients whose seizures are associated with widespread cerebral damage.

(3) *Ictal generalized asynchronous slow waves* are very rare.

21.5.7 *Infectious diseases:*

(1) *High fever* can lead to generalized asynchronous slow waves and slowing of alpha rhythm in keeping with a reduction of alertness. However, slow waves in patients with only moderate fever may be the expression of a cerebral infection.

(2) *Meningitis* is more likely to produce EEG abnormalities if it extends into the brain; generalized slow waves are more common in children than in adults.

(3) *Encephalitis* of most causes produce generalized asynchronous slow waves as a signal of widespread involvement of cerebral structure or function. Bisynchronous slow waves may be added as the result of toxic or metabolic complications

or of predominant involvement of cortical and subcortical grey matter. Focal slow waves can appear when there is more localized damage, especially that produced by herpes simplex encephalitis and abscesses.

Subacute sclerosing panencephalitis, a late complication of measles infection, initially often produces generalized asynchronous slow waves as a background on which the characteristic periodic complexes later develop.

(4) *Progressive multifocal leukoencephalopathy,* a disease of probably viral cause, produces generalized asynchronous slow waves; they may be preceded by a stage of focal slow waves.

(5) *Sydenham's chorea* associated with streptococcal infections, in many cases produces asynchronous generalized slow waves in excess of those of normal children at the same age and in some cases produces bisynchronous slow waves or spikes and sharp waves.

(6) *General paresis* produces asynchronous and, occasionally, bisynchronous slow waves in slightly over one-half of all cases whereas patients with other forms of neurosyphilis usually have a normal EEG.

(7) *AIDs dementia complex, or encephalopathy*, is characterized in the early stages by mild degrees of background slowing with widespread bisynchronous and asynchronous waveforms predominantly in the theta frequency range. This may occur at a time when neuroanatomical imaging studies and evoked potential studies are normal. As the disease progresses slowing becomes more prominent. A characteristic EEG pattern has not been identified. Milder degrees of background disorganization and slowing may be detectable with serial studies in patients at risk.

21.5.8 *Psychiatric diseases.* The incidence of generalized asynchronous slow waves is slightly higher in patients with various psychiatric diseases than in the general population (Fig. 21.1). This is most evident in schizophrenia where slow waves are seen most often in the catatonic form, least in the paranoid form. However, the slow waves are usually only mild or moderate and therefore do not help in the diagnosis except that (a) the absence of other abnormalities in the EEG may help to exclude gross organic disease and (b) the presence of marked generalized slow waves suggests organic disease.

See summary

REFERENCES

Brenner, R.P. (1985) The electroencephalogram in altered states of consciousness. In: Aminoff, M.J. (Ed.), Electrodiagnosis, Neurologic Clinics. Saunders, Philadelphia, pp. 615–629.

Courjon, J., Ed. (1972) Traumatic disorders. In: Rémond, A. (Ed.), Handbook of Electroenceph. clin. Neurophysiol., Vol. 14B. Elsevier, Amsterdam.

Farrell, D.F. (1969) The EEG in progressive multifocal leukoencephalopathy. Electroenceph. clin. Neurophysiol. 26: 200–205.

Giel, R., De Vlieger, M. and Van Vliet, A.G.M. (1966) Headache and the EEG. Electroenceph. clin. Neurophysiol. 21: 492–495.

Hansotia, P., Harris, R. and Kennedy, J. (1969) EEG changes in Wilson's disease. Electroenceph. clin. Neurophysiol. 27: 523–528.

Jóhannesson, G., Brun, A., Gustafson, L. and Ingvar, D.H. (1977) EEG in presenile dementia related to cerebral blood flow and autopsy findings. Acta Neurol. Scand. 56: 89–103.

Jóhannesson, G., Hagberg, B., Gustafson, L. and Ingvar, D.H. (1979) EEG and cognitive impairment in presenile dementia. Acta Neurol. Scand. 59: 225–240.

Kaszniak, A.W., Garron, D.C., Fox, J.H., Bergen, D. and Huckman, M. (1979) Cerebral atrophy, EEG slowing, age, education, and cognitive functioning in suspected dementia. Neurology 29: 1273–1279.

Kurtz, D. (1976) Section VII. The EEG in acute and chronic drug intoxications. In: Rémond, A. (Ed.), Handbook of Electroenceph. clin. Neurophysiol., Vol. 15C. Elsevier, Amsterdam, pp. 88–104.

Lević, Z.M. (1978) Electroencephalographic studies in multiple sclerosis. Specific changes in benign multiple sclerosis. Electroenceph. clin. Neurophysiol. 44: 471–478.

Mellerio, F. and Kubicki, S. (1977) Section VII. B. Encephalopathy due to poisoning. In: Rémond, A. (Ed.), Handbook of Electroenceph. clin. Neurophysiol., Vol. 15A. Elsevier, Amsterdam, pp. 108–135.

Radermecker, F.J., Ed. (1977) Infections and inflammatory reactions, allergy and allergic reactions; degenerative diseases. In: Rémond, A. (Ed.), Handbook of Electroenceph. clin. Neurophysiol., Vol. 15A. Elsevier, Amsterdam, pp. 1–108.

Radermecker, F.J. (1977) Degenerative diseases of the nervous system. In: Rémond, A. (Ed.), Handbook of Electroenceph. clin. Neurophysiol., Vol. 15A. Elsevier, Amsterdam, pp. 162–191.

Roberts, M.A., McGeorge, A.P. and Caird, F.I. (1978) Electroencephalography and computerised tomography in vascular and non-vascular dementia in old age. J. Neurol. Neurosurg. Psychiat. 41: 903–906.

Rumpl, E., Lorenzi, E., Hackl, J.M., Gerstenbrand, F. and Hengl, W. (1979) The EEG at different stages of acute secondary traumatic midbrain and bulbar brain syndromes. Electroenceph. clin. Neurophysiol. 46: 487–497.

Sharbrough, F.W. (1987) Nonspecific abnormal EEG patterns. In: Niedermeyer, E. and Lopes da Silva, F. (Eds.), Electroencephalography: Basic Principles, Clinical Applications and Related Fields. Urban and Schwarzenberg, Baltimore, pp. 163–182.

Silverman, D. (1975) Section VII. The electroencephalogram in anoxic coma. In: Rémond, A. (Ed.), Handbook of Electroenceph. clin. Neurophysiol., Vol. 12. Elsevier, Amsterdam, pp. 81–94.

Stevens, J.R., Sachdev, K. and Milstein, V. (1968) Behavior disorders of childhood and the electroencephalogram. Arch. Neurol. 18: 160–177.

Stigsby, B., Jóhannesson, G. and Ingvar, D.H. (1981) Regional EEG analysis and regional cerebral blood flow in Alzheimer's and Pick's diseases. Electroenceph. clin. Neurophysiol. 51: 537–547.

Tarrier, N., Cooke, E.C. and Lader, M.H. (1978) The EEG's of chronic schizophrenic patients in hospital and in the community. Electroenceph. clin. Neurophysiol. 44: 669–673.

Volavka, J., Feldstein, S., Abrams, R., Dornbush, R. and Fink, M. (1972) EEG and clinical change after bilateral and unilateral electroconvulsive therapy. Electroenceph. clin. Neurophysiol. 32: 631–639.

Westmoreland, B.F. (1987) The EEG in cerebral inflammatory processes. In: Niedermeyer, E. and Lopes da Silva, F. (Eds.), Electroencephalography: Basic Principles, Clinical Applications and Related Fields. Urban and Schwarzenberg, Baltimore, pp. 259–274.

Westmoreland, B.F. and Saunders, M.G. (1979) The EEG in the evaluation of disorders affecting the brain diffusely. In: Klass, D.W. and Daly, D. (Eds.), Current Practice of Clinical Electroencephalography, Raven, New York, pp. 307–342.

Bilaterally synchronous slow waves

22

SUMMARY

(22.1) *The pattern* of bisynchronous slow waves is characterized by waves which have a frequency of less than 8 Hz and occur on both sides of the head so that waves of the same frequency appear at the same time in corresponding areas. These waves may be distributed over the entire head or be limited to one or a few electrodes on each side; in many cases, their distribution shifts from one moment to the next. They usually appear as intermittent trains of waves on a background of lower amplitude. Bisynchronous slow waves commonly are regular and rhythmical in shape, but may be irregular and arrhythmical. These waves are reduced or blocked by eye opening or alerting; they are increased during hyperventilation and drowsiness. A characteristic variety of bisynchronous slow waves is frontal intermittent rhythmical delta activity (FIRDA), also called 'monorhythmic frontal delta' (MFD). This consists of bursts of sinusoidal 2–3 Hz waves of high amplitude and a bifrontal maximum.

(22.2) *The causes* of bisynchronous slow waves include several normal and abnormal conditions. Normal bisynchronous slow waves are seen in infants and children during wakefulness and sleep and in adults during drowsiness and sleep and during and after hyperventilation. Bisynchronous slow waves are abnormal in alert resting adults. Bisynchronous slow waves result from the projection of an abnormality from distant, subcortical structures, especially from the brainstem reticular system and its rostral connections deep at the midline of the posterior, middle and anterior fossa, to the site of EEG production in the cerebral cortex. These abnormalities include (1) diffuse encephalopathies involving subcortical and cortical cerebral grey matter more than cerebral white matter; (2) structural lesions which directly or indirectly involve the mesencephalon, diencephalon, orbital and mesial surfaces of the frontal lobe; and (3) metabolic, toxic and endocrine encephalopathies.

(22.3) *Other EEG abnormalities* include a background of generalized asynchronous slow waves from which bisynchronous slow waves are often difficult to distinguish; however, the special diagnostic implications of bisynchronous slow waves justify the attempt to discriminate between these two varieties of generalized slow waves.

(22.4) *Mechanisms* causing bisynchronous slow waves involve thalamocortical and interhemispheric interactions.

(22.5) *Specific disorders* include many diseases impairing structure and function of deep midline structures.

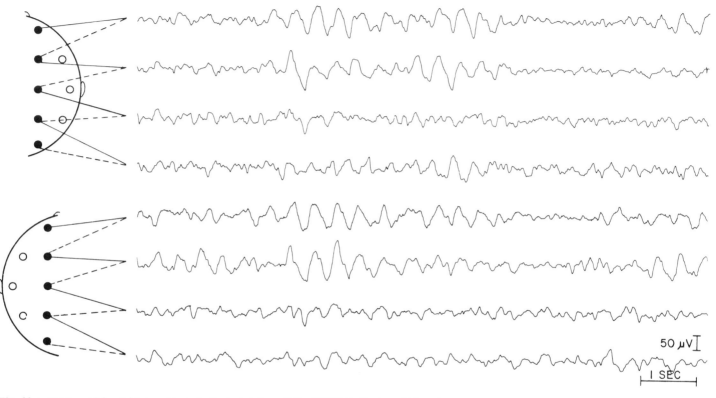

Fig. 22.1. Pattern of frontal intermittent rhythmical delta activity (FIRDA). Trains of bisynchronous slow waves of 2–3 Hz and of high amplitude appear with a maximum in the frontal regions on a background of diffuse slow waves of low to medium amplitude. The patient is an 18-year-old girl who sustained a severe head injury 2 weeks earlier. She had been in coma initially, then was confused and irritated until 2 days before the recording. At the time of the recording, her neurological examination was normal; there were no gross mental symptoms. Followup EEGs 7 weeks and several months later were entirely normal; the patient recovered without deficit. The final diagnosis was brainstem contusion.

Bisynchronous slow waves have a frequency of less than 8 Hz and appear simultaneously in corresponding parts of the two hemispheres. Individual waves are commonly sinusoidal or at least regular (Fig. 22.1). They are usually rhythmical, i.e., they repeat at the same rate and vary by no more than a few hertz over the course of time. They are usually intermittent, lasting for a few seconds and forming trains which begin and end at about the same time on the two sides. The wave peaks in one area do not always coincide with the peaks in another area, but waves of the same frequency in different areas are usually synchronous on the two sides. In contrast to most other slow waves, bisynchronous slow waves of even high amplitude may occur sporadically, separated from each other by periods of entirely normal activity.

Bisynchronous slow waves may be generalized or restricted; they may have a maximum in the same portions of both hemispheres or may be more prominent on one side. Their distribution and prominence, in contrast to that of other slow waves, often varies from moment to moment and may shift from one area to another or from restricted to more generalized. They are abolished or reduced on both sides by eye opening or alerting; they are increased during eye closure, hyperventilation and drowsiness. Abnormal bisynchronous slow waves disappear in the background of normal bisynchronous slow waves during sleep stages I–IV, but may reappear in REM sleep.

Bisynchronous slow waves commonly have delta frequency, medium to high amplitude and are regular and rhythmical (Fig. 22.1); however, bisynchronous slow waves may have theta frequency, low to medium amplitude and be irregular and arrhythmical (Figs. 22.2, 22.3). Discrete trains of rhythmical delta waves, i.e. intermittent rhythmical delta activity ('IRDA') (Fig. 22.1) may occur maximally in the frontal areas (frontal intermittent rhythmical delta activity, 'FIRDA') or in the oc-

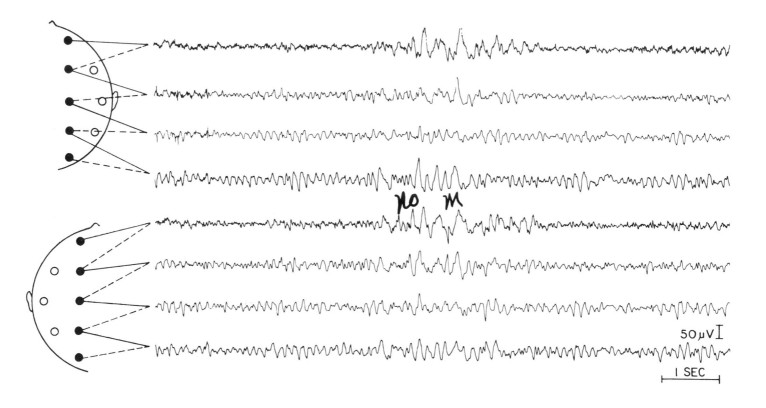

Fig. 22.2. Pattern of paroxysmal bisyncronous slow waves of irregular shape on a normal background. Technician's comment (NO M) means that the patient did not move during this paroxysm. This 58-year-old woman had a parathyroidectomy 18 years earlier. For several weeks before the recording she felt increasingly tired and experienced an episode of nearly fainting. Chvostek and Trousseau signs were positive, serum calcium was decreased at 5.6 mg % and phosphorus was increased at 6.3 mg %.

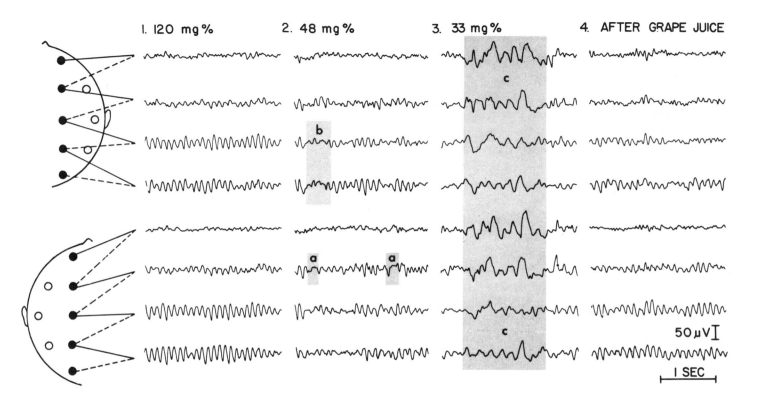

Fig. 22.3. Bisyncronous slow waves induced by hypoglycemia which developed during a glucose tolerance test. 1. Before the beginning of the test, the EEG was normal; 2. At a blood sugar level of 48 mg %, the EEG showed low to medium amplitude diffuse theta (a) and delta (b) waves of low to medium amplitude; 3. At a blood sugar level of 33 mg %, bursts of high amplitude bisynchronous delta and theta waves appeared with a maximum in the frontal regions (c); 4. After the patient drank some grapefruit-juice, the EEG returned almost completely to normal. This recording is of an 18-year-old boy with two episodes of nearly fainting several hours after the last meal.

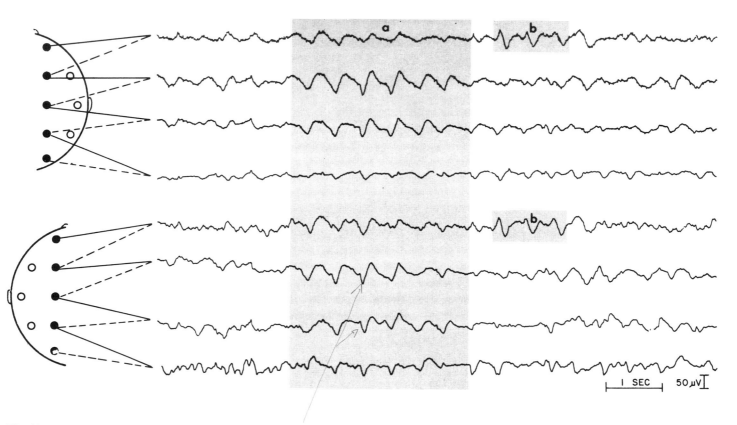

Fig. 22.4. Pattern of bisynchronous slow waves of the triphasic wave pattern demonstrating an apparent longitudinal time delay of the second phase (downgoing phase) over the more posterior head regions compared to the anterior head regions. The recording is from a 54 year-old in hepatic coma who died several days later.

446

cipital areas (occipital intermittent rhythmical delta activity, 'OIRDA'). Because these waves usually are of only a single frequency, they have also been called 'monorhythmic frontal delta' (MFD) activity. Other names, implicating their origin, are 'rhythmes à distance' or 'projected slow waves'.

22.2 CLINICAL SIGNIFICANCE OF BISYNCHRONOUS SLOW WAVES

22.2.1 *Normal bisynchronous slow waves* are seen (1) during drowsiness and sleep at any age; (2) during wakefulness in subjects under the age of 20 years; (3) in response to hyperventilation at any age, especially childhood; (4) in adults having the rare patterns of slow alpha variant and of posterior slow waves (11.7).

22.2.2 *Abnormal bisynchronous slow waves* are those occurring under conditions other than the ones listed above and usually reflect abnormalities located deeply in the brain and at some distance from the recording site. These abnormalities may be diffuse or circumscribed structural lesions, or disorders of cerebral function.

Diffuse structural damage may produce bisynchronous slow waves if it involves grey matter of subcortical structures alone or in combination with cortical grey matter, especially when the grey matter is damaged more than the hemispheric white matter. This is the presumed cause of bisynchronous slow waves in some degenerative encephalopathies.

Circumscribed structural lesions may cause bisynchronous slow waves either directly or indirectly. Lesions which are located near the midline at the base of the brain may directly involve the brainstem, diencephalon or the orbital and mesial surfaces of the frontal lobes (Fig. 22.1); lesions located near these structures may secondarily invade, compress, or distort them or render them ischemic or edematous (Fig. 20.3). While increased intracranial pressure by itself does not alter the EEG until it reaches the range of the arterial blood pressure, it can produce herniation of

447

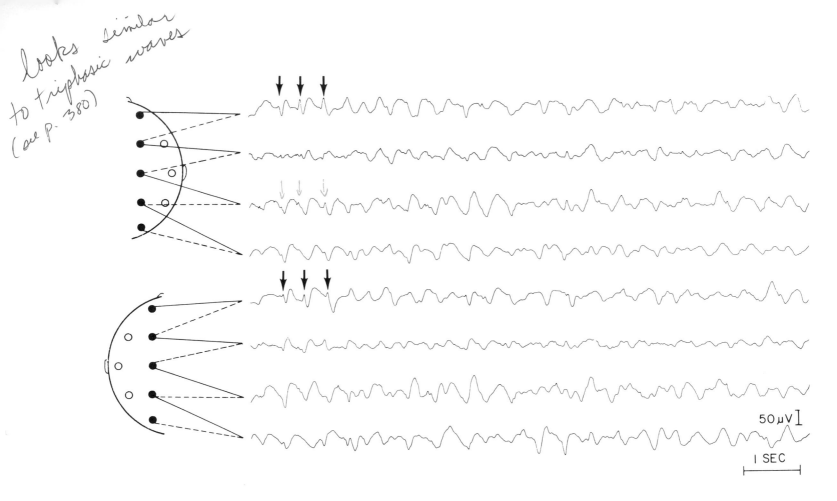

looks similar to triphasic waves (see p. 380)

50 μV

1 SEC

Fig. 22.5. Pattern of continuous bisynchronous slow waves mixed with sharp waves (arrows). This 26-year-old woman was in delirium due to water intoxication with metabolic acidosis and hyponatremia. Her EEG 5 days later was normal; she had completely recovered.

448

the uncus of the temporal lobe which distorts the brainstem and thereby induces bisynchronous slow waves.

Disorders of cerebral function include mainly encephalopathies of toxic and metabolic etiology (Figs. 22.2; 22.3; 22.4; 22.5). The bisynchronous slow waves in these encephalopathies may disappear when the underlying abnormality is reversed. Transient bisynchronous slow waves may also be seen during and after generalized seizures, in attacks of vertebral-basilar migraine or of vertebral-basilar ischemia, in syncope and in some cases of transient global amnesia.

22.3 OTHER EEG ABNORMALITIES ASSOCIATED WITH BISYNCHRONOUS SLOW WAVES

22.3.1 *Reduction, slowing and disorganization of alpha rhythm* may occur with mild or moderate bisynchronous slow waves (Fig. 22.3).

22.3.2 *Generalized asynchronous slow waves* may be so prominent as to obscure bisynchronous slow waves. They usually are not seen in cases of uncomplicated deep circumscribed lesions.

22.3.3 *Focal slow waves, local reduction of amplitude or focal epileptiform activity* suggest either a local lesion which primarily produces focal EEG abnormalities and secondarily involves subcortical structures producing bisynchronous slow waves (Fig. 20.3), or a metabolic or toxic encephalopathy which primarily produces bisynchronous slow waves and secondarily causes local cerebral damage producing focal EEG abnormalities.

The bilaterally synchronous appearance of slow waves, like that of bilaterally synchronous epileptiform activity, is commonly thought to be due to the faulty action of a central pacemaker which projects abnormal impulses diffusely to the cerebral cortex causing slow waves to be generated synchronously on both sides (1.2). The system responsible for the synchronization of the two hemispheres is unknown but is probably located in the brainstem and diencephalon and may be identical with part or all of the reticular formation. This hypothesis could explain why three very different types of basic cerebral pathology, namely diffuse damage to subcortical and cortical grey matter, local lesions near deep midline structures, and metabolic and toxic encephalopathies, all cause bisynchronous slow waves. Diffuse damage to subcortical and cortical grey matter may cause bisynchronous slow waves by damaging both the subcortical and cortical components of the reticulocortical system implicated in the production of this abnormality. Local damage to deep midline structures may directly or indirectly interfere with the reticular formation and its rostral projections to the cerebral cortex. Metabolic and toxic encephalopathies are known to preferentially affect the function of mesencephalic and diencephalic centers, especially those responsible for alertness.

22.5 SPECIFIC DISORDERS CAUSING BILATERALLY SYNCHRONOUS SLOW WAVES

22.5.1 *Degenerative, developmental and demyelinating diseases:*

(1) *Alzheimer's disease* is in some cases associated with bifrontal synchronous slow waves but asynchronous slow waves and slowing of the alpha rhythm are more common findings. Infrequently, sporadic bilateral triphasic waves occur.

(2) *Parkinson's disease* is rarely associated with bisynchronous slow waves; asynchronous slow waves are more common.

450

TABLE 22.1

	Decreased alpha frequency	Generalized asynchronous slow waves	Focal slow waves	Triphasic waves	Spikes
ACTH, cortisone Rx	+	+			(+)
Acute anoxia, pulmonary insufficiency	+	+		+ +	
Addison's disease	+	+			(+)
Cerebromacular degenerations		+ +			
CO poisoning		+		(+)	
Dialysis encephalopathy	+	+	(+)	+	+
Hepatic encephalopathy (Fig. 22.2)	+	+		+ +	
Hydration (Hyponatremia, Fig. 22.3)		+		+	+
Hyperglycemia without ketoacidosis					+
Hyperparathyroidism (Hypercalcemia)	+	+	(+)	+	
Hypoglycemia	+	+	+	+	+
Hypokalemia (alkalosis)	+	+			
Hypoparathyroidism pseudohypo- parathyroidism (Hypocalcemia, Fig. 22.4)	+	+			+
Hypopituitarism		+			
Porphyria	+	+	+		+
Renal encephalopathy		+	+	+ +	+
Thyrotoxicosis		+		+	+
Vitamin B-12 deficiency	+	+	+		
Wernicke's encephalopathy	+	+			
Wilson's disease		+	+	(+)	

451

(3) *Progressive supranuclear palsy* may produce bisynchronous slow waves, usually after the sleep EEG has become abnormal.

(4) *Other diseases* may induce bisynchronous slow waves in some cases: Leber's hereditary optic atrophy, Ramsey-Hunt's cerebellar myoclonic dyssynergia, myotonic dystrophy, tuberous sclerosis, hydrocephalus, and others.

(5) *Multiple sclerosis* causes bisynchronous slow waves in some patients, often in combination with asynchronous slow waves.

22.5.2 *Metabolic and toxic encephalopathies. Bisynchronous slow waves* occur in the mild or moderate stages of many of these disorders (Table 22.1 and Figs. 22.2; 22.3, Part 3) and are commonly associated with other abnormalities, namely slowing of the alpha rhythm and generalized asynchronous slow waves, and less often with focal slow waves, triphasic waves, and generalized or focal spikes and sharp waves.

In acute encephalopathies, EEG abnormalities appear in a sequence which roughly parallels the severity of the disorder. At the mildest stage, bisynchronous slow waves do not appear spontaneously but may be induced by hyperventilation; at this stage, photic stimulation may produce an increased or abnormal response. The alpha rhythm decreases in frequency and may decrease in prominence (Fig. 22.3, Part 2). Spontaneous bisynchronous slow waves appear first in short bursts (Fig. 22.3, Part 3, Fig. 22.2), later in long trains or continuously (Fig. 22.1). Asynchronous generalized slow waves may appear as soon as the alpha rhythm becomes disorganized; these slow waves become prominent and replace the alpha rhythm when alertness becomes impaired. Other abnormalities which may appear at this stage are focal slow waves and focal, unilateral or generalized spikes or sharp waves. With increasing severity, generalized asynchronous slow waves obscure all other abnormalities; the patient then is usually in deep coma. Death is often preceded by activity of low amplitude which may be interrupted by bursts of slow waves to form suppression burst patterns. If the underlying metabolic or toxic abnormality is reversed at any point, the EEG abnormalities may regress in reverse sequence except that generalized slow waves may persist to indicate that widespread cerebral damage has resulted, or focal slow waves may appear while generalized slow waves are present or as they disappear to indicate that local structural damage has occurred. (as in hypoglycemia)

Most chronic metabolic encephalopathies produce bisynchronous slow waves, slowing of alpha rhythm and generalized asynchronous slow waves. One or more of these abnormalities are seen in vitamin B12 deficiency, Wilson's disease, metachromatic leukodystrophy, Krabbe's disease, Wernicke's encephalopathy and dialysis encephalopathy; dialysis encephalopathy may also produce repetitive bisynchronous spike-and-wave complexes. However, a few metabolic encephalopathies produce bisynchronous slow waves only rarely and are characterized mainly by other abnormalities: Hypothyroidism decreases the frequency and amplitude of the alpha rhythm, hyperthyroidism increases alpha frequency, the lipidoses and other metabolic derangements, when seen in infants and young children, produce hypsarrhythmia, slow spike-and-waves and multifocal independent spikes (19.2).

22.5.3 *Cerebrovascular diseases:*

(1) *Transient ischemia* of the brain in general and of the brainstem in particular. as seen in syncope, in attacks of transient brainstem ischemia and of basilar artery migraine, can lead to bisynchronous slow waves which appear when consciousness begins to fade and abate when consciousness is regained. If they do not completely disappear in a few days, lasting damage is likely to have occurred.

(2) *Strokes* due to thrombosis, embolism or hemorrhage involving the central parts of the upper midbrain and diencephalon can lead to bisynchronous slow waves, often associated with asynchronous slow waves. Large hemispheric strokes, especially hypertensive hemorrhages, may lead to edema and to com-

pression of the brainstem and thereby produce bisynchronous slow waves mixed with focal and asynchronous generalized slow waves. Even strokes in the distribution of the anterior cerebral artery, causing damage to deep parts of the frontal lobe, are capable of producing bisynchronous intermittent frontal delta activity.

(3) *Postanoxic encephalopathy* may be associated with bisynchronous slow waves as one of many abnormalities and indicate involvement of deep structures of the brain.

(4) *Chronic subdural hematoma* may produce intermittent bisynchronous slow waves, especially in cases with fluctuating levels of consciousness; focal slow waves and amplitude changes are more common and more characteristic of subdural hematoma.

(5) *Subarachnoid hemorrhage* may be associated with bisynchronous slow waves in addition to asynchronous slow waves in patients with impaired consciousness; focal slow waves may be present and reflect local damage.

(6) *Moyamoya disease in children* may be associated with bisynchronous posterior slow waves.

22.5.4 *Cerebral trauma:*

(1) *Head injury* may produce bisynchronous slow waves either at the onset of unconsciousness when the EEG shows reduction of amplitude, or as patients emerge from deep coma when the EEG shows asynchronous slow waves and other abnormalities due to local or widespread cerebral damage. Bisynchronous slow waves indicate a relatively light stage of post-traumatic coma. Intermittent bisynchronous slow waves may persist for days or weeks nor only after severe (Fig. 22.1) but also after fairly mild head injuries.

(2) *Epidural and acute subdural hematoma* may initially produce bisynchronous slow waves; focal delta waves and reduction of amplitude follow.

(3) *Functional neurosurgery*, for instance coagulation of the anterior parts of the

internal capsule or of the thalamus and internal globus pallidus may produce bisynchronous frontal intermittent delta activity, presumably by interrupting subcortical
connections to the frontal cortex.

(4) *Progressive traumatic encephalopathy* may produce bisynchronous slow
waves in addition to asynchronous slow waves.

22.5.5 *Brain tumors:*

(1) *Infratentorial tumors* may cause bisynchronous slow waves if they invade or
compress the midbrain or distort the diencephalon. These slow waves are thus often
produced by tumors which arise within or near the central structures of the midbrain, for instance ependymomas and pineal tumors. In contrast, tumors located at
some distance from these structures, for instance cerebellar tumors and
meningiomas of the posterior fossa, may grow to considerable size without compressing the brainstem and producing bisynchronous slow waves. Tumors of the
lower brainstem, such as pontine gliomas, do not usually cause EEG abnormalities.

(2) *Supratentorial tumors* are likely to cause bisynchronous slow waves if they are
located in or near the diencephalon or the mesial and orbital parts of the frontal
lobe. Tumors in other locations may cause bisynchronous slow waves by secondarily
involving the deep midline structures. Other associated EEG abnormalities are
described above (22.3). Combinations of bisynchronous slow waves with focal slow
waves (Fig. 20.3) and focal epileptiform activity are particularly suggestive of deeply
located supratentorial tumors. Bisynchronous slow waves as a manifestation of
supratentorial tumor are more likely to be found in old persons than in young
adults.

(3) *Pseudotumor cerebri* or benign intracranial hypertension shares with cerebral
tumors only the name but not the pathology or EEG abnormalities. In contrast to
obstructive hydrocephalus, it produces no EEG abnormality in most patients,
but mild or moderate bisynchronous slow waves may occasionally be seen.

455

22.5.6 *Seizure disorders:*

(1) *Interictal* bisynchronous slow waves appear in some patients with primary generalized seizures. In particular, patients with absence attacks often show interictal bisynchronous rhythmical waves of 3 Hz. Interictal slow waves may be only indirectly related to seizures: They may be the manifestation of diseases causing seizures, for instance metabolic encephalopathies or myoclonus epilepsy, or they may be the result of disorders caused by seizures, for instance subdural hematomas or brainstem contusions.

(2) *Ictal* bisynchronous slow waves are rarely the only manifestation of a seizure. Bisynchronous slow waves in combination with generalized spikes or sharp waves form part of spike-and-waves of many epileptiform patterns.

(3) *Postictal* bisynchronous slow waves, including triphasic waves, may occur in addition to asynchronous postictal slow waves.

22.5.7 *Infectious diseases:*

(1) *Fever, reduced alertness, metabolic abnormalities* and electrolyte imbalances associated with infections may cause bisynchronous slow waves even if the brain is not infected.

(2) *Meningitis and encephalitis* may cause bisynchronous slow waves in conditions in which they cause asynchronous slow waves.

(3) *Sydenham's chorea* causes bisynchronous slow waves in many cases; asynchronous slow waves may also appear.

22.5.8 *Psychiatric diseases:*

(1) *Personality disorders, behavior disturbances and schizophrenia* are occasionally associated with bisynchronous slow waves. However, this abnormality, like other abnormal EEG patterns, is not very common in psychiatric diseases. Therefore, organic causes for this abnormality have to be excluded, particularly

456

treatable conditions such as metabolic and toxic encephalopathies, frontal, hypo-
thalamic and pituitary tumors which all may cause psychiatric symptoms.

(2) *Kleine-Levin syndrome* during attacks may be associated with bursts of bisynchronous slow waves on a background of asynchronous slow waves; these abnormalities are not entirely explained by drowsiness and sleep.

see summary

REFERENCES

Allen, E.M., Singer, F.R. and Melamed, D. (1970) Electroencephalographic abnormalities in hypercalcemia. Neurology 20: 15–22.

Bingley, T. and Persson, A. (1978) EEG studies on patients with chronic obsessive-compulsive neurosis
before and after psychosurgery (stereotaxic bilateral anterior capsulotomy). Electroenceph. clin.
Neurophysiol. 44: 691–696.

Dow, R.S. (1961) The electroencephalographic findings in acute intermittent porphyria. Electroenceph.
clin. Neurophysiol. 13: 425–437.

Gastaut, H. and Fischer-Williams, M. (1957) Electro-encephalographic study of syncope. Its differentiation from epilepsy. Lancet 2: 1018–1025.

Glaser, G.H., Ed. (1976) Metabolic, endocrine and toxic diseases. In: Rémond, A. (Ed.), Handbook of
Electroenceph. clin. Neurophysiol., Vol. 15C, Elsevier, Amsterdam.

Gloor, P., Kalaby, O. and Giard, N. (1968) The electroencephalogram in diffuse encephalopathies: Electroencephalographic correlates of grey and white matter lesions. Brain 91: 779–802.

Gloor, P. (1976) Section IV. Generalized and widespread bilateral paroxysmal activities. In: Rémond,
A. (Ed.), Handbook of Electroenceph. clin. Neurophysiol., Vol. 11B, Elsevier, Amsterdam, pp.
52–87.

Harner, R.N. and Katz, R.I. (1975) Section IV. Electroencephalography in metabolic coma. In: Rémond, A. (Ed.), Handbook of Electroenceph. clin. Neurophysiol., Vol. 12, Elsevier, Amsterdam, pp.
47–62.

Hasegawa, K. and Aird, R.B. (1963) An EEG study of deep-seated cerebral and subtentorial lesions in
comparison with cortical lesions. Electroenceph. clin. Neurophysiol. 15: 934–946.

Heller, G.L. and Kooi, K.A. (1962) The electroencephalogram in hepato-lenticular degeneration
(Wilson's disease). Electroenceph. clin. Neurophysiol. 14: 520–526.

Jóhannesson, G., Brun, A., Gustafson, L. and Ingvar, D.H. (1977) EEG in presenile dementia related
to cerebral blood flow and autopsy findings. Acta Neurol. Scand. 56: 89–103.

Martinius, J., Matthes, A. and Lombroso, C.T. (1968) Electroencephalographic features in posterior
fossa tumors in children. Electroenceph. clin. Neurophysiol. 25: 128–139.

Schaul, N., Gloor, P. and Gotman, J. (1981) The EEG in deep midline lesions. Neurology 31: 157–167.

Schaul, N., Lueders, H. and Sachdev, K. (1981) Generalized bilaterally synchronous bursts of slow waves in the EEG. Arch. Neurol. 38: 690–692.

Sharbrough, F.W. (1987) Nonspecific abnormal EEG patterns. In: Niedermeyer, E. and Lopes da Silva, F. (Eds.), Electroencephalography: Basic Principles, Clinical Applications and Related Fields, Urban and Schwarzenberg, Baltimore, pp. 163–182.

Sidell, A.D. and Daly, D.D. (1961) The electroencephalogram in cases of benign intracranial hypertension. Neurology 11: 413–417.

Su, P.C. and Goldensohn, E.S. (1973) Progressive supranuclear palsy. Arch. Neurol. 29: 183–186.

van der Drift, J.H.A. and Magnus, O. (1962) The EEG with space occupying intracranial lesions in old patients. Electroenceph. clin. Neurophysiol. 14: 664–673.

Wallace, P.W. and Westmoreland, B.F. (1976) The electroencephalogram in pernicious anemia. Mayo Clin. Proc. 51: 281–285.

Westmoreland, B.F. and Saunders, M.G. (1979) The EEG in the evaluation of disorders affecting the brain diffusely. In: Klass, D.W. and Daly, D. (Eds.), Current Practice of Clinical Electroencephalography. Raven, New York, pp. 307–342.

Wilkus, R.J. and Chiles, J.A. (1975) Electrophysiological changes during episodes of the Kleine-Levin syndrome. J. Neurol. Neurosurg. Psychiat. 38: 1225–1231.

Localized and lateralized changes of amplitude: Asymmetries

23

SUMMARY

(23.1)   Asymmetry is characterized by differences in amplitude of the EEG recorded from the two sides of the head. Differences in amplitude may involve the entire background or only some background patterns. Local reduction of the amplitude of alpha rhythm in some cases is associated with reduction of alpha frequency.

(23.2)   *Causes* of asymmetry are unilateral lesions, most of which are superficial. The amplitude of acitivity in the alpha and beta frequency range is usually reduced on the side of the lesion, rarely increased. Amplitude may be reduced by local cortical damage, for instance by superficial infarctions, tumors and head injuries, or by transient disturbances of cerebral function, for instance by attacks of transient ischemia and migraine. Extracerebral lesions can also change EEG amplitude. Subdural hematomas may reduce it and skull defects may increase it. The alpha rhythm may be reduced by lesions of thalamocortical connections, i.e. lesions not located at the cortex of the posterior head regions where the alpha rhythm is produced. In some instances, the alpha rhythm is reduced by lesions in the anterior head regions.

(23.3)   *Other EEG abnormalities,* if limited to one side, may further help to indicate the site of the underlying cerebral abnormality.

(23.4)   *Mechanisms* of asymmetries involve either changes of cortical EEG production as in the case of structural or functional cortical lesions, or alterations of the media between cortex and recording electrodes such as fluid collections or skull defects.

(23.5)   *Specific disorders* causing asymmetries include many clinically important diseases.

(23.6)   *Asymmetries of alpha, beta, mu and other rhythms* are seen in a variety of clinical conditions.

23.1   DESCRIPTION OF PATTERN

Asymmetry consists of a difference in the amplitude of activity recorded from corresponding areas on the two sides of the head (Figs. 23.1; 23.2; 23.3). Asymmetries usually affect all types of background activity during wakefulness and sleep

459

(Fig. 23.1); occasionally they involve only the alpha rhythm, beta rhythm, mu rhythm, responses to photic stimulation and hyperventilation, or sleep patterns. A local decrease in the amplitude of alpha rhythm is often associated with a decrease of alpha frequency. Lesions which cause an asymmetry of normal background activity may also cause an asymmetry of abnormal activity. This can produce *e.g. subdural* difficulties in identifying the side of the abnormality. For instance, a superficial lesion reducing the amplitude of the EEG on the same side may also cause bilateral abnormalities such as slow waves or epileptiform activity. This combination makes the abnormal activity appear with a higher amplitude on the uninvolved side and falsely suggests that the uninvolved side is the abnormal one (Fig. 23.2). To correctly identify the involved side in these cases, the EEG reader must carefully search for: (1) normal patterns which should be reduced in amplitude on the abnor-

TABLE 23.1
Asymmetries

Abnormal patterns	Causes	Mechanisms	Examples of diseases
Decreased amplitude of all types of activity	Local cortical damage	Decreased cortical EEG production	Cortical infarct, Sturge-Weber syndrome
	Local disorder of cortical function	As above	Local cortical ischemia
	Unilateral increase of media between cortex and recording electrodes	Decreased electrical impedance within the conducting media *≈ Shunting*	Subdural hematoma
		Increased electrical impedance between cortex and recording electrodes	Skull hyperostosis
Of alpha, beta, mu rhythm, sleep patterns	Defect may be distant, at presumed site of pacemaker *	Decreased rhythmical input to cortex	Cerebral infarcts, tumors, injuries, without reliable relation to location of rhythm
Increased amplitude	Skull defects	Decreased electrical impedance between cortex and electrodes	Postoperative skull defect

460

＊ thalamus for alpha + sleep spindles

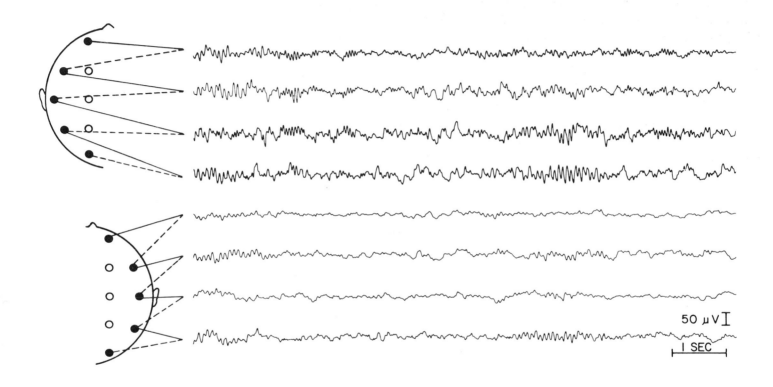

Fig. 23.1. Pattern of asymmetry of normal background activity. Sleep spindles and slow waves of sleep
are attenuated over the right side. This 7-year-old boy has signs characteristic of Sturge-Weber syndrome:
a right facial naevus, cerebral calcifications extending into the parietal and temporal areas, and left-sided
and generalized motor seizures.

461

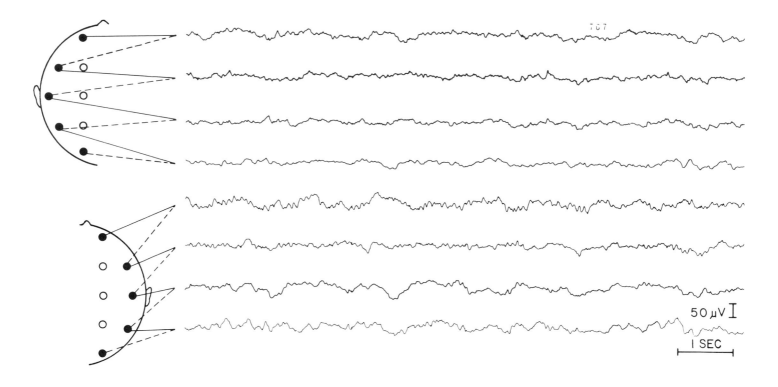

Fig. 23.2. Pattern of asymmetry combined with generalized asynchronous slow waves. The reduction of amplitude on the left side attenuates the generalized slow waves on that side and thereby makes them appear with higher amplitude on the right side, falsely suggesting a right-sided cerebral abnormality. The correct localization of an abnormality on the left side is suggested by the circumstance that the faster frontal rhythms are also reduced on the left side. The patient is a 37-year-old chronic alcoholic in coma. A large chronic subdural hematoma on the left side was evacuated a few hours after this EEG recording.

mal side (Fig. 23.1); (2) subtle (1–2 Hz) differences in the peak frequency of the background rhythm (with the slower frequency indicating the more abnormal side); (3) reduced reactivity on the abnormal side; and (4) additional abnormalities that may be limited to the abnormal side.

Asymmetries of activity in large parts of the hemispheres can be recognized with referential recordings. However, asymmetries between small areas are better detected with bipolar linkages between closely spaced electrodes. Asymmetry of amplitude can be accepted as having an intracranial cause only if asymmetries in electrode placement, electrode impedance imbalances, differences in gain and filter settings, skull defects, and scalp edema have been excluded.

23.2 CLINICAL SIGNIFICANCE OF ASYMMETRIES

23.2.1 *Normal asymmetries* are those described earlier for the alpha rhythm and for photic driving. The mu rhythm typically occurs bilaterally with similar amplitude over the two hemispheres. But asymmetry of photic driving or the mu rhythm alone, in the absence of other abnormalities, is of little clinical significance. A consistent asymmetry of beta activity of greater than 35% is considered abnormal and an asymmetry of greater than 50% is considered abnormal for the alpha rhythm.

23.2.2 *Abnormal asymmetries* are usually due to a decrease of amplitude on the side of the cerebral abnormality. Only rarely is the amplitude increased on the involved side causing activity of lower amplitude to appear on the normal side. However, in the absence of associated localizing abnormalities, or in the presence of bilateral abnormal EEG activity, it may be difficult to decide which side is abnormal (see above).

Asymmetries of all background activity.   A decrease of amplitude of all types of

463

activity in one area is due either to a reduction of cortical EEG production or to an increase of the media separating the cortex from the recording electrodes. Reductions of cortical electrogenesis may be long-lasting and due to structural lesions such as cortical strokes, tumors and injuries; transient reductions may follow focal seizures or be due to reversible conditions such as transient local ischemia or migraine. An increase of material between cortex and recording electrodes explains reduction of amplitude seen in many cases of subdural hematoma.

An increase of amplitude of all types of activity in one area is much rarer than a decrease of amplitude. It is usually due to a local skull defect.

Asymmetry of alpha rhythm has little localizing value. A local decrease of the amplitude in the posterior head regions may be due (a) to a lesion of the underlying cortex; (b) to a lesion of the thalamus or its connections to the underlying cortex; or (c) to a lesion in the frontal and central regions.

Asymmetry of beta rhythm may be the earliest and most sensitive indicator of a local lesion: An increase may be seen as the first sign of a superficial brain tumor, a decrease may be the last evidence of a long-standing atrophic scar.

Asymmetry of other activities include hyperventilation responses and sleep patterns. They may occur in an isolated fashion or in association with asymmetries of other patterns. When present they suggest a lesion of the hemisphere with lower amplitude.

23.3 OTHER ABNORMALITIES ASSOCIATED WITH ASYMMETRIES

23.3.1 *Focal slow waves* may appear in an area of reduced amplitude suggesting that white matter under the cortex is involved as well as the cortex itself and that the cortical function is not completely abolished. The center of the lesion may show waves of the slowest frequencies and of the lowest amplitude.

464

23.3.2 *Focal epileptiform activity* may appear in or near the area of depressed amplitude suggesting local irritation of the cortex. The combination of focal epileptiform activity and reduced amplitude may be the manifestation of a cortical epileptogenic lesion or the result of a very recent focal seizure.

23.3.3 *Generalized asynchronous and bisynchronous slow waves and generalized epileptiform activity* may be attenuated on the side of a lesion causing a reduction of amplitude and thus falsely suggest a lesion on the opposite side (see above).

23.4 MECHANISMS CAUSING LOCAL CHANGES OF AMPLITUDE

23.4.1 *Decreases of amplitude* are due to mechanisms which vary with the type of underlying lesion:

(1) *Reduction of cortical EEG production* may be due to structural damage reducing the total area of functioning membrane of cortical nerve cells, particularly of the large pyramidal neurons which are the major generators of the EEG (1.1). A temporary reduction of electrocortical potential changes may be due to a transient decrease of regional cerebral blood flow resulting in local hypoxia and hypoglycemia. These conditions may completely depolarize cortical neurons and make their membrane incapable of responding to excitatory and inhibitory input.

(2) *Interposition of material* between the cortical generators and the recording electrodes can attenuate the EEG by one of two mechanisms; the effect depends on the electrical properties of the interposed material. Substances of high impedance such as thickened skull or greasy scalp act as insulators and partly isolate the electrocortical potentials from the recording electrodes. Substances of low impedance such as subdural blood or spinal fluid act as conductors within the volume under the electrodes and shunt the potential differences before they reach the electrodes.

(3) *Selective decreases of alpha rhythm* may be due to derangements of thalamo-

465

cortical networks producing the impulses which synchronize the potential changes in cortical neurons in the posterior head regions (1.2). The mechanisms whereby frontal and central lesions reduce posterior alpha rhythm is unknown but may be related to the production of ischemia in structures engaged in the production of this rhythm.

23.4.2 *Increases of amplitude* are commonly seen after craniotomy and are partly due to reduced impedance between the EEG generator and the recording electrodes; in addition, local cortical excitability may produce local increases in amplitude.

Seemingly paradoxical asymmetric increases in background activity amplitude may occur, particularly in middle cerebral artery territory infarctions, but they are often accompanied by a 1–2 Hz reduction in peak frequency or less well sustained alpha and beta activity (23.1).

23.5 SPECIFIC DISORDERS CAUSING ASYMMETRIES OF AMPLITUDE

23.5.1 *Developmental, degenerative and demyelinating diseases:*

(1) *Porencephaly, holoprosencephaly and other defects* due to developmental malformation, perinatal injury or disease may show reduced EEG amplitude in addition to focal slow waves and focal epileptiform activity over areas of atrophic brain defects.

(2) *Sturge-Weber syndrome* is commonly associated with a decrease of amplitude on the side of the naevus (Fig. 23.1). This decrease may be found in infancy before cortical calcium deposits develop. The EEG may also show focal slow waves and focal epileptiform activity in the same area; bilateral synchronous slow waves and widespread epileptiform activity may be present.

(3) *Paget's disease* may cause a local increase in the thickness of the skull and thereby decrease the amplitude of the EEG over the involved area.

(4) *Multiple sclerosis* may produce a local decrease of EEG amplitude with or without other abnormalities.

23.5.2 *Metabolic and toxic encephalopathies.* A local or unilateral decrease of amplitude is not a direct result of these diseases but may occur as the result of complications, especially of cortical infarcts in renal, hypertensive, hypoglycemic and anoxic encephalopathy, and of subdural hematoma in hepatic and Wernicke's encephalopathy.

23.5.3 *Cerebrovascular diseases:*
(1) *Attacks of transient ischemia* involving the cortex of parts of the cerebral hemispheres may cause a local decrease of amplitude. The effects of acute local ischemia can be observed when EEG monitoring is used during carotid endarterectomies: A local reduction of amplitude, usually preceded by slow waves, may occur after clamping of the internal carotid artery.
(2) *Strokes* involving the cortex may cause a prolonged reduction of amplitude over the infarcted area. Focal slow waves may be present in the same area or in the surrounding parts during the acute stage but a reduction of amplitude may outlast other EEG abnormalities in the chronic stage.

Less often middle cerebral artery territory infarctions may produce a widespread increase in background activity. This is often accompanied by other findings that include: (1) irregularities in amplitude and frequency; (2) a 1–2 Hz reduction in the peak background rhythm compared to homotopic head regions; and (3) less well sustained rhythmic alpha and beta activity.
(3) *Chronic subdural hematoma* causes a unilateral or focal decrease of background amplitude in about one-half of all cases; alpha rhythm may be depressed more than other background activity. Focal slow waves are even more common than a decrease of amplitude in chronic subdural hematoma, but the decrease of

467

amplitude is an important signal of a superficial lesion and should always raise the suspicion of a subdural hematoma.

(4) *Subarachnoid hemorrhage* may produce amplitude asymmetry especially if there is local cortical damage or significant vasospasm.

(5) *Migraine* may cause unilateral reduction of amplitude during attacks. Between attacks, patients with migraine may show persistent reductions of background amplitude, especially of alpha rhythm, possibly representing residues of vascular damage incurred during an attack.

23.5.4 *Cerebral trauma:*

(1) *Head injuries* that are mild may lead to an immediate and transient decrease of amplitude which does not indicate definite cerebral damage. Severe head injuries can cause various EEG abnormalities initially and may later be followed by a long-lasting decrease of amplitude indicating residual structural damage due to contusions, intracerebral hemorrhage, epidural and acute subdural hematomas. Traumatic hemorrhages of newborn infants may be characterized by large areas of depressed amplitude.

(2) *Subgaleal hematoma,* a collection of blood between skull and scalp occurring mainly in infants with linear skull fractures, acts like a subdural or epidural hematoma in that it attenuates the amplitude of the EEG locally.

(3) *Scalp edema,* often caused by infiltration of intravenous fluids given through scalp veins to newborn infants, is a possible source of local attenuation of EEG amplitude.

(4) *Cranial defects* such as burrholes or larger defects remaining after neuro-surgical operations are characterized by a local increase of background amplitude. These asymmetries appear not only in recordings from electrodes placed over the defect but also in recordings from electrodes on bone near the edges of the defect. Alpha rhythm of higher amplitude may be recorded on the side of bony defects near

the posterior head regions. Beta activity may be found near bone defects in any part of the head; contralateral beta activity may be either absent or of lower amplitude. Bone defects near the central regions are often associated with a mu-like rhythm, local slow waves and sharp waves, all of which block like mu rhythm (11.3); mu rhythm of lower amplitude is not always present on the other side (Fig. 23.3). The appearance of these unilateral rhythms near a bone defect raises the question whether they are due only to the bone defect which may cause a fairly selective reduction of electrical impedance for fast EEG rhythms or to a change in the electrical activity produced by underlying cortex. A cerebral abnormality is more likely if (a) the activity on the two sides differs not only in amplitude but also in wave form and frequency, (b) recording from electrodes at some distance from the edge of the bone defect also shows abnormalities, and (c) differences of amplitude develop gradually after removal of the bone. While the reduction of an asymmetry after replacement of the bone (Fig. 23.3) suggests that the asymmetry was due to the bone defect, its persistence does not necessarily indicate that it is due to a cerebral abnormality because persisting gaps between skull and replacement may cause persistent asymmetries of impedance. Moreover, even if asymmetries are due to a cerebral abnormality, the abnormality may consist of no more than local meningo-cortical adhesions and cortical gliosis; only in the case of clearcut focal slow waves and spikes would one suspect the recurrence of an underlying cerebral lesion such as a tumor or a subdural hematoma, or the development of an epilepto-genic focus.

(5) *Hemispherectomy,* i.e. the partial or complete removal of a hemisphere reduces the amplitude of the EEG on the operated side in most cases but causes little change in some. The EEG on the operated side is probably generated by the opposite hemisphere and by deep remnants of the operated hemisphere and volume conducted to the recording electrodes on the operated side. The volume con-ducted EEG is attenuated by the electrical shunting effect of cerebrospinal fluid which usually accumulates in the operated space.

469

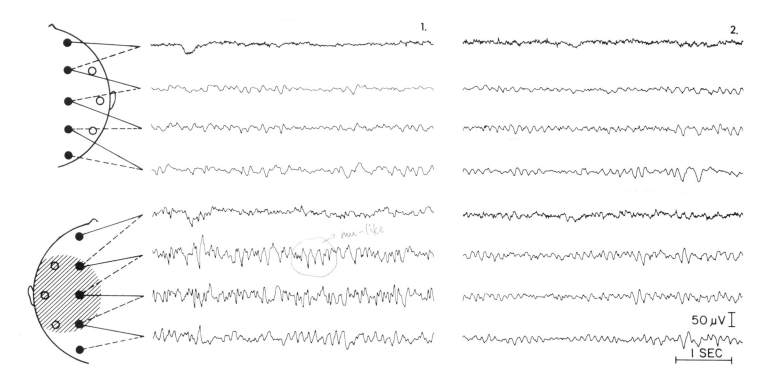

mu-like

50 μV

I SEC

Fig. 23.3. Pattern of local amplitude changes due to a skull defect. 1. Theta waves resembling mu rhythm appear at the left central electrode which is located over a skull defect indicated by the hatched area in the diagram on the left. Frontal beta rhythm and occipital alpha rhythm are also larger on the left than on the right side.* 2. After repair of the skull defect, both sides show symmetrical activity. This 48-year-old woman had an acute traumatic subdural hematoma evacuated 2 months before the recording in part 1; part 2 was recorded 3 months after repair of the skull defect. She had no neurological abnormalities at the time of either recording.

470

* away from the skull defect

23.5.5 *Brain tumors.* *Primary and metastatic brain tumors* sometimes, although rarely, first manifest by an asymmetry of amplitude in general or of alpha, beta or mu rhythm in particular.

23.5.6 *Seizure disorders:*

(1) *Postictal* local reduction of amplitude commonly appears immediately and only for a few minutes after a focal seizure discharge.

(2) *Interictal asymmetry* is usually due to the lesion causing the seizures, for instance an old cerebral infarct, residual damage after a head injury, Sturge-Weber syndrome or porencephaly.

(3) *Ictal* decreases of amplitude (19.4) are usually bilateral, even in partial complex seizures. However, a local reduction of amplitude often briefly precedes focal seizure discharges.

23.5.7 *Infectious diseases:*

(1) *Encephalitis* of any etiology can produce a local reduction of amplitude in the area of maximum involvement. A lasting reduction may indicate residual local damage.

(2) *Abscesses* can decrease the amplitude of all background activity or of alpha, beta or mu rhythms only.

(3) *Progressive multifocal leukoencephalitis* in its early stages may reduce the amplitude of background activity locally before causing generalized asynchronous slow waves.

(4) *Thrombophlebitis* of the cerebral venous sinuses may reduce the amplitude of all activity locally or unilaterally, especially in the acute phase when unilateral seizure discharges or status epilepticus are also likely to occur.

23.5.8 *Psychiatric diseases* without gross organic abnormalities are not associated with localized or lateralized reductions of EEG amplitude. Therefore, the finding of an asymmetry in a patient with psychiatric disease should raise the suspicion of an organic cerebral lesion.

23.6 ASYMMETRIES OF ALPHA, BETA, MU AND OTHER RHYTHMS

A decrease of the amplitude of one of these rhythms is usually part of an amplitude reduction involving all types of activity in one area. However, in a few conditions, the amplitude of one of these rhythms is reduced on one side or in one area while the amplitude of other activity remains symmetrical or is not reduced to the same extent. To be abnormal, an asymmetry of these rhythms must exceed their normal range of asymmetry (23.2.1). A selective asymmetry of one of these rhythms, without other associated abnormalities, may represent either a decrease of amplitude on one side or an increase of amplitude on the other and therefore does not indicate the abnormal side. However, clinically important asymmetries are often associated with a decrease of the frequency of that rhythm, or with other unilateral or focal EEG abnormalities which help to lateralize the underlying lesion correctly. In most instances, an asymmetry of the alpha rhythm is due to a posterior lesion and asymmetries of central beta and of mu rhythms are due to anterior lesions.

23.6.1 *Asymmetries of the alpha rhythm:*
(1) *Chronic subdural hematoma* may show a preferential depression of alpha rhythm. This is seen more commonly with posterior than with anterior hematomas.
(2) *Hemispheric infarcts* may reduce the amplitude of alpha rhythm more than that of other activity; a decrease of alpha activity may be the last residual abnormality of old infarcts.
(3) *Migraine* may reduce alpha rhythm unilaterally acutely during the attack;

472

alpha rhythm may be found to be asymmetrical in the interval between attacks without other evidence for infarction.

(4) *Head injuries* can lead to a unilateral decrease of the amplitude of alpha rhythm acutely. Asymmetry of alpha rhythm may be present while other EEG abnormalities due to the injury are also present; the alpha asymmetry may persist and be the last residual of severe head injuries or the only effect of mild head injuries.

(5) *Brain tumors and abscesses* involving the hemispheres, the thalamus or the floor of the third ventricle may selectively decrease alpha amplitude.

23.6.2 *Asymmetries of the beta and mu rhythms:*

(1) *Developmental lesions* reduce beta activity if they lead to cortical defects such as those seen in porencephaly or local atrophy.

(2) *Degenerative diseases* may produce an asymmetrical reduction of beta and mu before producing generalized reductions of amplitude.

(3) *Vascular diseases* may cause atrophic lesions producing selective reductions of the beta and mu rhythms; *central fast activity activated by movement* may be seen in postanoxic action myoclonus.

(4) *Cerebral trauma, and brain operations* leading to skull defects, are followed by a local increase of fast activity or mu rhythm, often associated with other abnormalities.

(5) *Brain tumors and abscesses* may cause a reduction or an increase of beta activity and the mu rhythm as the earliest EEG abnormality.

(6) *Ictal and interictal* beta activity may be produced by epileptogenic foci (19.4).

23.6.3 *Asymmetry and asynchrony* of sleep activity may persist in infants and children with perinatal cerebral abnormalities, particularly those with hydrocephalus. An asymmetry of sleep spindles can occur at any age as the result of hemispheric tumors, infarcts, Sturge-Weber's syndrome, leucotomy or other conditions, which involve either: (1) the nonspecific thalamic nuclei which generate sleep spindles, (2) the thalamocortical projections of the nonspecific nuclei, or (3) the cortex which receives those projections.

REFERENCES

Binnie, C.D. (1987) Recording techniques: Montages, electrodes, amplifiers and filters. In: Halliday, A.M., Butler, S.R. and Paul, R. (Eds.), A Textbook of Clinical Neurophysiology, Wiley, Chichester, pp. 3–22.

Chatrian, G.E., Somasundaram, M. and Foltz, E.L. (1969) EEG changes in subgaleal hematomas. Electroenceph. clin. Neurophysiol. 26: 524–527.

Cobb, W. and Sears, T.A. (1960) A study of the transmission of potentials after hemispherectomy. Electroenceph. clin. Neurophysiol. 12: 371–383.

Cobb, W.A., Guiloff, R.J. and Cast, J. (1979) Breach rhythm: The EEG related to skull defects. Electroenceph. clin. Neurophysiol. 47: 251–271.

Coull, B.M. and Pedley, T.A. (1978) Intermittent photic stimulation: Clinical usefulness of nonconvulsive responses. Electroenceph. clin. Neurophysiol. 44: 353–363.

Fisch, B.J. and Pedley, T.A. (1985) Evaluation of focal cerebral lesions. Role of electroencephalography in the era of computerized tomography. In: Aminoff, M.J. (Ed.), Electrodiagnosis, Neurologic Clinics, Saunders, Philadelphia, pp. 649–662.

Fukuyama, Y. and Tsuchiya, S. (1979) A study on Sturge-Weber syndrome. Report of a case associated with infantile spasms and electroencephalographic evolution in five cases. Eur. Neurol. 18: 194–204.

Goldensohn, E.S., O'Brien, J.L. and Ransohoff, J. (1961) Electrical activity of the brain. In patients treated with hemispherectomy or extensive decortication. Arch. Neurol. 5: 210–220.

Green, R.L. and Wilson, W.P. (1961) Asymmetries of beta activity in epilepsy, brain tumor, and cerebrovascular disease. Electroenceph. clin. Neurophysiol. 13: 75–78.

Homan, R.W., Herman, J. and Purdy, P. (1987) Cerebral localization of international 10–20 system electrode placement. Electroenceph. clin. Neurophysiol. 66: 376–382.

Jaffe, R. and Jacobs, L. (1972) The beta focus: Its nature and significance. Acta Neurol. Scand. 48: 191–203.

Kellaway, P. (1979) An orderly approach to visual analysis: parameters of the normal EEG in adults and children. In: Klass, D.W. and Daly, D.D. (Eds.), Current Practice of Clinical Electroencephalography, Raven, New York, pp. 69–147.

Kelly, J.J., Sharbrough, F.W. and Westmoreland, B.F. (1978) Movement-activated central fast rhythms: An EEG finding in action myoclonus. Neurology 28: 1037–1040.

Leissner, P., Lindholm, L.-E. and Petersen, I. (1970) Alpha amplitude dependence on skull thickness as measured by ultrasound technique. Electroenceph. clin. Neurophysiol. 29: 392–399.

Marshall, C. and Walker, A.E. (1950) The electroencephalographic changes after hemispherectomy in man. Electroenceph. clin. Neurophysiol. 2: 147–156.

Nealis, J.G.T. and Duffy, F.H. (1978) Paroxysmal beta activity in the pediatric electroencephalogram. Ann. Neurol. 4: 112–116.

Generalized changes of amplitude: Symmetrically high and low amplitude

SUMMARY

(24.1)   *The patterns* of generalized changes of amplitude consist of a bilateral symmetrical decrease or increase of amplitude of all types of normal activity or of specific patterns only. Such changes of amplitude are best recognized by comparison with previous recordings from the same subject because the amplitude of normal patterns differs widely in the general population. While abnormally low amplitude can be defined by voltage criteria, there is practically no upper limit for the amplitude of normal patterns. Instead the amplitude of activity in a given frequency range is judged as normal or abnormal according to its distribution and its amplitude in comparison to the activity in the other frequency bands.

(24.2)   *Causes* of bilateral abnormally low amplitude are similar to those producing unilateral reductions of amplitude, namely bilateral superficial lesions which reduce cortical function transiently or in a lasting manner or which change the media between cortex and recording electrodes. Bilateral reductions of amplitude may also be due to widespread cerebral disorders such as Huntington's chorea, postanoxic encephalopathy, cerebral death or severe changes in cortical function caused by toxic and metabolic diseases.

(24.3)   *Other EEG abnormalities* include generalized asynchronous slow waves and periodic complexes.

(24.4)   *Mechanisms* causing bilateral amplitude reductions consist of either decreased cortical activity or an alteration of the electrical impedance of the media between cortex and recording electrodes. Selective changes of the amplitude of specific rhythms are probably due to selective involvement of distant structures controlling the production of these rhythms by the cortex.

(24.5)   *Specific disorders* reducing overall amplitude include those associated with a wide variety of structural and functional abnormalities.

(24.6)   *A bilateral decrease of the alpha rhythm* may result from toxic and metabolic conditions or simply from anxiety.

(24.7)   *Generalized increased beta activity* is seen mainly as a result of tranquilizers and sedatives.

(24.8)   *Sleep patterns* may be changed in amplitude by drugs and metabolic disorders.

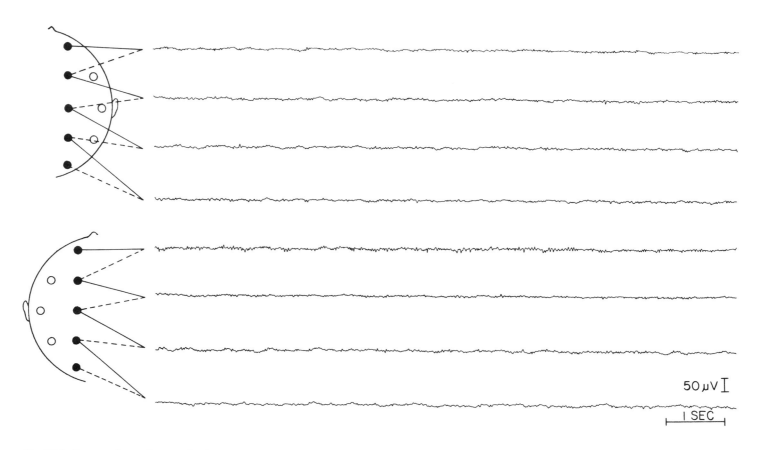

Fig. 24.1. Pattern of very low amplitude. There is no activity over 10 μV. The patient is a 66-year-old woman with a family history of Huntington's disease who has had progressive chorea and dementia for over 12 years.

24.1.1 *Abnormally low amplitude in general* consists of activity not exceeding 20 µV in any channel during relaxed wakefulness while the eyes are closed (Figs. 24.1; 24.2). The low amplitude must be sustained: Transient reductions of amplitude due to transient anxiety, mental effort, eye opening or intermittent increase or decrease of alertness are not abnormal. Because amplitude increases with interelectrode distances up to about 10 cm, the diagnosis of abnormally low amplitude requires the use of such long interelectrode distances. Correct gain settings, calibration signals and electrode impedances are essential to make the diagnosis of low amplitude. Special recording methods are needed to establish the absence of all electrocerebral activity (5.3).

24.1.2 *Abnormally low amplitude of specific patterns* can be diagnosed only by comparison with previous recordings from the same subject because of the great variability of the amplitude of normal patterns between subjects. A complete absence of the alpha rhythm in children and teenagers or an absence of sleep spindles between the ages of 6 and 8 months is abnormal.

24.1.3 *Abnormally high amplitude* of all types of activity cannot be well defined. Even though activity of 100 µV is uncommon in wakeful adults, it is only considered abnormal on the basis of frequency, morphology, or distribution rather than amplitude alone.

24.1.4 *Abnormally high amplitude of specific patterns* can usually be determined only by comparison with previous records from the same individual. The common exception is prominent, sustained, rhythmic, generalized beta activity.

* as in brain death
▷ but not in adults

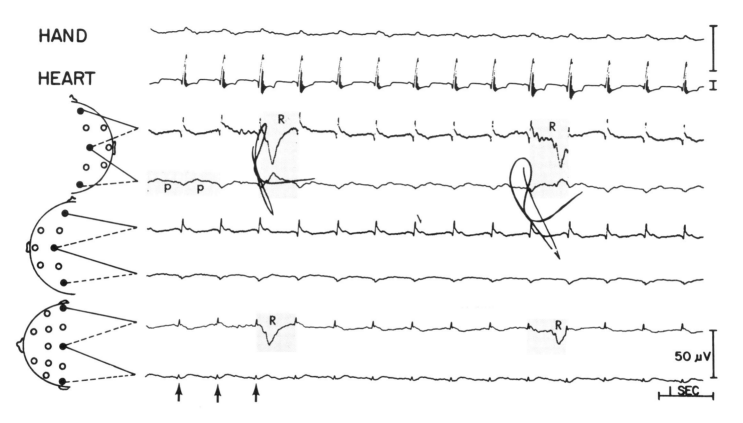

HAND

HEART

R R

p p

R R

50 μV

1 SEC

Fig. 24.2. Pattern of electrocerebral silence. The recording is made with widely spaced electrodes and high sensitivity. The artifacts commonly seen in this type of recording are due to heart beat (arrows), pulse waves (p) and movement by artificial respiration (R). This recording is from a 65-year-old woman who had a cardiac arrest 3 days earlier and was in postanoxic coma without spontaneous respiration and brainstem mediated reflexes since then. EEG and clinical condition did not change over the next 24 hours and she was pronounced cerebrally dead.

24.2.1 *Normal* high amplitude occurs in the waking record of children and in deep stages of sleep at any age. Normal low amplitude of under 20 μV occurs transiently as a result of eye opening, mental effort, anxiety, alerting or drowsiness.

24.2.2 *Abnormally low amplitude of all activity.* *Low amplitude in normal subjects* can be seen in about 5–10% of adults but is not acceptable as normal in younger persons. The reduction of amplitude is usually mild in degree, i.e. the waking record contains some activity of 10–20 μV. Such low voltage patterns (11.8) in adults are similar to slight excesses of generalized asynchronous slow waves in that they do not sharply distinguish between normal and abnormal subjects. This does not affect the significance of a moderate and marked reduction of overall amplitude which is abnormal at any age.

Abnormally low amplitude in abnormal conditions may be either transient and due to acute anoxic, toxic and metabolic factors, head injury, postictal state, or permanent and due to lasting damage resulting from these conditions or from other diseases significantly involving the cortex, such as Huntington's chorea. An increase of the material between cortex and recording electrodes such as that caused by bilateral subdural hematoma may produce a bilateral reduction of amplitude.

24.2.3 *Abnormal reduction of specific patterns* are presumably due to abnormalities involving the afferent input to the cortex which is normally responsible for the production of these patterns. For instance, interruption of thalamocortical connections may attenuate or abolish the alpha rhythm or sleep spindles.

24.2.4 *Abnormal increases of specific patterns* of clinical importance are the increases of beta rhythms produced by toxic and metabolic conditions, especially by

barbiturates, benzodiazepenes, high dose chloral hydrate and other sedatives, tranquilizers and by hyperthyroidism.

24.3 OTHER EEG ABNORMALITIES ASSOCIATED WITH HIGH AND LOW AMPLITUDE

24.3.1 *Generalized asynchronous slow waves* are often produced by the same
conditions which reduce amplitude.

24.3.2 *Bursts of periodic sharp waves and slow waves* may alternate with activity
of low amplitude in burst-suppression and other special patterns (19.3).

24.4 MECHANISMS CAUSING GENERALIZED CHANGES OF AMPLITUDE

24.4.1 *Reduction of cortical potentials* may be caused by structural abnormalities
(e.g., infarction, trauma, tumor), or by metabolic abnormalities (e.g., ischemia,
hypoglycemia, renal or hepatic failure, post-ictal depression, general anesthesia).

24.4.2 *Reduced amplitude is* also caused by other mechanisms which cause local
decreases of amplitude when they involve both sides of the head (23.4.1).

24.4.3 *Selective decreases of amplitude of patterns* over both sides of the head may
be due to interference with distant structures which control the production of these
patterns in the cortex. Thus, bilateral reduction of alpha rhythm may be due to
bilateral interruption of the input from thalamic nuclei which modulates the alpha
rhythm in the cortex or to an increase in the activity of diencephalic and
mesencephalic structures which normally abolishes alpha rhythm under conditions
of increased and decreased alertness. A reduction of sleep spindles may also be due
to an abnormality of thalamic or thalamocortical pathway function.

482

The term 'desynchronization' is sometimes used to describe replacement of widespread activity of medium or high amplitude, for instance the alpha rhythm or slow waves, by low amplitude irregular activity. It is thought that the disappearance of these patterns, which often occurs in response to alerting stimuli, may be due to a failure in the synchronization of the underlying neuronal potentials (1.2). However, because the mechanisms reducing the amplitude of the EEG are not precisely known, the reduction of amplitude is best described in terms which do not make any implications regarding an underlying mechanism.

24.4.4 *High amplitude of all types of activity* may, in some cases, be due to relatively short distances between cortex and recording electrodes or to thin skull. Other causes for high amplitude of normal activity in adults are unknown. Although abnormally low cerebral metabolism causes low amplitude and normal metabolism is required for maintenance of normal amplitude, an increase of metabolism does not increase the amplitude of activity under 13 Hz.

24.4.5 *High amplitude beta activity* seen in some toxic and metabolic conditions is poorly understood.

24.5 SPECIFIC DISORDERS CAUSING A GENERALIZED DECREASE OF AMPLITUDE OF ALL TYPES OF ACTIVITY

24.5.1 *Degenerative, developmental and demyelinating diseases:*

(1) *Huntington's chorea* is characterized by activity of very low amplitude which correlates with the cortical atrophy observed in this disease (Fig. 24.1). In the early stages of the disease when background features are still distinguishable, alpha rhythm becomes disorganized, asynchronous generalized slow waves appear, and sleep spindles and K complexes disappear. The EEG of family members at risk does not predict later development of the disease.

483

(2) *Jakob-Creutzfeldt disease* leads to a decrease of overall amplitude in the advanced stages, i.e. after generalized asynchronous slow waves have vanished. Activity of very low amplitude is also present during the intervals between periodic generalized sharp waves.

(3) *Senile and presenile dementia (Alzheimer's disease)* is associated with a decrease of background amplitude in some cases; alpha and beta activity are usually affected most. Generalized slow waves are a more reliable indicator of dementia.

(4) *Microcephaly* may cause low amplitude of the EEG in addition to other abnormalities.

(5) *Multiple sclerosis* in malignant, progressive cases may be associated with a generalized reduction of amplitude although generalized asynchronous slow waves are a more common abnormality in this disease.

24.5.2 *Metabolic and toxic encephalopathies.* Many of these encephalopathies reduce the amplitude of the EEG by reducing cerebral blood flow, oxygen supply and metabolism. Hypo- or hyperthermia can also decrease EEG amplitude.

(1) *Acute cerebral anoxia* leads first to asynchronous and bilaterally synchronous slow waves which may be followed by a generalized decrease of amplitude and electrocerebral silence if anoxia persists.

(2) *Hypothermia* leads to a decrease of EEG amplitude and frequency beginning at about 25 °C. Electrocerebral activity disappears completely at 10–20 °C. Because reduction of amplitude even after long periods of hypothermia is reversible, hypothermia must be excluded as a cause or contributing factor in cases of electrocerebral silence in the determination of cerebral death. It is generally accepted that EEGs for this purpose be recorded only if the body temperature is above 90°F (32.2°C).

(3) *Hyperthermia* of over 42 °C reduces the amplitude of the EEG. Moderate hyperthermia can increase the amplitude of background activity; slow waves appear when consciousness becomes clouded.

(4) *Hypothyroidism* usually reduces the frequency and organization of alpha rhythm and characteristically leads to an overall reduction of amplitude. Generalized asynchronous slow waves may also be present and sleep spindles are often reduced or absent.

(5) *Hypoparathyroidism and pseudohypoparathyroidism* may lead to a reduction of amplitude in general and of the alpha rhythm in particular as one of several abnormalities.

(6) *Renal and hepatic encephalopathy* may reduce the amplitude of all activity or of the alpha rhythm in the intermediate stages; in advanced hepatic encephalopathy, an acute decrease of amplitude is often associated with sudden clinical deterioration. Bisynchronous slow waves and other abnormalities are most common in the intermediate stages (Table 24.1).

(7) *Intoxication with barbiturates and other drugs* depressing the central nervous system leads to loss of amplitude preterminally. However, electrocerebral silence may develop fairly long before cerebral death: Partial or complete recovery of EEG and cerebral function is possible even after more than 24 hours of electrocerebral silence. Intoxication with barbiturates and other central nervous system depressant drugs must therefore be excluded in the evaluation of electrocerebral silence as an indicator of cerebral death.

24.5.3 *Cerebrovascular diseases:*

(1) *Syncope,* Stokes-Adams attacks and other conditions producing a generalized reduction of cerebral blood flow, like acute anoxia from other causes, produce first generalized slow waves and then a generalized decrease of amplitude.

(2) *Postanoxic encephalopathy* causes generalized asynchronous slow waves

TABLE 24.1
Generalized changes of amplitude

Abnormal patterns	Causes	Mechanisms	Examples of diseases
Decreased amplitude of all types of activity	Bilateral cortical damage	Decreased cortical EEG production	Bilateral cortical infarcts, postanoxic encephalopathy
	Widespread cerebral damage, involving cortex and subcortex	Decreased cortical EEG production, decreased rhythmical input to cortex	Huntington's chorea, Jakob-Creutzfeldt disease, postanoxic encephalopathy
	Widespread disturbance of cortical function	Same as above	Anoxia, hypothermia, hypothyroidism, preterminal toxic-metabolic encephalopathies, head injury, postictal coma, anxiety
	Bilateral increase of media between cortex and recording electrodes	Decreased electrical impedance within the conducting media	Bilateral subdural hematomas
		Increased electrical impedance between cortex and recording electrodes	Dry scalp, Paget's disease
of alpha rhythm	Mild metabolic disturbances	Decreased cortical EEG production	Early hepatic, hypothyroid, hypoparathyroid encephalopathy
	Functional subcortical disturbance	Decreased rhythmical input to cortex	Anxiety
of sleep patterns	Structural brainstem damage	As above	Progressive supranuclear palsy, pontine lesions
	Functional brainstem disturbance	As above	Phenylketonuria, hypothyroidism, uremia
Increased amplitude of all types of activity	No known pathological cause		
of beta rhythm	Functional disturbance	Unknown	Sedatives and tranquilizers, hyperthyroidism, anxiety
of sleep patterns	As above	Increased input to cortex	Tricyclic antidepressants, flurazepam

486

and other EEG abnormalities. Low amplitude may occur either early, i.e. during the first few hours or days, or late, i.e. as a residual after other EEG abnormalities have abated. If low amplitude of early onset persists, the prognosis is poor.
poor.

(3) *Cerebral death* is often the immediate result of cerebral anoxia which is most often caused by cardiac or respiratory arrest; toxic, metabolic and traumatic disorders can cause cerebral death directly or through cardiorespiratory arrest and

(4) *Bilateral subdural hematomas* may reduce the amplitude of the EEG over wide parts of both hemispheres and are often associated with focal slow waves.

(5) *Vertebro-basilar insufficiency* seems to be associated with an increase in the incidence of low voltage EEG patterns between attacks.

(6) *Air embolism* may suddenly reduce the amplitude of the EEG or induce generalized slow waves, occasionally more on the right side than the left, possibly because of the more direct arterial pathway.

24.5.4 *Cerebral trauma. Head injury*, if mild, may produce a brief decrease of amplitude with or without loss of consciousness. Severe head injuries that lead to coma may be associated with prolonged or progressive reduction of amplitude which carries a poor prognosis. A decrease of amplitude may occur during recovery in comatose patients who initially demonstrated high amplitude generalized slow waves.

24.5.5 *Brain tumors.* Tumors do not reduce overall amplitude directly; pituitary tumors may cause low amplitude by producing hypothyroid encephalopathy.

24.5.6 *Seizure disorders:*

(1) *Ictal decreases of amplitude* may occur at the beginning of a generalized seizure. A reduction of amplitude may be the only ictal manifestation in some forms

of seizures (for example, electrodecremental electrographic seizures). Flattening of the EEG, or low amplitude fast activity, also occurs during 'cerebellar fits' which, despite their name and paroxysmal character, are not seizures but attacks of decerebration; the underlying mechanisms are not yet fully understood but probably involve a sudden increase in intracranial pressure, generalized cortical ischemia, or an abrupt change of the function of the brainstem reticular formation.

(2) *Postictal depression* of amplitude appears immediately after most generalized seizures and lasts a few minutes until slow waves supervene.

24.5.7 *Infectious diseases:*

(1) *Encephalitis and meningitis* can reduce overall EEG amplitude during the acute phase of the disease. Persistence of reduced amplitude indicates residual widespread cerebral damage.

(2) *Progressive multifocal leukoencephalopathy* may reduce amplitude widely or induce generalized asynchronous slow waves.

24.5.8 *Psychiatric diseases.* Anxiety reduces overall amplitude mainly by reducing alpha rhythm.

24.6 GENERALIZED DECREASE OR ABSENCE OF ALPHA RHYTHM

24.6.1 *Normal attenuation of alpha rhythm* occurs with eye opening, alerting, mental effort, anxiety, and decrease of alertness to the level of drowsiness. A slight degree of anxiety is a normal reaction of many subjects to their first EEG recording and usually disappears during the course of the recording. The transient nature of these normal patterns of alpha attenuation distinguishes them from the low voltage patterns and from the effects of pathological anxiety. (For the normal limits of the amplitude of the alpha rhythm see 10.4.)

24.6.2 *Acute and chronic anxiety reactions* of psychiatric relevance produce commonly a persistent reduction of alpha rhythm leaving mainly beta activity. In the absence of beta activity, the results of anxiety reactions may be identical with the low voltage pattern.

24.7 GENERALIZED INCREASE OF BETA RHYTHM

24.7.1 *Normal* prominence of beta activity varies widely; beta activity is very prominent in some normal subjects and absent in others. However, the persistence of increased beta activity throughout the recording is an EEG abnormality.

24.7.2 *Hyperthyroidism* produces prominent fast activity either in the central regions or in a wide distribution. This activity mixes with, or replaces alpha rhythm. The frequency of alpha rhythm is often increased.

en bolines

24.7.3 *Barbiturates, benzodiazepines, other sedatives and tranquilizers* acutely induce widespread fast activity with a maximum in the central and frontal regions. This persists during wakefulness and becomes more conspicuous during drowsiness when the alpha rhythm disappears. Barbiturates in doses producing coma may cause nonreactive frontal or widespread 10–12 Hz rhythms (25.3.2). Many patients chronically taking barbiturates lose this fast activity.

alpha coma-like (?)

24.7.4 *Acute and chronic anxiety* are usually associated with an increase of fast activity in addition to the reduction of alpha activity. In many cases, however, this activity may be largely due to muscle artifact.

24.8.1 *Phenylketonuria* may be associated with absent, jagged or sharp spindles and K complexes during sleep while the waking record may show hypsarrhythmia, multifocal independent spikes or slow spike-and-waves.

24.8.2 *Progressive supranuclear palsy* may cause reduction of sleep spindles, V waves and K complexes and disturbances of sleep cycles (25.4.5) even before the waking record shows abnormalities.

24.8.3 *Hypothyroidism, hypoparathyroidism, uremia and chlorpromazine intake* are among other conditions which reduce sleep spindles more than overall amplitude.

— Dalmane (?)

24.8.4 *Tricyclic antidepressants and hypnotics,* notably flurazepam, increase sleep spindles.

see table + sum.

REFERENCES

Alvarez, L.A., Moshe, S.L., Belman, A.L., Maytal, J., Resnick, T.J. and Keilson, M. (1988) EEG and brain death determination in children. Neurology 38: 227–230.

Arfel, G., Casanova, C., Naquet, R., Passelecq, J. and Dubost, C. (1967) Étude électro-clinique de l'embolie gazeuse cérébrale en chirurgie cardiaque. Electroenceph. clin. Neurophysiol. 23: 101–122.

Bauer, G. (1987) Coma and brain death. In: Niedermeyer, E. and Lopes da Silva, F. (Eds.), Electroencephalography: Basic Principles, Clinical Applications and Related Fields. Urban and Schwarzenberg, Baltimore, pp. 391–404.

Beecher, H.K. (1968) A definition of irreversible coma. JAMA 205: 337–340.

Brenner, R.P., Schwartzman, R. and Richey, E. (1975) Prognostic significance of episodic low amplitude or relatively isoelectric EEG patterns. Dis. Nerv. Syst. 36: 582.

Cabral, R., Prior, P.F., Scott, D.F. and Brierley, J.B. (1977) Reversible profound depression of cerebral electrical activity in hyperthermia. Electroenceph. clin. Neurophysiol. 42: 697–701.

Celesia, G.G. and Andermann, F. (1964) Some observations on the electrographic correlates of the decerebrate attack. Electroenceph. clin. Neurophysiol. 16: 295–300.

Chatrian, G.E. (1986) Electrophysiologic evaluation of brain death: A critical appraisal. In: Aminoff, M.J. (Ed.), Electrodiagnosis in clinical neurology. Churchill/Livingstone, New York, pp. 669–736.

Jørgensen, E.O. (1974) EEG without detectable cortical activity and cranial nerve areflexia as parameters of brain death. Electroenceph. clin. Neurophysiol. 36: 70–75.

Leestma, J.E., Hughes, J.R. and Diamond, E.R. (1984) Temporal correlates in brain death. Arch. Neurol. 41: 147–152.

Niedermeyer, E. (1963) The electroencephalogram and vertebrobasilar artery insufficiency. Neurology 13: 412–422.

Schultz, M.A., Schulte, F.J., Akiyama, Y. and Parmalee, A.H. (1968) Development of electroencephalographic sleep phenomena in hypothyroid infants. Electroenceph. clin. Neurophysiol. 25: 351–358.

Scott, D.F., Heathfield, K.W.G., Toone, B. and Margerison, J.H. (1972) The EEG in Huntington's chorea: A clinical and neuropathological study. J. Neurol. Neurosurg. Psychiat. 35: 97–102.

Sishta, S.K., Troupe, A., Marszalek, K.S. and Kremer, L.M. (1974) Huntington's chorea: An electroencephalographic and psychometric study. Electroenceph. clin. Neurophysiol. 36: 387–393.

Trewby, P.N., Casemore, C. and Willians, R. (1978) Continuous bipolar recording of the EEG in patients with fulminant hepatic failure. Electroenceph. clin. Neurophysiol. 45: 107–110.

Deviations from normal patterns

SUMMARY
Several patterns are abnormal due to features other than those described in the preceding chapters. These patterns include: (1) abnormal slowing of the alpha rhythm; (2) abnormal reactivity of the alpha rhythm; (3) activity of theta, alpha and beta frequency in coma and seizures; and (4) abnormal timing and incidence of sleep patterns.

25.1 ABNORMAL FREQUENCY OF THE ALPHA RHYTHM

25.1.1 *Description of patterns.* A unilateral decrease in the frequency of the alpha rhythm is abnormal if it results in a consistent left−right difference of over 0.5 Hz. Left−right differences in alpha frequency of less than 1 Hz are difficult to appreciate by routine visual inspection but can be detected in some cases by computerized analysis. The underlying abnormality is always located on the side with the lower alpha frequency.

A bilateral increase or decrease in the frequency of the alpha rhythm can be diagnosed with certainty only by comparing records from the same patient. To qualify as abnormal, the alpha frequency should be consistently lowered by more than 2 Hz between recordings performed with the patient in a similar level of alertness. The chances of reliably detecting such changes in older children and adults are considerably increased by the routine practice of asking specific alerting questions during the recording (e.g., time, date, mental calculation, etc.). It is obvious, however, that without a previous record for comparison many patients with an abnormal reduction of the alpha frequency will escape detection, since significant decreases in frequency may occur without exceeding the lower normal value of 8 Hz. Even so, it is important to be aware that an alpha rhythm of 8–8.5 Hz is likely to represent an abnormal decline in frequency, even in elderly individuals. A bilateral increase of the frequency of alpha rhythm beyond the upper limit of 13 Hz transforms the alpha rhythm into fast alpha variant, i.e. a beta rhythm which has

TABLE 25.1

Deviations from normal patterns

Abnormal patterns	Causes	Examples of diseases
1. Bilateral decrease of alpha frequency	Generalized disturbance of cerebral function:	
	Metabolic disorders	Hypothyroidism, hepatic and renal encephalopathy
	Change of rhythmical input to cortex	Reduced alertness
	Bilateral structural damage to occipital cortex or its thalamic input	Alzheimer's disease, multiple infarcts, subdural hematoma
2. Unilateral decrease of alpha frequency	Unilateral disturbance of function of occipital cortex or its thalamic input	Transient ischemic attack, condition after mild head injury
	Unilateral structural damage to occipital cortex or its thalamic input	Unilateral chronic subdural hematoma, condition after severe head injury, cerebral infarct
3. Bilateral increase of alpha frequency	Metabolic disorders	Hyperthyroidism, fever
4. Unilateral failure of alpha blocking✱	Parietal or temporal lobe lesions	Tumors, infarcts
5. Bilateral failure of alpha blocking on monocular input	Disorders of one eye or optic nerve	Monocular blindness
6. Absence of alpha rhythm, presence of occipital spikes (Table 19.4)	Long-standing diseases of both eyes or central visual path	Congenital or early acquired binocular blindness
7. Alpha frequency coma	Central pontine lesions	Infarcts, head injuries
	Widespread cerebral damage	Postanoxic encephalopathy
8. Ictal activity of alpha or beta frequency (Table 19.3)	Local or widespread cerebral damage in newborns	Infantile partial or generalized seizures or status epilepticus
	Irritative temporal lobe lesions	Partial complex seizure activity

✱ Bancaud's phenomenon

a similar distribution and reactivity as the alpha rhythm and which is important only
if it represents a significant increase in comparison with a recent control recording
from the same subject.

25.1.2 *Clinical significance of frequency changes of alpha rhythm. Bilateral
decrease of alpha frequency* is often due to conditions which slow the metabolism of
the brain. Many of these conditions are associated with a decrease of alertness,
memory, awareness and orientation. Some of these conditions are transient, for
instance toxic or metabolic encephalopathies; others are associated with long-
standing damage, for instance cerebral atrophy or bilateral subdural hematomas.
Generalized slowing of alpha rhythm may be an early signal of various types of abnormalities which later produce other, more specific, abnormalities.

Unilateral decrease of alpha frequency occurs in conditions which also cause a
unilateral decrease of the amplitude of alpha rhythm. Such decreases may be the
only residual EEG abnormality in mild or old vascular or traumatic lesions of the
posterior head regions, but they occasionally appear early in expanding tumors and
in lesions of the central and frontal areas.

Bilateral increase of alpha frequency occurs in some conditions of increased
cerebral metabolism.

25.1.3 *Other EEG abnormalities associated with abnormal frequency of alpha
rhythm. Abnormal amplitude of alpha rhythm* may appear in the same distribution as abnormal frequency of alpha rhythm, especially in unilateral changes.

Bisynchronous and asynchronous generalized slow waves often appear on a background of slow alpha frequency.

25.1.4 *Mechanisms causing an abnormal frequency of the alpha rhythm* are probably similar to those mechanisms which cause an attenuation in amplitude by interrupting normal thalamocortical function.

25.1.5 *Specific disorders causing unilateral or bilateral decrease of alpha frequency:*

(1) *Degenerative, developmental and demyelinating diseases. Senile and presenile dementia (Alzheimer's disease)* causes abnormal slowing of alpha rhythm which is of less diagnostic importance than are asynchronous generalized slow waves.

Myotonic dystrophy may cause slowing of alpha rhythm; this is probably due to the endocrine disturbances characteristic of this disease.

(2) *Metabolic and toxic encephalopathies.* Many of these encephalopathies produce early slowing of alpha frequency before causing other abnormalities and disappearance of alpha rhythm. The most important encephalopathies in this group are due to acute anoxia, hyponatremia, Vitamin B12 deficiency, hypoglycemia, hepatic and renal failure, porphyria, Addison's disease, hyper- and hypoparathyroidism, Wernicke's disease, acute intoxication with barbiturates, phenytoin, alcohol, antipsychotics, amphetamines, lithium and other psychotropic drugs. Hypothyroidism may cause slowing of alpha rhythm often followed by reduction of amplitude without other abnormalities.

(3) *Cerebrovascular diseases.* Local or generalized slowing of alpha rhythm occurs temporarily in transient local or generalized cerebral ischemia. Persistent slowing of alpha rhythm may be seen in bilateral or multiple cerebral infarcts, lacunar state of hypertensives, unilateral and bilateral subdural hematomas, thalamic infarcts, mesencephalic infarcts, postanoxic encephalopathy, subarachnoid hemorrhage with obtundation and in conditions associated with reduced cardiac output (e.g. coronary artery disease and congestive heart failure).

(4) *Cerebral trauma.* *Head injuries* of mild intensity may produce no more EEG abnormalities than a slowing of alpha rhythm, with or without a reduction of its amplitude. Patients recovering from more severe head injuries may show a decrease of alpha frequency, amplitude, or both as the last residual EEG abnormality.

Repeated head injuries, for instance those of boxers, may produce lasting and progressive reduction of the frequency of alpha rhythm in addition to generalized slow waves.

(5) *Brain tumors.* *Infratentorial tumors* may reduce alpha frequency and amplitude on both sides in addition to producing bisynchronous slow waves and other abnormalities.

Supratentorial tumors, especially those in the parietal or occipital lobes or the thalamus, may decrease alpha frequency and amplitude on the side of the tumor in addition to producing focal or lateralized slow waves.

(6) *Seizure disorders.* *Ictal discharges* sometimes consist of rhythmical waves of alpha or slower frequency which are usually easily distinguished from alpha rhythm.

Postictal slowing in the alpha frequency range may persist longer than other postictal changes.

(7) *Infectious diseases.* *Non-specific slowing of the alpha rhythm* may occur in many infectious diseases including those not directly involving the brain; this slowing is commonly associated with fever and mental status changes.

Cerebral infections causing widespread cerebral damage may produce slowing of the alpha rhythm in addition to other abnormalities.

25.1.6 *Specific disorders causing a bilateral increase of the alpha frequency:*

(1) *Hyperthyroidism,* including that induced by treatment, is commonly associated with an increase in alpha frequency; the absolute amount of the alpha rhythm may also be reduced. Other abnormalities are often present. Many patients show increased beta activity, some have diffuse spikes and sharp waves, and a few have prominent generalized asynchronous slow waves. Treatment of the hyperthyroidism gradually reverses all abnormalities except for the asynchronous slow waves.

(2) *Fever* may transiently increase the alpha rhythm frequency.

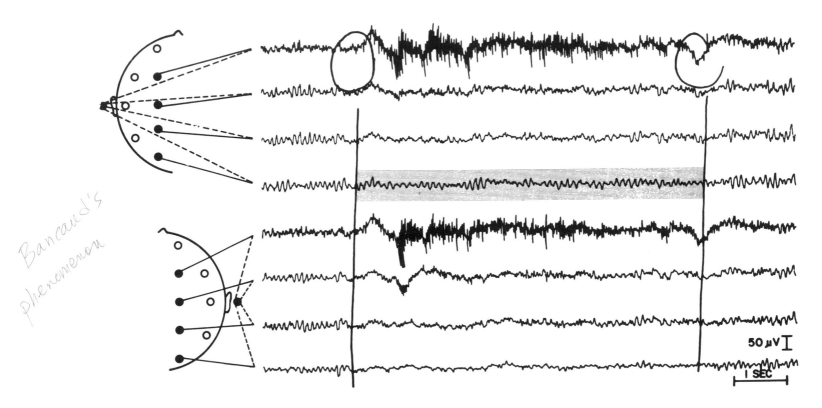

Bancaud's phenomenon

Fig. 25.1. Unilateral failure of blocking of alpha rhythm. Before eye opening (O) and after eye closing (C), alpha rhythm is present and symmetrical on the two sides. While the eyes are open, alpha rhythm is blocked normally on the right side but persists on the left (shaded). This 32-year old woman sustained a head injury without loss of consciousness 9 days before the EEG recording and had some receptive aphasia which cleared gradually.

498

25.2.1 *Unilateral failure of alpha blocking* on eye opening, often referred to as *Bancaud's phenomenon*, may occur with lesions of the parietal and temporal lobe on the side which fails to block (Fig. 25.1). This sign may be present in the absence of any other EEG abnormality and therefore may be the earliest indicator of lesions in those areas. More often, other obvious background abnormalities are present or a careful inspection of the record reveals a slight reduction in the peak frequency of alpha activity on the abnormal side.

25.2.2 *Bilateral failure of alpha blocking:*

(1) *Normal subjects* show great variability of alpha blocking (Fig. 13.2) and may have only very brief reductions of alpha amplitude in response to eye opening and alerting.

(2) *Unilateral cerebral lesions* located in the frontal or temporal lobes that abolish the blocking of alpha activity are usually associated with an impairment of consciousness, prominent neurological deficits, or both. In contrast, lesions located in the parietal or occipital lobes that abolish blocking of the alpha rhythm are often not associated with impaired consciousness or severe deficits.

(3) *Binocular blindness* when acquired after the development of alpha leads to a loss of the reactivity of alpha rhythm to eye opening. The alpha rhythm in this condition may have a central or unusually wide distribution. Like congenitally blind persons, persons with acquired blindness may have no alpha rhythm and may develop occipital spikes even in the absence of occipital lesions.

(4) *Monocular blindness* or loss of discriminative vision can cause failure of alpha blocking in both hemispheres when the blind eye is opened; opening of the seeing eye produces normal bilateral alpha blocking.

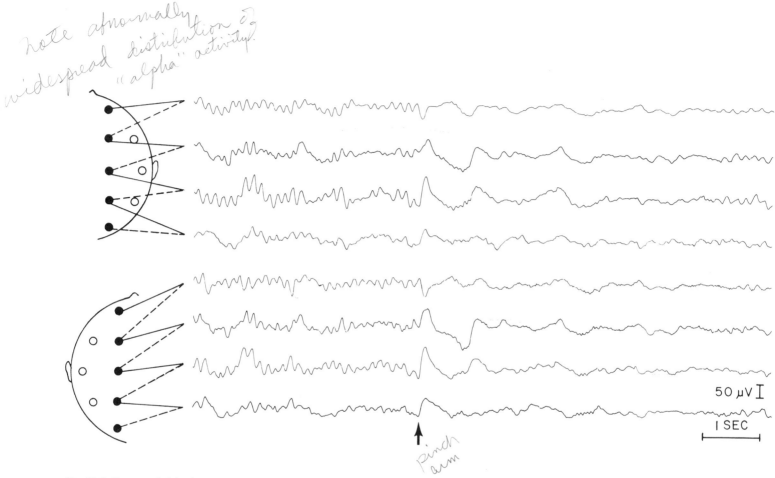

note abnormally widespread distribution of "alpha" activity.

50 µV

1 SEC

pinch arm

Fig. 25.2. Pattern of alpha frequency coma in a patient with a presumed pontine lesion. Sinusoidal 7 Hz waves, superimposed on delta waves, are seen in a wide distribution in the left part of the figure. Pinching of the left arm (arrow) blocks the sinusoidal waves promptly for several seconds. This 25-year-old woman sustained a severe head injury in a motorcycle accident 3 days before this recording and was in coma since then with pupillary and other signs suggestive of a pontine contusion.

500

25.3.1 The terms *theta coma, alpha coma, beta coma and spindle coma* are often used to denote patterns of rhythmical waves which have theta, alpha or beta frequency but differ from normal rhythms in that they occur in comatose patients. In addition, they usually do not attenuate with alerting maneuvers but do have abnormal topographic distributions. In some cases, these waves show little variation in frequency and are the only activity present; in other cases, their frequency varies by several hertz, and generalized slow waves may be present.

25.3.2 Two kinds of *alpha coma pattern* have been distinguished which loosely correspond with different anatomical distributions of pathological involvement.

(1) *The posterior dominant alpha coma pattern* shows either no reaction, or, rarely, a variable attenuation or increase in amplitude following alerting maneuvers. This pattern is usually encountered in patients with brainstem lesions, particularly pontine infarction (Fig. 25.2). It is important to attempt to differentiate patients with similarly located lesions who are in the so-called 'locked in state' from those who are comatose. A posterior dominant alpha background activity that attenuates with alerting in patients with little other evidence of response to stimulation (or in some cases only vertical eye movements) is indicative of the 'locked in state'. Such patients may have nearly complete awareness, but are immobilized by an interruption of corticospinal motor pathways.

(2) *Generalized or predominantly frontal alpha activity* without reaction to alerting stimuli can be seen in patients with widespread cerebral damage, especially that following cardiac or respiratory arrest, prolonged hypoglycemia or bilateral destruction of midline thalamic nuclei (Fig. 25.3). Focal or generalized slow waves or amplitude abnormalities are sometimes also present. This alpha pattern is usually

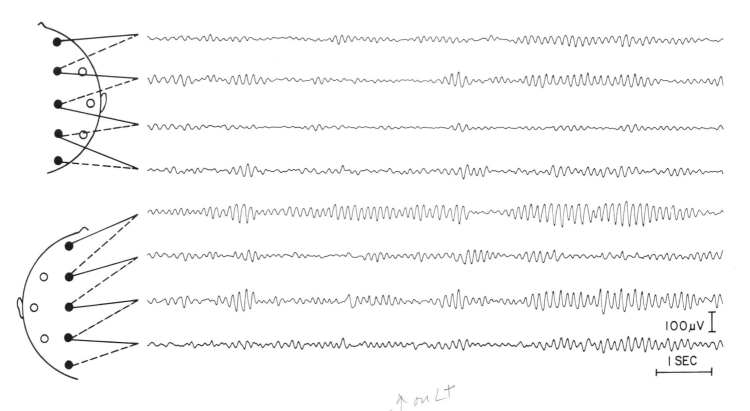

100μV

1 SEC

Fig. 25.3. Pattern of alpha frequency coma in a patient with widespread cerebral damage after cardiac arrest. Sinusoidal 8 Hz waves appear in a wide and asymmetrical distribution. They did not react to loud noises or noxious stimuli. This 27-year-old man was in postanoxic coma for 2 days after a cardiac arrest. A followup EEG 9 days later showed generalized slow waves of very low amplitude. The patient then was unresponsive and in a decerebrate posture and had roving vertical eye movements. He died 3 weeks later without regaining consciousness.

502

seen for up to four days after the insult and is then replaced by other abnormalities. The prognosis for complete recovery or survival is generally considered to be poor, particularly in cases of anoxic encephalopathy. However, complete recovery has been reported to occur frequently in cases of electrical injury and sedative intoxication uncomplicated by anoxia.

25.3.3   The *theta coma pattern* is characterized by generalized monorhythmic activity in the theta frequency range that shows little or no evidence of either spontaneous variability or reactivity to noxious stimulation. The clinical correlates of the theta coma pattern are similar to those of the generalized or frontal dominant alpha coma pattern. Interestingly, it is not unusual for the alpha coma pattern to be replaced by the theta coma pattern. Such transitions indicate a poor prognosis for normal recovery or survival.

25.3.4   The *beta coma pattern* consists of a generalized, sometimes frontal dominant, pattern of mainly rhythmic beta waveforms. It usually occurs in coma caused by or complicated by barbiturate or benzodiazepene intoxication. Unlike the alpha and theta coma patterns, the beta coma pattern is usually associated with a favorable outcome, probably because in most cases it is a demonstration of the ability of cortical structures to generate a 'normal' response to pharmacological stimulation.

25.3.5   The *spindle coma pattern* is so named because it consists of recognizable sleep spindles occurring in patients who are either in a vegetative state or in coma. Like the beta coma pattern, it is usually associated with a favorable outcome. It is often seen following head trauma but has also been observed in patients recovering from anoxic encephalopathy or encephalitis.

503

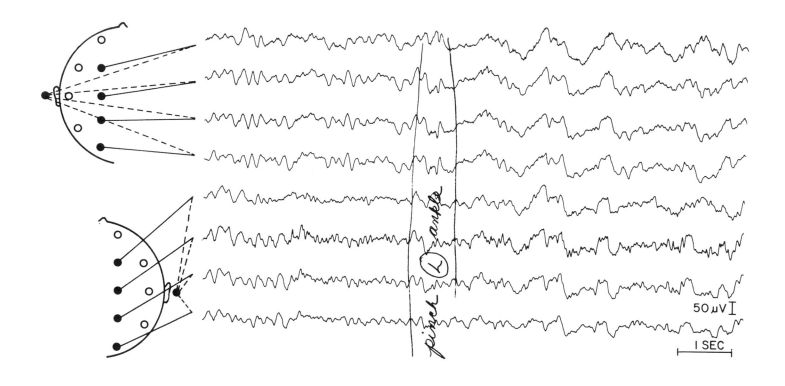

Fig. 25.4. Paradoxical slow wave response to alerting stimuli in an obtunded patient. Rhythmical 4–5 Hz waves at rest are replaced by generalized delta waves after pinching of the left ankle. This 70-year-old woman had repeated subarachnoid hemorrhages from an aneurysm on the left posterior communicating artery 2–3 weeks before this recording and began to recover from coma at the time of the recording.

25.4 ABNORMAL TIMING AND INCIDENCE OF SLEEP PATTERNS

25.4.1 *Sleep activity in comatose patients* is occasionally superimposed on the slow waves or the alpha activity which characterize coma due to various structural lesions or toxic and metabolic encephalopathies. Sleep activity seems inappropriate in these patients insofar as they do not exhibit cycles of wakefulness and sleep. However, the appearance of sleep activity in such patients indicates a better prognosis than does the absence of sleep activity.

25.4.2 *Paradoxical slow wave response to alerting stimuli* consists of a transient increase or appearance of generalized slow waves on a background of slow waves of lower amplitude or of alpha activity in patients with reduced alertness most often due to head injuries (Fig. 25.4).

25.4.3 *Sleep onset REM periods (SOREMPs) and short latency to sleep onset* of less than 5 minutes on the multiple sleep latency test occurs in patients with narcolepsy, and Kleine-Levin syndrome.

25.4.4 *Reduction of REM sleep* can occur as the result of diseases causing structural damage, for instance mongolism, and Pelizaeus-Merzbacher disease, and as an effect of various drugs, for instance alcohol, barbiturates, tricyclic antidepressants and various other neuroleptic drugs.

25.4.5 *Disordered sleep cycles* occur in sleep apnea, progressive supranuclear palsy and children with episodic sleep disturbances.

505

25.5 IMMATURE PATTERNS

Immature patterns are those found at an age when these patterns normally have disappeared. In neonates a retrogression of EEG patterns occurs as a nonspecific response to transient or longlasting cerebral disorders. In older individuals the persistence of immature patterns (e.g. posterior slow waves of youth seen in adults) is of uncertain clinical significance.

REFERENCES

Austin, E.J., Wilkus, R. and Longstreath, W.T. (1988) Etiology and prognosis of alpha coma. Neurology 38: 773–777.

Bancaud, J., Hacaen, H. and Lairy, G.C. (1955) Modifications de la réactivité EEG, troubles des fonctions symboliques et troubles confusionnels dans les lésions hémisphériques localisées. Electroenceph. clin. Neurophysiol. 7: 179–192.

Bauer, G. (1987) Coma and brain death. In: Niedermeyer, E. and Lopes da Silva, F. (Eds.), Electroencephalography: Basic Principles, Clinical Applications and Related Fields, Urban and Schwarzenberg, Baltimore, pp. 391–404.

Benoit, O., Goldenberg-Leygonie, F., Lacombe, J. and Marc, M.E. (1978) Sommeil de l'enfant presentant des manifestations episodiques du sommeil: Comparaison avec l'enfant normal. Electroenceph. clin. Neurophysiol. 44: 502–512.

Brenner, R.P. (1985) The electroencephalogram in altered states of consciousness. In: Aminoff, M.J. (Ed.), Electrodiagnosis, Neurologic Clinics, Saunders, Philadelphia, pp. 615–629.

Britt Jr., C.W., Raso, E. and Gerson, P. (1980) Spindle coma, secondary to primary traumatic midbrain hemorrhage. Electroenceph. clin. Neurophysiol. 49: 406–408.

Cadilhac, J. (1976) Section V. EEG in thyroid dysfunction. In: Rémond, A. (Ed.), Handbook of Electroenceph. clin. Neurophysiol., Vol. 15C. Elsevier, Amsterdam, pp. 70–76.

Carroll, W.M. and Mastaglia, F.L. (1979) Alpha and beta coma in drug intoxication uncomplicated by cerebral hypoxia. Electroenceph. clin. Neurophysiol. 46: 95–105.

Chatrian, G.E. (1975) Section V. Electrographic and behavioral signs of sleep in comatose states. In: Rémond, A. (Ed.), Handbook of Electroenceph. clin. Neurophysiol., Vol. 12, Elsevier, Amsterdam, pp. 63–77.

Chokroverty, S. (1975) 'Alpha-like' rhythms in electroencephalograms in coma after cardiac arrest. Neurology 25: 655–663.

Fukuyama, Y. and Hayashi, M. (1979) Sleep electroencephalograms and sleep stages in hypoparathyroidism. Eur. Neurol. 18: 38–48.

Glass, J.D. (1977) Alpha blocking: Absence in visuobehavioral deprivation. Science 198: 58–60.

Gross, R.A., Spehlmann, R. and Daniels, J.C. (1978) Sleep disturbances in progressive supranuclear palsy. Electroenceph. clin. Neurophysiol. 45: 16–25.

Gurvitch, A.M., Zarzhetsky, Y.V., Trush, V.D. and Zonov, V.M. (1984) Experimental data on the nature of post-resuscitation alpha frequency activity. Electroenceph. clin. Neurophysiol. 58: 426–437.

Harner, R.N. (1975) EEG evaluation of the patient with dementia. In: Benson, D.F. and Blumer, D. (Eds.), Psychiatric Aspects of Neurological Disease. Grune and Stratton, New York, pp. 63–82.

Homan, R.W. and Jones, M.G. (1981) Alpha coma pattern in a 2-month-old child. Ann. Neurol. 9: 611–613.

Jeavons, P.M. and Harding, G.F.A. (1975) Photosensitive epilepsy: A review of the literature and a study of 460 patients. Clin. Dev. Med. 56: 1–121.

Knauss, T.A. and Carlson, C.B. (1978) Neonatal paroxysmal monorhythmic alpha activity. Arch. Neurol. 35: 104–107.

Laffont, F., Autret, A., Minz, M., Beillevaire, T., Gilbert, A., Cathala, H.P. and Castaigne, P. (1979) Étude polygraphique du sommeil dans 9 cas de maladie de Steele-Richardson. Rev. Neurol. 135: 127–142.

Newmark, M.E. and Penry, J.K. (1979) Photosensitivity and Epilepsy: A Review. Raven, New York.

Pfurtscheller, G., Maresch, H. and Schuy, S. (1977) Inter- and intrahemispheric differences in the peak frequency of rhythmic activity within the alpha band. Electroenceph. clin. Neurophysiol. 42: 77–83.

Schwartz, M.S. and Scott, D.F. (1978) Pathological stimulus-related slow wave arousal responses in the EEG. Acta Neurol. Scand. 57: 300–304.

Stockard, J.J., Werner, S.S., Aalbers, J.A. and Chiappa, K.H. (1976) Electroencephalographic findings in phencyclidine intoxication. Arch. Neurol. 33: 200–203.

Sørenson, K., Thomassen, A. and Wernberg, M. (1978) Prognostic significance of alpha frequency EEG rhythm in coma after cardiac arrest. J. Neurol. Neurosurg. Psychiat. 41: 840–842.

Van Hufflen, A.C., Poortvliet, D.C.J. and Van der Wulp, C.J.M. (1984) Quantitative electroencephalography in cerebral ischemia. Detection of abnormalities in 'normal' EEGs. In: Pfurtscheller, G., Jonkman, E.J. and Lopes da Silva, F.H. (Eds.), Brain Ischemia: Quantitative EEG and Imaging Techniques, Elsevier, Amsterdam, pp. 3–28.

Westmoreland, B.F., Klass, D.W., Sharbrough, F.W. and Reagan, T.J. (1975) Alpha-coma. Electroencephalographic, clinical, pathologic, and etiologic correlations. Arch. Neurol. 32: 713–718.

Zander Olsen, P., Støier, M., Siersbaek-Nielsen, K., Mølholm Hansen, J., Schiøler, M. and Kristensen, M. (1972) Electroencephalographic findings in hyperthyroidism. Electroenceph. clin. Neurophysiol. 32: 171–177.

Zaret, B.S. (1985) Prognostic and neurophysiological implications of concurrent burst suppression and alpha patterns in the EEG of post-anoxic coma. Electroenceph. clin. Neurophysiol. 61: 199–209.

The EEG report

SUMMARY

The EEG report should include:

(26.1)   *A simple brief description* of the essential features of normal and abnormal activity observed under various conditions of recording, namely resting wakefulness, hyperventilation, photic stimulation and sleep;

(26.2)   *An EEG summary* listing the major significant abnormal findings and events;

(26.3)   *An interpretation* that includes the EEG impression and clinical correlation in the light of the patient's problems and referring physician's queries.

26.1   DESCRIPTION OF THE RECORD

The report should describe the essential normal and abnormal patterns appearing under the various recording conditions so that a person with some knowledge of EEG can envisage the findings on which diagnosis and interpretation are based. Sufficient detail should be given to enable the reader of a later EEG to estimate whether the major features of the two recordings are similar or different. The report should not be exhaustive in describing normal detail but should include those rare or unusual features in the record which may have clinical significance. As far as possible, the report should use the terms defined in the glossary of the International Federation of Societies for EEG and Clinical Neurophysiology (9). Judgements like 'good' and 'poor' should be used only sparingly and only to characterize the overall composition of a record, but not to rate individual rhythms: Persons not familiar with the EEG cannot know that 'poor' driving has no different clinical significance than has 'good' or even 'excellent' driving.

Patterns should be described by indicating the frequency, amplitude and distribution of the component waves. Wave shape, rhythmicity, symmetry, synchrony, persistence, reactivity and periodicity may be important for the description of abnormal patterns. Because the frequency of a rhythm often varies, it is usually indicated in terms of a frequency range or band of a few hertz in width rather than in terms of a single frequency. In most instances, it is not sufficient to use only the wide bands of delta, theta, alpha and beta frequency to describe the frequencies of waves in a record; the frequency of alpha and beta rhythms and of theta and delta waves observed in a recording should be specified in narrower bands in every case. Amplitude may be reported in absolute or relative measurements. Absolute units must be used in the diagnosis of electrocerebral silence which requires that no electrocerebral activity of over 2 μV is present. Even if activity of very low amplitude is found in these cases, the amplitude may be specified to indicate the severity of the abnormality and to give the basis for comparison with subsequent recordings. In most other instances, it is sufficient to characterize amplitude as low, medium or high.

To avoid omitting important features in the report, one should adhere to a standard sequence of reporting.

26.1.1 *The opening statement* should describe the general level of consciousness of the patient. In particular, it should mention behavioral abnormalities such as somnolence, coma, lack of cooperation, or persistent movement and muscle artifacts. All these factors could render the record technically unsatisfactory or reduce the length of the readable EEG to a sample shorter than the minimum required for reliable interpretation (5.1). The opening statement should indicate any unusual recording conditions, for instance recordings made at the bedside or in an intensive care unit, or the use of special recording techniques such as nasopharyngeal electrodes or other special monitors.

26.1.2 *The resting record:*

(1) *Description of normal background. Alpha, beta, mu and other rhythms and patterns,* if present, are described in terms of their frequency range, relative amplitude and distribution. Wave shape, rhythmicity, symmetry, distribution, persistence and reactivity should be mentioned if they are abnormal. Excessive beta activity and unilateral blocking of the alpha rhythm must be reported.

(2) *Description of abnormal patterns. Epileptiform activity* is characterized by its shape, amplitude, repetition rate, persistence, distribution, synchrony, symmetry, relationship between focal and generalized discharges and any other feature of possible clinical significance including the association with behavioral seizure manifestations.

Slow waves are described in terms of frequency, amplitude, shape, rhythmicity, regularity, persistence, distribution, symmetry, synchrony and any other parameter of clinical importance. If more than one type of slow wave is present, the specifications for each type must be given. Abnormal generalized asynchronous slow waves must be distinguished by amplitude, frequency, distribution and persistence from the range of asynchronous slow waves normally seen at the age of the patient.

Asymmetries and generalized changes of amplitude are usually noted when describing the normal background.

Deviations from normal must be described by indicating the specific features which make a pattern abnormal, for instance the appearance of alpha activity which has a frontal maximum, lacks reactivity and is associated with coma.

26.1.3 *Hyperventilation. Normal responses* can be described in one short sentence, for instance 'Hyperventilation produced no change' or 'Hyperventilation produced bilaterally synchronous slow waves'. The performance of the patient may be mentioned. Symptoms induced by hyperventilation should be reported, particularly if the symptoms resemble episodic symptoms for which the patient is ex-

511

amined. Changes in the patient's behavior, such as jerking movements or loss of responsiveness must be reported.

Abnormal responses such as an asymmetrical buildup, enhancement of abnormalities of the resting record and induction of new abnormalities must be described in detail.

26.1.4 *Photic stimulation.* Normal responses can be described briefly by stating 'Photic stimulation did not elicit a driving response' or 'Photic stimulation elicited a symmetric driving response'.

Abnormal responses such as significant asymmetries and photoconvulsive responses must be described.

26.1.5 *Sleep.* It is helpful to either briefly describe the major EEG findings during sleep or simply list the deepest stage of sleep that occurred. If the patient was referred for the evaluation of a possible seizure disorder and epileptiform activity did not occur, then the depth and duration of sleep will be of particular importance. The report should also indicate whether sleep was induced with a sedative or occurred spontaneously.

Abnormalities during sleep should be described in detail. Most important is the appearance of epileptiform activity. Other abnormalities of clinical significance include persistence of abnormal patterns seen in the waking record, abnormal sleep patterns and sleep onset REM periods. Patterns of doubtful clinical significance such as 6 Hz spike-and-slow-wave, 14 and 6 Hz positive bursts, small sharp spikes and rhythmical midtemporal discharges may be mentioned, but their uncertain significance must be stressed in the description and summary to avoid confusion with clinically significant EEG abnormalities.

It is helpful to summarize the diagnostically important features of the EEG under a separate heading. This serves several purposes. First, it allows individuals with some understanding of electroencephalography to quickly review the relevant findings. Second, it allows the electroencephalographer to quickly review the salient features of prior recordings. Third, it forces the reader to focus clearly on the major findings and summarize them succinctly. Summary writing is therfore an extremely useful teaching exercise for residents and fellows who are learning to read EEGs. Finally, the summary can be used in combination with the interpretation to form a preliminary report that can be read over the phone or sent out in typewritten form. In some laboratories a purely descriptive summary is replaced by a graded classification system. This, of course, requires that the referring physicians be familiar with the grading system.

EEG summaries should be stated with the least number of terms needed to describe the major findings. It is helpful to organize the findings in the following order: *major finding; amplitude; persistence, reactivity, or activation; location;* and *behavioral state.* For example, an EEG that contains: (1) focal left anterior temporal continuous irregular delta activity that does not disappear with alerting and persists during wakefulness and sleep; and (2) left anterior temporal epileptiform spikes during sleep, could be summarized as follows:

Summary of findings:
   (1) Epileptiform spikes; left anterior temporal; during sleep only.
   (2) Focal irregular delta activity; moderate amplitude; continuous, non-reactive; left anterior temporal maximal.

In the interpretation the reader may choose to refer to the summary and then state the clinical correlation. For example, in the EEG described above the interpretation might read as follows:

Interpretation: The EEG is moderately abnormal due to the above summarized findings. These findings indicate the presence of a potentially epileptogenic focal cerebral dysfunction involving the left anterior temporal area and strongly suggests the presence of an underlying structural abnormality. These findings are consistent with the clinical impression of a partial seizure disorder.

26.3 CLINICAL CORRELATION

26.3.1   *Normal records* generally do not need an interpretation. Exceptions should be made in cases of apparent discrepancies between the EEG and the clinical condition of the patient. This is especially true if the patient has clinical abnormalities during the recording as in the example of a report given above. Other interpretations of normal reports may be of interest to some, but not all recipients of EEG reports; the EEG reader should try to tailor his reports to the needs of the referring physician. Thus, in the case of a patient with dementia, the interpretation may include the statement that 'a normal EEG may be seen in mild or even moderately advanced cases of Alzheimer's dementia'. The proper use of the terms *cerebral dysfunction, indicative, suggestive*, and *consistent* are discussed in the Guidelines for Writing EEG Reports in Appendix II.

26.3.2   *Abnormal findings* must be interpreted. Without interpretation, the report of an abnormal EEG finding is as meaningless as an X-ray report that lists opacities and translucencies but does not say whether they indicate a fracture. To interpret an abnormal EEG, the reader should take into consideration each abnormal pattern and mentally scan its general pathological and specific clinical correlates as outlined in the preceding chapters and tables. To arrive at a meaningful interpretation, he must compare the many possible clinical correlates of the EEG patterns with the clinical presentation of the case and must select the diagnoses most likely to satisfy both (15.3). Clearly, the interpretation will improve with the amount of clinical information given to the EEG reader and with the reader's ability to match the abnormal patterns with the clinical presentation.

26.3.3 *Recommendations for further diagnostic work* may be appropriate in some cases. Repeat EEG recordings may help to answer questions whether focal slow waves are postictal, i.e. whether they disappear after several days without seizures. The failure to obtain a sleep recording in a patient suspected of having partial complex seizures may lead to the suggestion to have the patient return sedated. A patient with a suspected seizure disorder who shows no epileptiform activity in his first EEG including a sleep recording may show epileptiform discharges in a second or third EEG recording. Repeat recordings may better evaluate the condition of patients with acute and transient changes resulting from head injuries, cardiorespiratory arrest or drug effects. The presence of muscle artifact preventing the interpretation of an EEG of a patient with suspected cerebral death may lead to the proposal to use neuromuscular blocking agents during the recording. The multiple sleep latency test may be indicated for patients with a possible diagnosis of narcolepsy or simultaneous respiratory monitoring during sedated sleep may be indicated for those suspected of having sleep apnea. Unexplained focal slowing may prompt the recommendation of further diagnostic studies.

26.3.4 *The following sample EEG report* is based on the recording of a 15-year-old boy referred with a history of four attacks of dizziness during the preceding three months. The referring physician requested the EEG to investigate the possibility of a convulsive disorder.

Description: The EEG during wakefulness contains an approximately symmetric, moderate amplitude, 10–11 Hz, posterior dominant activity that attenuates with eye opening. During eye closure at rest a moderate amplitude intermittent 9.5–10.5 Hz mu rhythm is present. Occasional randomly distributed 5–7 Hz theta waves are present over most head regions.

Hyperventilation did not elicit any abnormalities. During hyperventilation the patient complained of feeling dizzy and faint in a manner similar to that experienced during his recent attacks.

Photic stimulation elicited a symmetric driving response.

Sleep occurred following sedation with chloral hydrate and was characterized by the appearance of generalized slowing, vertex waves, POSTs, and sleep spindles.

Summary of findings:

(1) Hyperventilation induced a sensation of dizziness characteristic of the patient's attacks.

Interpretation: The EEG is normal with the patient recorded in the awake and sleep states. Hyperventilation produced a sensation of dizziness which the patient describes as similar to that which he experiences during his attacks. The absence of epileptiform activity at that time suggests that his dizziness is not a seizure manifestation. If a chronic seizure disorder is strongly suspected, then a repeat recording in the awake and sleep states may provide additional information.

26.3.5 The Guidelines for Writing EEG Reports recommended by the American EEG Society complement the information provided in this Chapter and the reader is encouraged to review them. They are reproduced in Appendix II.

REFERENCES

American EEG Society Guidelines in EEG and Evoked Potentials. Guideline 8: Guidelines for writing
EEG reports. (1986) J. Clin. Neurophysiol. 3 (Suppl. 1): 34–37.

Schneider, J. (1977) Section IV. The EEG report. In: Rémond, A. (Ed.), Handbook of Electroenceph.
clin. Neurophysiol., Vol. 11A, Elsevier, Amsterdam, pp. 97–109.

Appendix I

A GLOSSARY OF TERMS MOST COMMONLY USED BY CLINICAL ELECTROENCEPHALOGRAPHERS[1,2,3,4]

G.E. CHATRIAN (CHAIRMAN), L. BERGAMINI, M. DONDEY, D.W. KLASS, M. LENNOX-BUCHTHAL AND I. PETERSÉN

Absence. Use of term discouraged when describing EEG patterns. Terms suggested, whenever appropriate: 3 Hz spike-and-slow-waves; atypical repetitive spike-and-slow-waves.

Abundance. Use of term discouraged. Term suggested: quantity (not a synonym).

Activation. (1) Any procedure designed to enhance or elicit normal or abnormal EEG activity, especially paroxysmal activity. Examples: hyperventilation; photic stimulation; sleep; injection of convulsant drugs. (2) EEG pattern consisting of a low voltage record which becomes apparent upon blocking of EEG rhythms by physiological or other stimuli such as electrical stimulation of the brain (use discouraged).

Active electrode. Use of term discouraged. *Cf.,* exploring electrode (not a synonym).

Activity, EEG. Any EEG wave or sequence of waves.

After-discharge. (1) EEG seizure pattern following repetitive electrical stimulation of a discrete area of the brain via cortical or intracerebral

---

[1] The following annotations are used throughout the glossary:

*American.

**British.

****Cf.* Report of the Committee on Methods of Clinical Examination in electroencephalography. *Electroenceph. clin. Neurophysiol.*, **1958**, *10:* 370–375

*****Cf.* Report of the Committee on EEG Instrumentation Standards. *Electroenceph. clin. Neurophysiol.*, **1974**, *37:*549–553.

[2] The Report of the Committee on Terminology, page 529, to which this glossary is an appendix, should be consulted.

[3] Enquiries regarding reprints should be addressed to the President of the Federation, Dr. R.J. Ellingson, Nebraska Psychiatric Institute, 602 South 44th Avenue, Omaha, Nebr. 68105, U.S.A.

[4] This Appendix is an official document of the International Federation of Societies for Electroencephalography and Clinical Neurophysiology. As such it has not been subject to editorial review, nor are the editors of the EEG Journal responsible for its contents.

electrodes. (2) Burst of rhythmic activity following a transient such as an evoked potential or a spike.

Alpha band. Frequency band of 8–13 Hz. Greek letter: *a*.

Alpha rhythm. Rhythm at 8–13 Hz occuring during wakefulness over the posterior regions of the head, generally with higher voltage over the occipital areas. Amplitude is variable but is mostly below 50 μV in the adult. Best seen with the eyes closed and under conditions of physical relaxation and relative mental inactivity. Blocked or attenuated by attention, especially visual, and mental effort. Comment: use of term alpha rhythm must be restricted to those rhythms which fulfil all these criteria. Acitivities in the alpha band which differ from the alpha rhythm as regards their topography and/or reactivity either have specific appellations (for instance, the mu rhythm) or should be referred to as *rhythms of alpha frequency*. *Cf.*, rhythm of alpha frequency.

Alpha variant rhythms. Term applies to certain characteristic EEG rhythms which are recorded most prominently over the posterior regions of the head and differ in frequency but resemble in reactivity the alpha rhythm. *Cf.*, fast alpha variant rhythm; slow alpha variant rhythms.

Alpha wave. Wave with duration of 1/8–1/13 sec.

Alphoid rhythm. Use of term discouraged.

Amplitude. Voltage of EEG waves. Generally expressed in microvolts (μV). Measured peak-to-peak. Comment: amplitude of EEG waves recorded from the surface of the head is influenced to a major degree by extracerebral factors including the impedances of the meninges, cerebrospinal fluid, skull, scalp and electrodes.

Antiphase signal**. *Cf.*, out-of-phase signal*.

Aperiodic. Applies to: (1) EEG waves or complexes occurring in a sequence at an irregular rate. (2) EEG waves or complexes occurring intermittently at irregular intervals.

Apotentiality, Record of cerebral. Use of term discouraged. Term suggested: record of electrocerebral inactivity. *Cf.*, inactivity, record of electrocerebral.

Application, Electrode. The process of establishing connection between an electrode and the subject's scalp or brain.

Arceau rhythm. Use of term discouraged. Term suggested: mu rhythm.

Arousal. Use of term discouraged when describing EEG pattern.

Array. A regular arrangement of electrodes over the scalp or brain or within the brain substance.

Arrhythmic activity. A sequence of waves of inconstant period. *Cf.*, rhythm.

Artifact (artefact). Any potential difference due to an extracerebral source, recorded in EEG tracings. (2) Any modification of the EEG caused by extracerebral factors such as alterations of the media surrounding the brain, instrumental distortion or malfunction, and operational errors.

Asymmetry. (1) Unequal amplitude and/or form and frequency of EEG activities over homologous areas on opposite sides of the head. (2) Unequal development of EEG waves about the baseline.

Asynchrony. The non-simultaneous occurrence of EEG activities over regions on the same or opposite sides of the head.

Attenuation. (1) Reduction in amplitude of EEG activity. May occur transiently in response to physiological or other stimuli, such as electrical stimulation of the brain, or result from pathological conditions. *Cf.*, blocking. (2) Reduction of sensitivity of an EEG channel, *i.e.*, decrease in output pen deflection by operation or sensitivity or filter controls. Customarily expressed as relative reduction of sensitivity at certain stated frequencies. *Cf.*, sensitivity; high frequency filter; low frequency filter****.

Atypical repetitive spike-and-slow-waves. Term refers to paroxysms consisting of a sequence of spike-and-slow-wave complexes which occur bilaterally synchronously but do not meet one or more of the criteria of 3 Hz spike-and-slow-waves. *Cf.*, 3 Hz spike-and-slow-waves.

Augmentation. Increase in amplitude of electrical activity.

Average potential reference. Average of the potentials of all or many EEG electrodes, used as a reference. Synonym: Goldmann-Offner reference (use discouraged).

Background activity. Any EEG activity representing the setting in which a given normal or abnormal pattern appears and from which such pattern is distinguished. Comment: not a synonym of any individual rhythm such as the alpha rhythm.

Balanced amplifier. An amplifier which consists essentially of two identical single-ended amplifiers operated as a pair and in opposite phases.

Band. Portion of EEG frequency spectrum. *Cf.,* delta, theta, alpha, beta bands.

Bandwidth, EEG channel. Range of frequencies between which the response of an EEG channel is within stated limits. Determined by the frequency response of the amplifier-writer combination and the frequncy filters used. Comment: the manner in which the EEG channel bandwidth is specified by different manufacturers is not standardized at present. For instance, in a given instrument, a bandwidth of 0.5–50 Hz may indicate that frequencies of 0.5 and 50 Hz are attenuated 30% (3 dB), or another stated per cent, with intermediate frequencies being attenuated less****.

Basal electrode. Any electrode located in proximity to the base of the skull. *Cf.,* nasopharyngeal electrode; sphenoidal electrode.

Baseline. (1) Strictly: line obtained when an identical voltage is applied to the two input terminals of an EEG amplifier or when the instrument is in the calibrate position but no calibration signal is applied. (2) Loosely: imaginary line corresponding to the approximate mean values of the EEG activity assessed visually in an EEG derivation over a period of time.

Beta band. Frequency band over 13 Hz. Greek letter: β. Comment: practically, most electroencephalographs using pen writers appreciably attenuate frequencies higher than 75 Hz. The customary use of relatively slow paper speeds further limits the electroencephalographer's ability to resolve visually waves of frequencies higher than 35 Hz. However, this does not justify limiting unduly the high frequency response of the EEG channels for EEG waves include transients such as spikes and sharp waves with components at frequencies above 50 Hz.

Beta rhythm. In general: any EEG rhythm over 13 Hz. Most characteristically: a rhythm from 13 to 35 Hz recorded over the fronto-central regions of the head during wakefulness. Amplitude of fronto-central beta rhythm is variable but is mostly below 30 μV. Blocking or attenuation by contralateral movement or tactile stimulation is especially obvious in electrocorticograms. Other beta rhythms are most prominent in other locations or are diffuse.

Bilateral. Involving both sides of the head.

Biparietal hump. Use of term discouraged. Term suggested: vertex sharp transient.

Biphasic wave. Use of term discouraged. Term suggested: diphasic wave.

Bipolar depth electrode. Use of term discouraged. Term suggested: dual-electrode (or multi-electrode) lead.

Bipolar derivation. Recording from a pair of exploring electrodes ***. *Cf.,* exploring electrode; bipolar montage.

Bipolar montage. Multiple bipolar derivations, with no electrode being common to all derivations. In most instances, bipolar derivations are linked, *i.e.,* adjacent derivations from electrodes along the same array have one electrode in common, connected to the input terminal 2 of one amplifier and to the input terminal 1 of the following amplifier***. *Cf.,* referential montage.

Bisynchronous. Abbreviation for: bilaterally synchronous (use discouraged).

Black lead*.** Use of term discouraged. Term suggested: input terminal 1.

Blocking. (1) Apparent, temporary obliteration of EEG rhythms in response to physiological or other stimuli such as electrical stimulation of the brain. *Cf.,* attenuation. (2) A condition of temporary unresponsiveness of the EEG amplifier, caused by major overload. Manifested initially by extreme, flat-topped pen excursion(s) lasting up to a few seconds. *Cf.,* overload; clipping.

Brain wave. Use of term discouraged. Term suggested: EEG wave.

Buffer amplifier. An amplifier, generally with a voltage gain of 1, a high input impedance and a low output impedance, used to isolate the input signal from the loading effects of an immediately following circuit. In some electroencephalographs, each input is connected to a buffer amplifier located in the jack box to reduce cable artifact and interference.

Build-up. Colloquialism. Employed to describe progressive increase in voltage of the EEG or appearance of waves of increasing amplitude, frequently associated with decrease in frequency. Sometimes applied to hyperventilation or seizure discharges (use discouraged).

Burst. A group of waves appear and disappear abruptly and are distinguished from background activity by differences in frequency, form and/or amplitude. Comments: (1) Term does not imply abnormality. (2) Not a synonym of paroxysm. *Cf.,* paroxysm.

Burst-suppression. Pattern characterized by burst of theta and/or delta waves, at times intermixed with faster waves, and intervening periods of relative quiescence. Comment: term should be used to describe the EEG effects of some anesthetic drugs at certain levels of anesthesia.

Calibration. (1) Procedure of testing and recording the responses of EEG channels to voltage differences applied to the input terminals of their respective amplifiers. Comment: DC (usually) or AC voltages of magnitude comparable to the amplitudes of EEG waves are used in this procedure***·*****. (2) The procedure of testing the accuracy of paper speed by means of a time marker. Comment: some electroencephalographs provide time marks throughout recording. *Cf.,* common EEG input test.

Cap, Head. A cap which is fitted over the head to hold pad electrodes in position.

Channel. Complete system for the detection, amplification and display of potential differences between a pair of electrodes. Comment: electroencephalographs generally consist of several EEG channels***·****.

Chopper. A device consisting of a mechanical or electronic switch used in some EEG amplifiers for interrupting (chopping) DC, and low frequency AC, signals and converting them into square waves of relatively high frequence. The same device may provide synchronous rectification of these square waves after amplification to reconvert them to the form of the original signal at the output.

Chopper amplifier. A direct current amplifier in which a chopper interrupts DC, and low frequency AC, signals and converts them into square waves of relatively high frequency. These are magnified by an AC amplifier and then reconverted by synchronous rectification to the form of the original signal at the output.

Circumferential bipolar montage. A montage consisting of derivations from pairs of electrodes along circumferential arrays.

Clipping. Distortion of EEG waves which makes them appear flat-topped in the write-out. Caused by overload.

Comb rhythm. Use of term discouraged. Term suggested: mu rhythm.

Common EEG input test. Procedure in which the same pair of EEG electrodes is connected to the two terminals of all channels of the electroencephalograph ***. Comment: used as adjunct to calibration procedure. *Cf.,* calibration.

Common mode rejection. A characteristic of differential amplifiers whereby they provide markedly reduced amplification of common mode signals, compared to differential signals. Expressed as common mode rejection ratio, *i.e.,* ratio of amplifications of differential and common mode signals. Example:

$$\frac{\text{amplification, differential}}{\text{amplification, common mode}} = \frac{20.000}{1} = 20{,}000{:}1.$$

Common mode signal. Common component of the two signals applied to the two respective input terminals of a differential EEG amplifier. Comment: in EEG recording, external interference frequently occurs as common mode signal.

Common reference electrode. A reference electrode connected to the input terminal 2 of several or all EEG amplifiers.

Common reference montage. Several referential derivations sharing a single reference electrode***. *Cf.,* referential derivation; reference electrode.

Complex. A sequence of two or more waves having a characteristic form or recurring with a fairly consistent form, distinguished from background acitivity.

Coronal bipolar montage. A montage consisting of derivations from pairs of electrodes along coronal (transverse) arrays. Synonym: transverse bipolar montage***.

Cortical electrode. Electrode applied directly upon or inserted in the cerebral cortex.

Cortical electroencephalogram. *Cf.,* electrocorticogram.

Cortical electroencephalography. *Cf., electrocorticography.*

Corticogram. Abbreviation for: electrocorticogram (use discouraged).

Corticography. Abbreviation for: electrocorticography (use discouraged).

Cycle. The complete sequence of potential changes undergone by individual components of a sequence of regularly repeated EEG waves or complexes.

Cycles per second. Unit of frequency. Abbreviation: c/sec. Synonym: hertz (Hz) preferred.

c/sec. Abbreviation for cycles per second. Equivalent: Hz preferred.

DEEG. Abbreviation for: depth electroencephalogram and depth electroencephalography.

Delta band. Frequency band under 4 Hz. Greek letter δ. Comment: DC potential differences are not monitored in conventional EEGs.

Delta rhythm. Rhythm under 4Hz.

Delta wave. Wave with duration over 1/4 sec.

Depression. Use of term discouraged when describing EEG patterns.

Depth electrode. Electrode implanted within the brain substance.

Depth electroencephalogram. Record of electrical activity of the brain by means of electrodes implanted within the brain substance itself. Abbreviation: DEEG. *Cf.,* stereotactic (stereotaxic) depth electroencephalogram.

Depth electroencephalography. Technique of recording depth electroencephalograms. Abbreviation: DEEG.

Derivation. (1) The process of recording from a pair of electrodes in an EEG channel. (2) The EEG record obtained by this process.

Desynchronization. Use of term discouraged when describing EEG change. Terms suggested: blocking; attenuation.

Desynchronized. Use of term discouraged when describing EEG pattern. *Cf.,* low voltage EEG.

Diffuse. Occuring over large areas of one or both sides of the head. *Cf.,* generalized.

Differential amplifier. An amplifier whose output is proportional to to the voltage difference between its two input terminals. Comment: electroencephalographs make use of differential amplifiers in their input stages.

Differential signal. Difference between two unlike signals applied to the respective two input terminals of a differential EEG amplifier.

Diphasic wave. Wave consisting of two components developed on alternate sides of the baseline.

Direct-coupled amplifier. An amplifier in which successive stages are connected (coupled) by devices which are not frequency-dependent.

Direct current amplifier. An amplifier which is capable of magnifying DC (zero frequency) voltages and slowly varying voltages. Comment: the direct-coupled amplifier and the chopper amplifier are direct current amplifiers. *Cf.,* direct-coupled amplifier; chopper amplifier.

Disk electrode. Metal disk attached to the scalp with an adhesive such as collodion, a paste or wax***.

Discharge. Interpretive term commonly used to designate such paroxysmal patters as epileptiform patterns and seizure patterns. *Cf.,* epileptiform pattern; seizure pattern, EEG.

Disorganization. Gross alteration in frequency, form, topography and/or quantity of physiologic EEG rhythms in an individual record, relative to previous records in the same subject or the rhythms of homologous regions on the opposite side of the head.

Distortion. An instrument alteration in wave form. *Cf.,* artifact.

Duration. (1) The interval from beginning to end of and individual wave or complex. Comment: the duration of the cycle of individual components of a sequence of regularly repeating waves or complexes is referred to as the period of the wave or complex. (2) The time that a sequence of waves or complexes or any other distinguishable feature lasts in an EEG record.

Dysrhythmia. Use of term discouraged.

Earth connection.** *Cf.,* synonym: ground connection*.

ECoG. Abbreviation for: electrocorticogram and electrocorticography.

EEG. Abbreviation for: electroencephalogram and electroencephalography.

Electrocorticogram. Record of EEG activity obtained by means of electrodes applied directly over or inserted in the cerebral cortex. Abbreviation: ECoG.

Electrocorticography. Technique of recording electrical activity of the brain by means of electrodes applied over or implanted in the cerebral cortex. Abbreviation: ECoG.

Electrode, EEG*.** Strictly: a conducting device applied over or inserted into a region of the scalp or brain. Loosely: synonym of lead.

Electrode impedance. Opposition to the flow of an AC current through the interface between an electrode and the scalp or brain. Measured between pairs of electrodes or, in some electroencephalographs, between each individual electrode and all other electrodes connected in parallel. Expressed in ohms (generally kilohms, $k\Omega$). Comments: (1) Over the EEG frequency range, because the capacitance factor is small, electrode impedance is usually numerically equal to electrode resistance. (2) Not a synonym of input impedance of EEG amplifier. *Cf.,* electrode resistance; input impedance.

Electrode resistance. Opposition to the flow of a DC current through the interface between an EEG electrode and the scalp or brain. Measured between pairs of electrodes or, in some electroencephalographs, between each individual electrode and all the other electrodes connected in parallel. Expressed in ohms (generally kilohms, $k\Omega$). Comment: measurement of electrode resistance with DC currents results in varying degrees of electrode polarization. *Cf.,* electrode impedance.

Electroencephalogram. Record of electrical activity of the brain taken by means of electrodes placed on the surface of the head, unless otherwise specified.

Electroencephalograph. Instrument employed to record electroencephalograms.

Electroencephalography. (1) The science relating to the electrical activity of the brain. (2) The technique of recording electroencephalograms. Abbreviation: EEG.

Electrogram. Use of term discouraged.

Electrography. Use of term discouraged.

Epidural electrode. Electrode located over the dural covering of the cerebrum.

Epileptic pattern. Use of term discouraged. *Cf.,* epileptiform pattern.

Epileptiform pattern. Interpretive term. Applies to distinctive waves or complexes, distinguished from background activity, and resembling those recorded in a proportion of human subjects suffering from epileptic disorders and in animals rendered epileptic experimentally. Epileptyform patterns include spikes and sharp waves, alone or accompanied by slow waves, occurring singly or in bursts lasting at most a few seconds. Comment: (1) Term refers to inter-ictal paroxysmal activity and not to seizure patterns. *Cf.,* seizure pattern. (2) Probability of association with clinical epileptic disorders is variable.

Epoch. A period of time in an EEG record. Duration of epochs is determined arbitrarily. Example: a 10 sec epoch.

Equipotential. Applies to regions of the head or electrodes which are at the same potential at a given instant in time.

Equipotential line. Imaginary line joining a series of points which are at the same potential at a given instant in time.

Evoked potential. Wave or complex elicited by and time-locked to a physiological or other stimulus, for instance an electrical stimulus, delivered to a sensory receptor or nerve, or applied directly to a discrete area of the brain. Comment: computer summation techniques are especially suited for the detection of these and other event-related potentials from the surface of the head.

Evoked response. Tautology. Use of term discouraged. Term suggested: evoked potential.

Exploring electrode. Any electrode over the scalp or brain or within the brain substance, intended to detect EEG activity. Such an electrode is customarily connected to either the input terminal 1 or the input terminal 2 of an EEG amplifier in bipolar derivations and to the input terminal 1 of an EEG amplifier in referential derivations. *Cf.,* bipolar derivation; referential derivation.

Extracerebral potential. Any potential which does not originate in the brain, referred to as an artifact in EEG. May arise from: electrical interference external to the subject and recording system; the subject; the electrodes and their connections to the subject and the electroencephalograph; and electroencephalograph itself. *Cf.,* artifact.

Fast activity. Activity of frequency higher than alpha, *i.e.,* beta activity.

Fast alpha variant rhythm. Characteristic rhythm at 14–20 Hz, detected most prominently over the posterior regions of the head. May alternate or be intermixed with alpha rhythm. Blocked or attenuated by attention, especially visual, and mental effort.

Fast wave. Wave with duration shorter than alpha waves, *i.e.,* under 1/13 sec.

Flat EEG. Use of term discouraged. *Cf.,* low voltage EEG; inactivity, record of electrocerebral.

Focus. A limited region of the scalp, cerebral cortex or depth of the brain displaying a given EEG activity, whether normal or abnormal.

Form. Shape of a wave. Synonym: wave form; morphology.

Fourteen and six Hz positive burst. Burst of arch-shaped waves at 13–17 Hz and/or 5–7 Hz but most commonly at 14 and/or 6 Hz, seen generally over the posterior temporal and adjacent areas of one or both sides of the head during sleep. The sharp peaks of its component waves are positive with respect to other regions. Amplitude varies but is generally below 75 μV. Comments: (1) Best demonstrated by referential recording using contralateral earlobe, or other remote, reference electrodes. (2) The clinical significance of this pattern, if any, is controversial.

Fourteen and six Hz positive spikes. Use of term discouraged. Term suggested: 14 and 6 Hz positive burst.

Frequency. Number of complete cycles of repetitive waves or complexes in one second. Measured in hertz (Hz), a unit preferred to its equivalent, cycles per second (c/sec).

Frequency response. *Cf.,* bandwidth; low frequency response; high frequency response****.

Frequency response curve. A graph depicting the relationships between output pen deflection or amplifier output and input frequency in an EEG channel, for a particular setting of low and high frequency filters****.

Frequency spectrum. Range of frequencies composing the EEG. Divided into 4 bands termed delta, theta, alpha and beta. *Cf.,* delta; theta; alpha; beta bands.

Frontal intermittent rhythmic delta activity. Fairly regular or approximately sinusoidal waves, mostly occurring in bursts at 1.5–3 Hz over the frontal areas of one or both sides of the head. Comment: caution should be exercised to differentiate this acitivity from potential changes generated by vertical eye movements.

G1*. Abbreviation for grid 1 (use of term discouraged).

G2*. Abbreviation for grid 2 (use of term discouraged).

Gain. Ratio of output signal voltage to input signal voltage of an EEG channel. Example:

$$\text{gain} = \frac{\text{output voltage}}{\text{input voltage}} = \frac{10 \text{ V}}{10 \ \mu\text{V}} = 1.000.000$$

often expressed in decibels (dB), a logarithmic unit. Example: a voltage gain of 10 = 20 dB, of 1000 = 60 dB, of 1,000,000 = 120 dB. *Cf.,* sensitivity.

Gamma rhythm. Use of term discouraged. *Cf.,* beta rhythm (not a synonym).

Generalization. Propagation of EEG activity from limited areas to all regions of the head.

Generalized. Occurring over all regions of the head.

Goldman-Offner reference. Use of term discouraged. Term suggested: average potential reference.

Grand mal. Use of term discouraged when describing EEG pattern.

Grid 1*. Use of term discouraged. Term suggested: input terminal 1****.

Grid 2*. Use of term discouraged. Term suggested: input terminal 2****.

Ground connection*. Conducting path between the subject and the electroencephalograph, and the electroencephalograph and earth****. Synonym: earth connection**.

Harness, Head. A combination of straps which are fitted over the head to hold pad electrodes in position.

Hertz. Unit of frequency. Abbreviation: Hz. Preferred to synonym: cycles per second.

High frequency filter. A circuit which reduces the sensitivity of the EEG channel to relatively high frequencies. For each position of the high frequency filter control, this attenuation is expressed as per cent reduction in output pen deflection at a given frequency, relative to frequencies unaffected by the filter, *i.e.*, in the mid-frequency band of the channel. Comment: at present, high frequency filter designations and their significance are not standardized for instruments of different manufacture. For instance, for a given instrument, a position of the high frequency filter control designated as 35 Hz may indicate a 30% (3 dB), or other stated per cent, reduction in sensitivity at 35 Hz, compared to the sensitivity, for example at 10 Hz***·****.

High frequency response. Sensitivity of an EEG channel to relatively high frequencies. Determined by the high frequency response of the amplifier-writer combination and the high frequency filter used. Expressed as per cent reduction in output pen deflection at certain specific high frequencies, relative to other frequencies in the mid-frequency band of the channel****.

High pass filter. *Cf.*, synonym: low frequency filter.

Hyperexcitability, Neuronal. Use of term discouraged when describing EEG patterns.

Hypersynchrony. Use of term discouraged when describing EEG patterns.

Hyperventilation. Deep and regular respiration performed for a period of several minutes***. Used as activation procedure. Synonym: overbreathing. *Cf.*, activation.

Hypsarrhythmia. Pattern consisting of high voltage arrhythmic slow waves interspersed with spike discharges, without consistent synchrony between the two sides of the head or different areas on the same side.

Hz. Abbreviation for hertz. Preferred to equivalent: c/sec.

Impedance meter. An instrument used to measure impedance. *Cf.*, electrode impedance.

Inactive electrode. Use of term discouraged. *Cf.*, reference electrode (not a synonym).

Inactivity, Record of electrocerebral. Absence over all regions of the head of indentifiable electrical activity of cerebral origin, whether spontaneous or induced by physiological stimuli and pharmacological agents. Comment: determination of electrocerebral inactivity requires advanced instrumentation and stringent technical precautions. Tracings of electrocerebral inactivity should be held in clear contradistinction to low voltage EEGs and records displaying delta activity of low amplitude. *Cf.*, low voltage EEG.

Independent (temporally). *Cf.*, Synonym: asynchronous.

Index. Per cent time an EEG activity is present in an EEG sample. Example: alpha index.

Indifferent electrode. Use of term discouraged. Term suggested: reference electrode (not a synonym).

In-phase discrimination. Use of term discouraged. Term suggested: common mode rejection (not a synonym).

In-phase signals. Waves with no phase difference between them. *Cf.*, common mode signal (not a synonym).

Input. The signal fed into an EEG amplifier. *Cf.*, input terminal 1; input terminal 2****.

Input terminal 1. The input terminal of the differential EEG amplifier at which negativity, relative to the other input terminal, produces an upward pen deflection****. Synonyms: "grid 1" (G1)*, black lead*** (use discouraged). Cf., polarity convention. Comment: in diagrams, the connection of an electrode to the input terminal 1 of the EEG amplifier is represented as a solid line.

Input terminal 2. The input terminal of the differential EEG amplifier at which negativity, relative to the other input terminal, produces a downward pen deflection****. Synonyms: "grid 2" (G2)*, white lead*** (use discouraged). Cf., polarity convention. Comment: in diagrams, the connection of an electrode to the input terminal 2 of the EEG amplifier is represented as a dotted or dashed line.

Input circuit. System consisting of the EEG electrodes and intervening tissues, the electrode leads, jack box, input cable and electrode selectors.

Input impedance. Impedance that exists between the two inputs of an EEG amplifier. Measured in ohms (generally megohms, $M\Omega$) with or without the additional specification of input shunt capacitance (measured in picofarads, pF)****. Comment: not a synonym of electrode impedance.

Input voltage. Potential difference between the two input terminals of a differential EEG amplifier.

Instrumental phase reversal. Simultaneous pen deflections in opposite directions caused by a wave in two bipolar derivations. This inversion is purely instrumental in nature, i.e., due to the same signal being simultaneously applied to the input terminal 2 of one differential amplifier and to the input terminal 1 of the other amplifier. Comment: when observed in two linked bipolar derivations, phase reversal indicates that the potential field is maximal or, less frequently, minimal at or near the electrode common to such derivations. Hence, this phenomenon is used to localize EEG activities, whether normal or abnormal. Cf., true phase reversal; bipolar montage; differential amplifier.

Inter-electrode distance. Spacing between pairs of electrodes. Comment: distances between adjacent electrodes placed according to the standard 10–20 system or more closely spaced electrodes are frequently referred to as short or small inter-electrode distances. Larger distances such as the double or triple distance between standard electrode placements are often termed long or large inter-electrode distances***.

Inter-hemispheric derivation. Recording between a pair of electrodes located on opposite sides of the head.

Intracerebral electrode. Cf., synonym depth electrode.

Intracerebral electroencephalogram. Cf., depth electroencephalogram.

Irregular. Applies to EEG waves and complexes of inconstant period and/or uneven countour

Isoelectric. (1) The record obtained from a pair of equipotential electrodes. Cf., equipotential. (2) Use of term discouraged when describing record of electrocerebral inactivity Cf., inactivity, record of electrocerebral.

Isolated. Occuring singly.

K complex. A burst of somewhat variable appearance, consisting most commonly of a high voltage diphasic slow wave frequently associated with a sleep spindle. Amplitude is generally maximal in proximity of the vertex. K complexes occur during sleep, apparently spontaneously or in response to sudden sensory stimuli, and are not specific for any individual sensory modality. Cf., vertex sharp transient.

Kappa rhythm. Rhythm consisting of bursts of alpha or theta frequency occurring over the temporal areas of the scalp of subjects engaged in mental activity. Comments: (1) Best recorded between electrodes located lateral to the outer canthus of each eye. (2) The cerebral origin of this rhythm is regarded as unproven.

Lambda wave. Sharp transient occurring over the occipital regions of the head of waking subjects during visual exploration. Mainly positive relative to other areas. Time-locked to saccadic eye movement. Amplitude varies but is generally below 50 μV. Greek letter λ.

Lambdoid wave. Use of term discouraged. Term suggested: positive occipital sharp transient of sleep.

Larval spike-and slow-waves. Use of term discouraged. Term suggested: 6 Hz spike-and-slow-waves.

Lateralized. Involving mainly the right or left side of the head. *Cf.*, unilateral.

Lead. Strictly: wire connecting an electrode to the electroencephalograph. Loosely: synonym of electrode.

Linkage. The connection of a pair of electrodes to the two respective input terminals of a differential EEG amplifier, *Cf.*, derivation.

Longitudinal bipolar montage. A montage consisting of derivations from pairs of electrodes along longitudinal, usually antero-posterior, arrays***.

Low frequency filter. A circuit which reduces the sensitivity of the EEG channel to relatively low frequencies***. For each position of the low frequency filter control, this attenuation is expressed as per cent reduction of output pen deflection at a given stated frequency, relative to frequencies unaffected by the filter, *i.e.*, in the mid-frequency band of the channel. Comment: at present, low frequency filter designations and their significance are not standardized for instruments of different manufacture. For instance, in a given instrument, a position of the low frequency filter control designated 0.5 Hz may indicate at 30% (3 dB) or other stated per cent, reduction in sensitivity at 0.5 Hz, compared to the sensitivity, for example, at 10 Hz. The same position of the low frequency filter control also may be designated by the time constant. Synonym: high pass filter. *Cf.*, time constant****.

Low frequency response. Sensitivity of an EEG channel to relatively low frequencies. Determined by the low frequency response of the amplifier and by the low frequency filter (time constant) used. Expressed as per cent reduction in output pen deflection at certain stated low frequencies, relative to other frequencies in the mid-frequency band of the channel. *Cf.*, low frequency filter; time constant****.

Low pass filter. *Cf.*, synonym: high frequency filter.

Low voltage EEG. A waking record characterized by activity of amplitude not greater than 20 μV over all head regions. With appropriate instrumental sensitivities this activity can be shown to be composed primarily of beta, theta and, to a lesser degree, delta waves, with or without alpha activity over the posterior areas. Comments: (1) Low voltage EEGs are susceptible to change under the influence of certain physiological stimuli, sleep, pharmacological agents and pathological processes. (2) They should be held in clear contradistinction to the tracings of electrocerebral inactivity, records which consist primarily of delta waves of relatively low voltage, and tracings which display low voltages over limited regions of the head.

Low voltage fast EEG. Use of term discouraged. Term suggested: low voltage EEG.

Machine, EEG. Use of term discouraged. Term suggested: electroencephalograph.

Monomorphic. Use of term discouraged when describing EEG patterns.

Monophasic wave. Wave developed on one side of the baseline.

Monopolar. Use of term discouraged. Term suggested: referential. *Cf.*, also unipolar.

Monorhythmic. Use of term discouraged when describing EEG patterns.

Monorhythmic sinusoidal delta activity. Use of term discouraged. *Cf.*, delta rhythm: frontal (occipital) intermittent rhythmic delta activity.

Montage. The particular arrangement by which a number of derivations are displayed simultaneously in an EEG record***.

Morphology. (1) The study of the form of EEG waves. (2) The form of EEG waves.

Mu rhythm. Rhythm at 7–11 Hz, composed of arch-shaped waves occurring over the central or centro-parietal regions of the scalp during wakefulness. Amplitude varies but is mostly below 50 μV. Blocked or attenuated most clearly by contralateral movement, thought of movement, readiness to move or tactile stimulation. Greek letter: μ. Synonyms: *arceau*, wicket, comb rhythms (use discouraged).

Multiple foci. Two or more spatially separated foci.

Multiple spike-and-slow-wave complex. A sequence of two or more spikes associated with one or more slow waves. Preferred to synonym: polyspike-and-slow-wave complex.

Multiple spike complex. A sequence of two or more spikes. Preferred to synonym: polyspike complex.

Nasopharyngeal electrode. Rod electrode introduced through the nose and placed against the nasopharyngeal wall with its tip lying near the body of the sphenoid bone.

Needle electrode. Small needle inserted into the subdermal layer of the scalp.

Neutral electrode. Use of term discouraged. Term suggested: reference electrode (not a synonym).

Noise, EEG channel. Small fluctuating output of an EEG channel recorded, when high sensitivities are used, even if there is no input signal. Measured in microvolts (μV), referenced to the input***·*****.

Notch filter. A filter which selectively attenuates a very narrow frequency band thus producing a sharp notch in the frequency response curve of an EEG channel. A 60 (50) Hz notch filter is used in some electroencephalographs to provide attenuation of 60 (50) Hz interference under extremely unfavorable technical conditions.

Occipital intermittent rhythmic delta activity. Fairly regular or approximately sinusoidal waves, mostly occurring in bursts at 2–3 Hz over the occipital areas of one or both sides of the head. Frequently blocked or attenuated by opening the eyes.

Ohmmeter. An instrument used to measure resistance. *Cf.*, electrode resistance.

Organization. The degree to which physiologic EEG rhythms conform to certain ideal characteristics displayed by a proportion of subjects in the same age group, free from personal and family history of neurologic and psychiatric diseases, and other illnesses that might be associated with dysfunction of the brain. Comments: (1) The organization of physiologic EEG rhythms progresses from birth to adulthood. (1) Poor organization of EEG rhythms such as the alpha rhythm does not necessarily imply abnormality.

Out-of-phase signals*. Two waves of opposite phases. *Cf.*, differential signal (not a synonym).

Output voltage. The voltage across the writer of an EEG channel.

Overbreathing. *Cf.*, synonym: hyperventilation.

Overload. Condition resulting from the application to the input terminals of an EEG amplifier of voltage differences larger than the channel is designed or set to handle. Causes clipping of EEG waves and/or blocking of the amplifier, depending on its magnitude. *Cf.*, clipping; blocking.

Pad electrode. Metal electrode covered with a cotton or felt and gauze pad, held in position by a head cap or harness.

Paper speed. Velocity of movement of EEG paper. Expressed in centimeters per second (cm/sec)***.

Paroxysm. Phenomenon with abrupt onset, rapid attainment of a maximum and sudden termination, distinguished from background activity. Comment: commonly used to refer to epileptiform patterns and seizure patterns. *Cf.*, epileptiform pattern; seizure pattern, EEG.

Pattern. Any characteristic EEG activity.

Peak. Point of maximum amplitude of a wave.

Pen galvanometer. *Cf.*, synonym: pen writer.

Pen motor. *Cf.*, synonym: pen writer.

Pen writer. A writer using ink delivered by a pen. Synonym: pen galvanometer; pen motor.

Period. Duration of complete cycle of individual component of a sequence of regularly repeated EEG waves or complexes. Comment: the period of the individual components of an EEG rhythm is the reciprocal of the frequency of the rhythm.

Periodic. Applies to: (1) waves or complexes occurring in a sequence at an approximately regular rate. (2) EEG waves or complexes occurring intermittently at approximately regular intervals, generally of 1 to several seconds.

Petit mal. Use of term discouraged when describing EEG patterns. Terms suggested, whenever appropriate: 3 Hz spike-and-slow-waves; Atypical repetitive spike-and-slow-waves; repetitive sharp-and-slow-waves.

Petit mal variant. Use of term discouraged when describing EEG patterns. Terms suggested whenever appropriate: atypical repetitive spike-and-slow-waves; repetitive sharp-and-slow-waves.

Phantom spike-and-waves. Use of term discouraged. Terms suggested: 6 Hz spike-and-slow-waves.

Phantom spike-and-slow-waves. Use of term discouraged. Term suggested: 6 Hz spike-and-slow-waves.

Phase. (1) Time or polarity relationships between a point on a wave displayed in a derivation and the identical point on the same wave recorded simultaneously in another derivation. (2) Time or angular relationships between a point on a wave and the onset of the cycle of the same wave. Usually expressed in degrees or radians****.

Phase reversal. *Cf.*, instrumental phase reversal; true phase reversal.

Photic driving. Physiologic response consisting of rhythmic activity elicited over the posterior regions of the head by repetitive photic stimulation at frequencies of about 5–30 Hz. Comments: (1) Term should be limited to activity time-locked to the stimulus and of frequency identical or harmonically related to the stimulus frequency. (2) Photic driving should be held in contradistinction to the visual evoked potentials elicited by isolation flashes of light or flashes repeated at very low frequencies.

Photic stimulation. Delivery of intermittent flashes of light to the eyes of a subject. Used as EEG activation procedure***.

Photic stimulator. Device for delivering intermittent flashes of light. Synonym: stroboscope (discouraged).

Photo-convulsive response. *Cf.*, synonym: photo-paroxysmal response (preferred).

Photo-myoclonic response. *Cf.*, synonym: photo-myogenic response (preferred).

Photo-myogenic response. A response to intermittent photic stimulation characterized by the appearance in the record of brief, repetitive muscular spikes over the anterior regions of the head. These often in-crease gradually in amplitude as stimuli are continued and cease promptly when the stimulus is withdrawn. Comment: this response is associated frequently with flutter of the eyelids and vertical oscillations of the eyeballs and sometimes with discrete jerking mostly involving the musculature of the face and head. Preferred to synonym: photo-myoclonic response.

Photo-paroxysmal response. A response to intermittent photic stimulation characterized by the appearance in the record of spike-and-slow-wave and multiple spike-and-slow-wave complexes. These are bilaterally synchronous, synnemtrical and generalized and may outlast the stimulus by a few seconds. Comment: this response may be associated with impairment of consciousness and brisk jerks involving the musculature of the whole body, most prominently that of the upper extremities and head. Preferred to synonym: photo-convulsive response.

Polarity convention. International agreement whereby differential EEG amplifiers are constructed so that negativity at the input terminal 1 relative to the input terminal 2 of the same amplifier produces an upward pen deflection***·****. Comment: this convention is contrary to that prevailing in some other biological and non-biological fields.

Polarity, EEG wave. Sign of potential difference existing at a given instant in time between an electrode affected by a given potential change and another electrode not appreciably, or less, affected by the same change. *Cf.*, polarity convention.

Polygraphic recording. Simultaneous monitoring of multiple physiological measures such as the EEG, respiration, electrocardiogram, electromyogram, eye movement, galvanic skin resistance, blood pressure, etc.

Polymorphic activity. Use of term discouraged when describing EEG pattern.

Polyphasic wave. Wave consisting of two or more components developed on alternating sides of the baseline. *Cf.*, diphasic wave; triphasic wave.

Polyrhythmic activity. Use of term discouraged when describing EEG pattern.

Polyspike-and-slow-wave complex. *Cf.*, synonym: multiple spike-and-slow-wave complex (preferred).

Polyspike complex. *Cf.*, synonym: multiple spike complex (preferred).

Positive occipital sharp transient of sleep. Sharp transient maximal over the occipital regions, positive relative to other areas, occurring apparently spontaneously during sleep. May be single or repetitive. Amplitude varies but is generally below 50 μV.

Positive occipital spike-like wave of sleep. Use of term discouraged. Term suggested: positive occipital sharp transient of sleep.

Potential. (1) Strictly: voltage. (2) Loosely: synonym of wave.

Potential field. Amplitude distribution of an EEG wave at the surface of the head or cerebral cortex or in the depth of the brain, measured at a given instant in time. Represented in diagrams by equipotential lines.

Projected patterns. Abnormal EEG activities believed to result from a disturbance at a site remote from the recording electrodes. Description of specific EEG patterns preferred.

Provocation procedure. Use of term discouraged. Term suggested: activation.

Pseudo-periodic. Use of term discouraged. Term suggested: quasi-periodic.

Psychomotor variant. Use of term discouraged when describing EEG pattern. Term suggested: rhythmic temporal theta burst of drowsiness.

Quantity. Amount of EEG activity with respect to both number and amplitude of waves.

Quasi-periodic. Applies to EEG waves or complexes occuring at intervals only approaching regularity.

R-C coupled amplifier. Abbreviation for: resistance-capacitance coupled amplifier.

Reactivity. Susceptibility of individual rhythms or the EEG as a whole to change following sensory stimulation or other physiologic actions.

Record. The end product of the EEG recording process.

Recording. (1) The process of obtaining an EEG record. Synonym: tracing. (2) The end product of the EEG recording process, most commonly traced paper. Synonyms: record; tracing.

Reference electrode. (1) In general: any electrode against which the potential variations of another electrode are measured. (2) Specifically: a suitable reference electrode is any electrode customarily connected to the input terminal 2 of an EEG amplifier and so placed as to minimize the likelihood of pickup of the same EEG activity recorded by an exploring electrode, usually connected to the input terminal 1 of the same amplifier, or of other activities. Comments: (1) Whatever the location of the reference electrode, the possibility that it might be affected by appreciable EEG potentials should always be considered. (2) A reference electrode connected to the input terminal 2 of all or several EEG amplifiers is referred to as a *common reference electrode*.

Referential derivation. Recording from a pair of electrodes consisting of an exploring electrode generally connected to the input terminal 1 and a reference electrode usually connected to the input terminal 2 of an EEG amplifier***. *Cf.*, exploring electrode; reference electrode; referential montage; common reference montage.

Referential montage. A montage consisting of referential derivations. Comment: a referential montage in which the reference electrode is common to multiple derivations is referred to as a common reference montage***. *Cf.*, referential derivation.

Regular. Applies to waves or complexes of approximately constant period and relatively uniform appearance.

Resistance-capacitance coupled amplifier. An amplifier in which succesive stages are connected (coupled) by networks consisting of capacitors and resistors. Abbreviation: R-C coupled amplifier.

Rhythm. EEG activity consisting of waves of approximately constant period.

Rhythm of alpha frequency. (1) In general, any rhythm in the alpha band. (2) Specifically: term should be used to designate those activities in the alpha band which differ from the *alpha rhythm* as regards their topography and/or reactivity and do not have specific appellations (such as mu rhythm). *Cf.*, alpha rhythm.

Rhythmic termporal theta burst of drowsiness. Characteristic burst of 4–7 Hz waves frequently notched by faster waves, occurring over the temporal regions of the head during drowsiness. Synonym: psychomotor variant pattern (use discouraged). Comment: the clinical significance of this pattern, if any, is controversial.

Run. Colloquialism. Use of term discouraged. Term suggested: montage.

Scalp electrode. Electrode held against, attached to or inserted into the scalp.

Scalp electroencephalogram. Record of electrical activity of the brain by means of electrodes placed on the surface of the head. Abbreviation: SEEG. Comment: term and abbreviations should be used only to distinguish between scalp and other electroencephalograms such as depth electroencephalograms. In all other instances, a scalp electroencephalogram should be referred to simply as an electroencephalogram (EEG).

Scalp electroencephalography. Technique of recording scalp electroencephalograms. Abbreviation: SEEG. Comment: term and abbreviation should be used only to distinguish between this and other recording techniques such as depth electroencephalography. In all other instances scalp electroencephalography should be referred to simply as electroencephalography (EEG).

SDEEG. Abbreviation for stereotactic (stereotaxic) depth electroencephalography.

SEEG. Abbreviation for scalp electroencephalogram and scalp electroencephalography.

Seizure pattern, EEG. Phenomenon consisting of repetitive EEG discharges with relatively abrupt onset and termination and characteristic pattern of evolution, lasting at least several seconds. The component waves or complexes vary in form, frequency and topography. They are generally rhythmic and frequently display increasing amplitude and decreasing frequency during the same episode. When focal in onset, they tend to spread subsequently to other areas. Comment: EEG seizure patterns unaccompanied by clinical epileptic manifestations detected by the recordist and/or reported by the patient should be referred to as "subclinical".*Cf.*, epileptiform pattern..

Sensitivity. Ratio of input voltage to output pen deflection in an EEG channel****. Sensitivity is measured in microvolts per millimeter (μv/mm)***. Example:

$$\text{sensitivity} = \frac{\text{input voltage}}{\text{output pen deflection}} = \frac{50\ \mu\text{V}}{10\ \text{mm}} = 5\ \mu\text{V/mm.}$$

Sharp wave. A transient, clearly distinguished from background activity, with pointed peak at conventional paper speeds and duration of 70–200 msec, *i.e.*, over 1/14–1/5 sec., approximately. Main component is generally negative relative to other areas. Amplitude is variable. Comments: (1) Term does not apply to (a) distinctive physiologic events such as vertex sharp transients, lambda waves and positive occipital sharp transients of sleep, (b) sharp transients poorly distinguished from background activity and sharp-appearing individual waves of EEG rhythms. (2) Sharp waves should be differentiated from spikes, *i.e.*, transients having similar characteristics but shorter duration. However, it is well to keep in mind that this distinction is largely arbitrary and serves primarily descriptive purposes. Practically, in ink-written EEG records taken at 3cm/sec, sharp waves occupy more than 2 mm of paper width and spikes 2 mm or less. *Cf.*, spike.

Sharp-and-slow-wave complex. A sequence of a sharp wave and a slow wave. Comment: hyphenation facilitates use of term in plural form: sharp-and-slow-wave complexes or sharp-and-slow-waves.

Sigma rhythm. Use of term discouraged. Term suggested: sleep spindles.

Silence, Record of electrocerebral. Use of term discouraged. Term suggested: record of electrocerebral inactivity. *Cf.*, inactivity record of electrocerebral.

Simultaneous. Occurring at the same time. Synonym: synchronous.

Sine wave. Wave having the form of a sine curve.

Single-ended amplifier. An amplifier that operates on signals which are asymmetric with respect to ground.

Sinusoidal. Term applies to EEG waves resembling sine waves.

Six Hz spike-and-slow-waves. Spike-and-slow-wave complexes at 4–7 Hz, but mostly at 6 Hz, occurring generally in brief bursts bilaterally synchronously, symmetrically or asymmetrically, and either confined to or of larger amplitude over the posterior or anterior regions of the head. Amplitude is variable but generally smaller than that of spike-and-slow-wave complexes repeating at slower rates. Comment: the clinical significance of this pattern, if any, is controversial.

Sleep spindle. Burst at 11–15 Hz, but mostly at 12–14 Hz, generally diffuse but of higher voltage over the central regions of the head, occuring during sleep. Amplitude is variable but is mostly below 50 μV in the adult. Synonym: sigma rhythm (use discouraged).

Sleep stages. Distinctive phases of sleep, best demonstrated by polygraphic recordings of the EEG and other variables, including at least eye movements and activity of certain voluntary muscles.

Slow alpha variant rhythms. Characteristic rhythms at 3.5–6 Hz but mostly at 4–5 Hz, recorded most prominently over the posterior regions of the head. Generally altenate, or are intermixed, with alpha rhythm to which they often are harmonically related. Amplitude is variable but is frequently close to 50 μV. Blocked or attenuated by attention, especially visual, and mental effort. Comment: slow alpha variant rhythms should be held in contradistinction to posterior slow waves characteristic of children and adolescents and occasionally seen in young adults.

Slow activity. Activity of frequency lower than alpha, *i.e.*, theta and delta activities.

Slow spike. Use of term discouraged. Term suggested: sharp wave.

Slow spike-and-wave complex. Use of term discouraged. Term suggested: sharp-and-slow-wave complex.

Slow wave. Wave with duration longer than alpha waves, *i.e.*, over 1/8 sec.

Special electrode. Any electrode other than standard scalp electrode.

Sphenoidal electrode. Needle or wire electrode inserted through the soft tissues of the face below the zygomatic arch with its tip lying near the base of the skull in the region of the foramen ovale.

Spike. A transient, clearly distinguished from background activity, with pointed peak at conventional paper speeds and a duration from 20 to under 70 msec, *i.e.*, 1/50–1/40 sec, approximately. Main component is generally negative relative to other areas. Amplitude is variable. Comments: (1) EEG spikes should be differentiated from sharp waves, *i.e.*, transients having similar characteristics but longer durations. However it is well to keep in mind that this distinction is largely arbitrary and serves primarily descriptive purposes. Practically, in ink-written EEG records taken at 3 cm/sec, spikes occupy 2 mm or less of paper width and sharp waves more than 2 mm. (2) EEG spikes should be held in clear contradistinction to the brief unit spikes recorded from single cells with micro-electrode techniques. *Cf.*, sharp wave.

Spike-and-dome complex. Use of term discouraged. Term suggested: spike-and-slow-wave complex.

Spike-and-slow-wave complex. A pattern consisting of a spike followed by a slow wave. Comment: hyphenation facilitates use of term in plural form: spike-and-slow-wave complexes or spike-and-slow-waves.

Spike-and-slow-wave rhythm. Use of term discouraged. Term suggested, whenever appropriate: 3 Hz spike-and-slow-waves; atypical repetitive spike-and-slow-waves.

Spindle. Group of rhythmic waves characterized by a progressively increasing, then gradually decreasing, amplitude. *Cf.*, sleep spindle.

Spread. Propagation of EEG waves from one region of the scalp and/or brain to another. *Cf.*, generalization.

Standard electrode. Conventional scalp electrode. *Cf.*, disk electrode; needle electrode; pad electrode; special electrode.

Standard electrode placement. Scalp electrode location(s) determined by the ten-twenty system. *Cf.*, Ten-twenty system.

Status epilepticus, EEG. The occurence of virtually continuous seizure activity in an EEG.

Stephenson-Gibbs reference. Use of term discouraged. Term suggested: sterno-spinal reference electrode.

Stereotactic (stereotaxic) depth electroencephalogram. Recording of electrical activity of the brain by means of electrodes implanted within the brain substance according to stereotactic (stereotaxic) measurements. Abbreviation: SDEEG.

Stereotactic (stereotaxic) depth electroencephalography. Technique of recording stereotactic (stereotaxic) depth electroencephalograms. Abbreviation: SDEEG.

Sterno-spinal reference. A non-cephalic reference achieved by interconnecting two electrodes placed over the right sterno-clavicular junction and the apophysis spinosa of the seventh cervical vertebra, respectively, and balancing the voltage between them by means of a potentiometer to reduce ECG artifact.

Stick-on electrode.** Colloquialism. Use of term discouraged. Term suggested: disk electrode.

Stigmatic electrode. Use of term discouraged. Term suggested: exploring electrode.

Subdural electrode. Electrode inserted under the dural covering of the cerebrum.

Suppression. Use of term discouraged when describing EEG patterns other than burst suppression pattern.

Symmetry. (1) Approximately equal amplitude, frequency and form of EEG activities over homologous areas on opposite sides of the head. (2) Approximately equal distribution of potentials of unlike polarity on either side of a zero isopotential axis. *Cf.*, true pase reversal. (3) Approximately equal distribution of EEG waves about the baseline.

Synchrony. The simultaneous occurence of EEG waves over regions on the same or opposite sides of the head. Comment: term *simultaneous* only implies lack of delay measurable with ink writers at customary paper speeds.

Ten-twenty system. System of standardized scalp electrode placement recommended by the International Federation of Societies for Electroencephalography and Clinical Neurophysiology***. According to this system, electrode placements are determined by measuring the head from external landmarks and taking 10% or 20% of such measurements. Comment: the use of additional scalp electrodes, such as true anterior temporal electrodes, is indicated in various circumstances.

Theta band. Frequency band from 4 to under 8 Hz. Greek letter: θ.

Theta rhythm. Rhythm with a frequency of 4 to under 8 Hz.

Theta wave. Wave with duration of 1/4 to over 1/8 sec.

Three Hz spike-and-slow-waves. Characteristic paroxysm consisting of a regular sequence of spike-and-slow-wave complexes which: (1) repeat at 3–3.5 Hz (measured during the first few seconds of the paroxysm), (2) are bilateral in their onset and termination, generalized and usually of maximal amplitude over the frontal areas, (3) are approximately synchronous and symmetrical on the two sides of the head throughout the paroxysm. Amplitude is variable but can reach values of 1000 μV (1 mV). *Cf.*, atypical repetitive spike-and-slow-waves.

Time constant, EEG channel. The product of the values of the resistance (in megohms, MΩ) and the capacitance (in microfarads, μF) which make up the time constant control of an EEG channel. This product represents the time required for the pen to fall to 37% of the deflection initially produced when a DC voltage difference is applied to the input terminals of the amplifier. Expressed in seconds (sec). Abbreviation: TC. Comment: for a simple R–C coupling network, the TC is related to the per cent reduction in sensitivity of the channel at a given stated low frequency by the equation $TC = 1/2\pi f$, where f is the frequency at which a 30% (3 dB) attenuation occurs. For instance, for a TC of 0.3 sec, an attenuation of 30% (3 dB) occurs at 0.5 Hz. Thus, either the time constant or the per cent attenuation at a given stated low frequency can be used to designate the same position of the low frequency filter of the EEG channel. *Cf.*, low frequency filter****.

Topography. Amplitude distribution of EEG activities at the surface of the head, cerebral cortex or in the depths of the brain.

Tracé alternant. EEG pattern of sleeping newborns, characterized by bursts of slow waves, at times intermixed with sharp waves, and intervening periods of relative quiescence.

Tracing. *Cf.,* synonyms: record; recording.

Transient, EEG. Any isolated wave or complex, distinguished from background activity.

Transverse bipolar montage. *Cf.,* synonym: coronal bipolar montage.

Triangular bipolar montage. A montage consisting of derivations from pairs of electrodes in a group of 3 electrodes arranged in a triangular pattern.

Triphasic wave. Wave consisting of 3 components alternating about the baseline.

True phase reversal. Simultaneous pen deflections in opposite directions occuring in two referential derivations using a suitable common reference electrode and displaying the same wave. Comments: (1) This phenomenon is rarely observed in scalp EEGs. (2) When demonstrated beyond doubt in appropriate recording conditions, it indicates a 180° change in phase of an EEG wave between adjacent areas of the brain, on either side of a zero isopotential axis. *Cf.,* instrumental phase reversal.

Unilateral. Confined to one side of the head. Comments: (1) Unilateral EEG activities may be focal or diffuse. (2) They are said to be lateralized to the right or left side of the head.

Unipolar. Use of term discouraged. Term suggested: referential.

Unipolar derivation. Use of term discouraged. *Cf.,* referential derivation.

Unipolar depth electrode. Use of term discouraged. Term suggested: single-electrode lead.

Unipolar montage. Use of term discouraged. Term suggested: referential montage.

Vertex sharp transient. Sharp potential, maximal at the vertex, negative relative to other areas, occurring apparently spontaneously during sleep or in response to a sensory stimulus during sleep or wakefulness. May be single or repetitive. Amplitude varies but rarely exceeds 250 μV. Abbreviations: V wave. *Cf.,* K complex.

Vertex sharp wave. Use of term discouraged when describing physiologic vertex sharp transient.

Voltage. *Cf.,* amplitude.

V wave. Abbreviation for: vertex sharp transient.

Wave. Any change of the potential difference between pairs of electrodes in EEG recording. May arise in the brain (EEG wave) or outside it (extracerebral potential).

Wave form. The shape of an EEG wave.

White lead*. Use of term discouraged. Term suggested: input terminal 2.

Wicket rhythm. Use of term discouraged. Term suggested: mu rhythm.

Writer. System for direct write-out of the output of an EEG channel. Most writers use ink delivered by a pen. In certain instruments, the ink is sprayed as a jet stream. In other recorders the pen writer uses carbon paper instead of ink****.

Zero potential reference electrode. Use of term discouraged. Term suggested: reference electrode (not a synonym).

Appendix II
American EEG Society Recording Guidelines

GUIDELINE ONE: MINIMUM TECHNICAL REQUIREMENTS FOR PERFORMING
CLINICAL ELECTROENCEPHALOGRAPHY

INTRODUCTION

Although no single best method exists for recording EEGs under all circumstances, the following standards are considered the minimum for the usual clinical recording of EEGs in all age groups except the very young (see Guideline Two: Minimum Technical Standards for Pediatric Electroencephalography).

Recording at minimum standards should not give prive to the EEG department working at this level and cannot ensure a satisfactory test. Minimum standards provide barely adequate fulfillment of responsibilities to the patient and the referring physician.

To the minimum standards have been added recommendations to improve standardization of procedures and also facilitate interchange of recordings and assessment among laboratories in North America.

1. Equipment

1.1 To find the distribution of EEG activity, it is necessary to record simultaneously from as many regions of the scalp as possible. When too few chan-

This material originally appeared in *J. Clin. Neurophysiol.* 1986;3(2):133–8. © 1986 American Electroencephalographic Society. Vol. 3, Suppl. 1, 1–37.

nels are used simultaneously, the chances of interpretive errors increase, and, conversely, when more channels are utilized, the likelihood of such errors decreases. This is particularly true for transient activity.

Eight channels of simultaneous recording are the minimum number required to show the areas producing most normal and abnormal EEG patterns, and 16 channels are now found to be necessary by most laboratories. Additional channels are often needed for monitoring other physiologic activities.

1.2 Alternating current (AC) wiring should meet the Underwriters Laboratories standards required for hospital service. Adequate grounding of the instrument must be provided by all AC receptacles. All equipment in each patient area in the EEG laboratory must be grounded to a common point.

1.3 In the usual clinical setting, electrical shielding of the patient and equipment is not necessary, and such shielding need not be installed unless proven necessary.

1.4 Ancillary equipment should include a device for delivering rhythmic, high-intensity flash stimuli to the patient.

2. Electrodes

2.1 Recording electrodes should be free of inherent noise and drift. They should not significantly attenuate signals between 0.5 and 70 Hz. Experimental evidence suggests that silver–silver chloride or gold disk electrodes held on by collodion are the best, but other electrode materials and electrode pastes have been effectively used especially with contemporary amplifiers having high input impedances. High-quality electrodes are available from several manufacturers and are generally preferable to homemade electrodes.

To decrease noise, electrodes must be kept clean, with appropriate precautions taken after recording from patients with contagious diseases (viral hepatitis, Creutzfeldt-Jakob disease, acquired immunodeficiency syndrome) (1).

2.2 Needle electrodes are not recommended. If circumstances necessitate their use, they must be completely sterilized, and the technologist who employs them should have been taught the exact techniques, as well as the disadvantages and hazards, of their use. Parallel anteroposterior alignment of the needles is important; misalignment may cause artifactual amplitude asymmetries or distortions.

It is rarely appreciated that proper use of needle electrodes requires more care and expertise than for any other type of electrode. However, needle electrodes can be effectively utilized in comatose patients, in whom pain responses are usually minimal or absent, and who are in medical settings requiring efficient recording with a minimum of delay.

2.3 All 21 electrodes and placements recommended by the International Federation of Societies for EEG and Clinical Neurophysiology (2,3) should be used. The 10–20 System is the only one officially recommended by the International Federation of Societies for EEG and Clinical Neurophysiology. It is the most commonly used existing system, and it should be used universally. The use of the term "modified 10–20 System" is undesirable when it means that head measurements have not been made and placements have been estimated. In this case, the term "estimated 10–20 placement" is more appropriate. (For neonates, refer to Guideline Two.)

An adequate number of electrodes is essential to ensure that EEG activity having a small area of representation on the scalp is recorded, and to analyze accurately the distribution of more diffuse activity. Occasionally, additional electrodes, placed between or below those representing the standard placements, are needed in order to record very localized activity.

A grounding electrode always should be used, except in situations (e.g., intensive care units, operating rooms) in which other electrical equipment is attached to the patient. In such cases, double grounding must be avoided.

2.4 Inter-electrode impedances should be checked as a routine pre-recording procedure. Ordinarily, electrode impedance should not exceed 5 kohms. 5,000 ohms

Electrode impedances should be rechecked during the recording when any pattern that might be artifactual appears.

3. Recordings

3.1 Montages should be designed in conformity with Guideline Seven: A Proposal for Standard Montages to Be Used in Clinical Electroencephalography. It is desirable that at least some montages in all laboratories be uniform to facilitate communication and comparison.

3.2 The record should have written on it as a minimum the name and age of the patient, the data of the recording, an identification number, and the name or initials of the technologist.

Identifications should be made at the time of recording. Failure to do so may result in errors that have adverse medical and legal consequences. A Basic Data Sheet, attached to every record, should include the time of the recording, the time and date of the last seizure (if any), the behavioral state of the patient, a list of all medications that the patient has been taking, including premedication given to induce sleep during EEG, and any relevant additional medical history.

3.3 Appropriate square-wave calibrations should be made at the beginning and end of every EEG recording. A recording with all channels connected to the same pair of electrodes should follow at the beginning (biologic calibration). At the outset, all channels should be adjusted, if necessary, so that they respond equally and correctly to the calibration signal. When doubt as to correct functioning of any amplifier exists, a repeat calibration run should be made.

The calibration is an integral part of every EEG recording. It gives a scaling factor for the interpreter, and tests the EEG machine for sensitivity, high and low frequency response, noise level, and pen alignment and damping. It also gives information about the competence and care of the technologist. Calibration voltages must be appropriate for the sensitivities used.

In addition to the standard square-wave calibration, a biologic calibration ("biocal") may at times be of additional help in detecting errors in the montage selection process or in the pen-writing mechanism. For this purpose, an anteroposterior (fronto-occipital) derivation should be used, since it can include fast and alpha range patterns as well as eye movement activity in the delta range.

3.4 The sensitivity of the EEG equipment for routine recording should be set in the range of 5–10 μV/mm of pen deflection.

Sensitivity is defined as the ratio of input voltage to pen deflection. It is expressed in microvolts per millimeter (μV/mm). A commonly used sensitivity is 7 μV/mm, which, for a calibration signal of 50 μV, results in a deflection of 7.1 mm.

If the sensitivity is decreased (for example, from 7 to 10 μV/mm), the amplitude of the writeout of a given EEG on the paper also decreases. Conversely, if the sensitivity is increased (for example, from 7 to 5 μV/mm), the amplitude of the writeout of a given EEG increases.

When the sensitivity is less than 10 μV/mm (for example, 20 μV/mm), significant low-amplitude activity may become indiscernible. If the sensitivity is greater than 5 μV/mm (for example, 3 μV/mm), normal EEG activity may overload the system, causing a squaring off of the peaks of the writeout onto the paper.

Note that a sensitivity of 5 μV/mm means that, to obtain a pen deflection of 1 mm, a 5-μV input voltage is required (and correspondingly, to obtain a 10 mm deflection, an input of 50 μV is required). If the sensitivity is decreased to 10 μV/mm, the same 1 mm pen deflection now requires a larger input, i.e., 10 μV rather than 5 μV (and correspondingly, a 10-mm pen deflection now requires an input of 100 μV rather than 50 μV). Thus, as the sensitivity is increased, its numerical value becomes smaller. Conversely, as the sensitivity is decreased, its numerical value becomes larger. This perhaps seemingly paradoxical relationship is actually a logical consequence of the definition of sensitivity as input voltage per unit of pen deflection.

During calibration for routine recordings, the recorded signals should not be distorted but should be large enough to permit measurement to better than $\pm 5\%$ between any of the signals on the different channels.

No matter which sensitivity (within the above limits) is chosen prior to the recording, appropriate adjustments should be made whenever EEG activity encountered is of too high or low amplitude to be recorded properly.

3.5 For standard recordings, the low-frequency filter should be no higher than 1 Hz (–3 dB) corresponding at a time constant of at least 0.16 s. The high-frequency filter should be no lower than 70 Hz (–3 dB).

A low-frequency filter setting higher than 1 Hz should not be used routinely to attenuate slow-wave artifacts in the record. Vital information may be lost when pathologic activity in the delta range is present. Similarly, a setting lower than 70 Hz for the high-frequency filters can distort or attenuate spikes and other pathologic discharges into unrecognizable forms and can cause muscle artifact to resemble spikes. Production of a record with lost or inaccurate information is poor medical practice.

It must be emphasized, however, that judicious use of the low- or high-frequency filters—with appropriate annotation on the record—can emphasize or clarify certain types of patterns in the record. These filter controls, therefore, should be used selectively and carefully.

3.6 The 60-Hz (notch) filter can distort or attenuate spikes; it therefore should be used only when other measures against 60 Hz interference fail.

3.7 A paper speed of 3 cm/s should be utilized for routine recordings. A paper speed of 1.5 cm/s is sometimes used for EEG recordings in newborns, during polysomnograms, or in other special situations.

3.8 When instrument settings (sensitivities, filters, paper speed, montage) are changed during the recording, the settings should be clearly identified on the record at the time of the change. The final calibration(s) should include each sensitivity and filter setting used in the recording, and should include calibration voltages appropriate to the sensitivities actually used. It is especially important to record calibration signals at very high sensitivities when these settings have been used.

3.9 The baseline record should contain at least 20 min of technically satisfactory recording. Longer recordings are often more informative.

The EEG is a short sample in time from the patient's life. Within reasonable limits, the longer the recording, the better the chance of recording an abnormality or abnormalities demonstrating the variability of these. Experience in many centers shows that a very minimum of 20 min of artifact-free recording is necessary to assess baseline waking EEG activity. The addition of photic stimulation, hyperventilation, and especially sleep—which should be recorded whenever possible—often requires an increase of recording time.

3.10 The recordings should include periods when the eyes are open and when they are closed.

Proper EEG recording requires examining the effect of stimuli upon the EEG. A comparison between the eyes-open and the eyes-closed condition constitutes one important means for assessment. Some rhythms can be masked by the alpha activity and are visibly only when the alpha rhythm has been attenuated by eye-opening. Certain forms of eye movement may appear to be frontal delta or theta activity but eye-opening and closing helps in differentiation. Finally, paroxysmal activity may appear only when the eyes are opened or only when the eyes are closed or at the times these conditions change. Thus, failure to record with eye-opening and closing as a routine procedure can reduce chances of obtaining potentially important information. This procedure is so simple that it is unjustifiable not to request eye-opening and close whenever paptient cooperation permits, or to manually open and close the eyes when it does not.

3.11 Hyperventilation should be used routinely unless medical or other justifiable reasons (e.g., a recent intracranial hemorrhage, significant cardiopulmonary disease, sickle cell disease or trait, or patient inability or unwillingness to cooperate) contraindicate it. It should be performed for a minimum of 3 min with continued recording for at least 1 min after cessation of overbreathing. At times, hyperventilation must be performed for a longer period in order to obtain adequate activation of the EEG. To evaluate the effects of this activation technique, at least 1 min of recording with the same montage should be obtained before overbreathing begins. The record should contain an assessment of the quality of patient effort during hyperventilation. It is often helpful to record electrocardiographic (EKG) activity directly on one EEG channel during this and other parts of the recording, particularly if spikes and sharp waves, or pulse or EKG artifact, are in question. With an additional (e.g., 17th) channel, the EKG can be monitored continuously.

3.12 Sleep recordings should be taken whenever possible but not to the exclusion of the waking record.

It is increasingly evident that considerable additional information can be added by recording during drowsiness and sleep. Some laboratories use sleep recording routinely. Sleep recording is usually essential for patients with suspected or known convulsive disorders.

3.13 The patient's level of consciousness (awake, drowsy, sleeping, or comatose), and any change thereof, should be noted by the technologist on the EEG recording. Any commands or signals to the patient, and any movement or clinical seizure activity or absence thereof, should also be noted on the recording. Careful observation of the patient with frequent notations is often essential, particularly when unusual waveforms are observed in the tracing. Abbreviations used should be standardized, with their definitions readily available to the reader.

In stuporous or comatose patients and those showing invariant EEG patterns of any kind, visual, auditory, and somatosensory stimuli should be applied

544

systematically during recording. The stimuli and the patient's responses or failure to respond should be noted on the recording paper as near as possible to their point of the occurrence.

It is the responsibility of the electroencephalographer to recognize the patterns usually associated with different states of consciousness. However, observations by the technologist about the patient's clinical status can be of considerable interpretative value, particularly when discrepancies or unusual correlations occur.

To facilitate assessing awake background activity, it is important for the technologist to ascertain that the patient is maximally alert for at least a portion of the record.

3.14 Special procedures that are of some risk to the patient should be carried out only in the presence of a qualified physician, only in a environment with adequate resuscitating equipment, and with the informed consent of the patient or responsible relative or legal guardian.

3.15 EEGs for the evaluation of cessation of cerebral function ("cerebral death") require special procedures and extraordinary precautions (see Guideline Three: Minimum Technical Standards for EEG Recording in Suspected Cerebral Death).

REFERENCES

1. American Electroencephalographic Society. Infectious Diseases Committee Report. *J Clin Neurophysiol* 1984;1:437–41.
2. Jasper HH. The ten-twenty electrode system of the International Federation. *Electroencephalogr Clin Neurophysiol* 1958;10:371–3.
3. Jasper HH. The ten-twenty electrode system of the International Federation. In: *International Federation of Societies for Electroencephalography and Clinical Neurophysiology: Recommendations for the practice of clinical electroencephalography*. Amsterdam: Elsevier, 1983:3–10.

INTRODUCTION

These guidelines for clinical pediatric EEG should be considered in conjunction with the more general Guideline One: Minimum Technical Requirements for Performing Clinical Electroencephalography (MTR).

The basic principles of clinical EEG outlined in the MTR also apply to the very young and are reaffirmed. However, special considerations are pertinent to pediatric recordings and are discussed below. The numbers in parentheses in this Guideline refer specifically to sections of the MTR that must be modified in these special situations. Where a subject is not covered here, the recommendations of Guideline One remain appropriate and should be consulted.

Emphasis here will be on EEG in neonates, infants, and young children, since recording the EEGs of older children and adolescents differs little from recording the EEGs of adults. Because EEG recording in the newborn presents a number of special problems, this Guideline is divided into two parts setting forth recommendations for children and for neonates separately.

1. Children

1.1 (MTR 2.1) Because children, especially young children, have a tendency to move a good deal during recording, electrode application should be performed with great care. Electrodes may be applied with paste or collodion, according to the preference of the laboratory, but their positions and impedances should be monitored carefully throughout the study. The inverted saucer-shaped silver–silver

This material originally appeared in *J. Clin. Neurophysiol.* 1986;3(2):139–43.

chloride electrode with a small hole for the injection of electrolyte solution is best. Needle electrodes are not needed and should not be used.

1.2 (MTR 2.3) All 21 electrodes of the International 10–20 System (1) should be used for most purposes. The standard montages used for adults should be used for children.

1.3 (MTR 3.2) Before recording the EEGs of young inpatients, especially those in so precarious a condition that the recordings must be done at bedside, the technician should consult with the nursing staff concerning the patient's condition and any limitations on recording procedures.

1.4 (MTR 3.4) The voltage of EEG activity in many young children is higher than that of older children and adults, and appropriate reduction of sensitivity (to 10 μV/mm or even 15 μV/mm) should be used. However, at least a portion of the record should be run at a sensitivity (such as 7 μV/mm) adequate to display low-voltage fast activity. Otherwise, for patients beyond infancy, the same instrument control settings can be used as for adults in the same laboratory.

1.5 (MTR 3.9) Photic stimulation over the frequency range of at least 1–20 flashes/s should be used during wakefulness in appropriate patients.

1.6 (MTR 3.10) Whenever possible, recordings should include periods when the eyes are open and when they are closed. In infants over 3 months of age, passive eye closure (by placing the technician's hand over the patient's eyes) is often successful in producing the dominant posterior rhythm, as is the playing of games such as peek-a-boo.

1.7 (MTR 3.12) Sleep recordings should be obtained whenever possible, but not to the exclusion of the awake record. The recording of the patient during drowsiness, initiation of sleep, and arousal is important. Natural sleep is preferred, but if the use of sedation is necessary, all efforts should still be made to record arousal at the end of the recording.

1.8 (MTR 3.13) The patient's condition should be clearly indicated at the beginning of the recording from every montage. Continuous observation by the technician, with frequent notations on the recording, is particularly important when recording young patients.

2. Neonates and Young Infants (Up to 4–8 Weeks Post-Term)

2.1 (MTR 1.1) Sixteen-channel instruments should be used. Two, and often more, channels must be devoted to recording non-EEG "polygraphic" variables, such as EKG and respiration. Consequently, the number of channels left for EEG recording on an 8-channel machine is unacceptable. Sixteen or more channels allow the necessary flexibility.

Because EEG patterns seen in the neonate are not as clearly related to stages of the wake–sleep cycle as are those of adults and older children, it is usually necessary to record polygraphic (non-EEG) variables along with the EEG in order to assess accurately the baby's state during the recording. Polygraphic recording is also helpful in identifying physiologic artifacts; for example, apparent monomorphic delta activity often turns out to be respiration artifact, since babies may have respiratory rates of up to 100/min. Moreover, variables other than the EEG may be directly pertinent to the patient's problems. For example, in those experiencing apneic episodes, breathing and heart rate changes are most relevant.

The parameters most frequently monitored along with EEG in infants are respirations, eye movements, and heartbeats. A recording of muscle movements, by submental electromyography (EMG) or movement transducer, also can be quite helpful.

Respirogram can be recorded by any of the following means: (1) abdominal and/or thoracic strain gauges, (2) changes in impedance between thoracic electrodes (impedance pneumogram), or (3) airway thermistors/thermocouples. In infants with respiratory problems, it is necessary to devote 3 or 4 channels to respiration in order to monitor both abdominal and thoracic movements, plus airflow in the upper airway. In infants without respiratory problems, one channel of abdominal or thoracic respirogram may be sufficient.

For recording eye movements, one electrode should be placed 0.5 cm above and slightly lateral to the outer canthus of one eye and another 0.5 cm below and slightly lateral to the outer canthus of the other eye. These can be designated E1 and E2. Both lateral and vertical eye movements can be detected by linking (referring) E1 to A1 hand E2 to A1 (or E1-A2, E2-A2).

EKG should be recorded routinely if there is an available channel and is particularly needed when there are cardiac or respiratory problems or when rhythmic artifacts occur.

2.2 (MTR 2.1) Electrodes may be applied with either collodion or paste. The inverted saucer-shaped silver–silver chloride electrode with a small hole for the injection of electrolyte solution is best. For neonates, the fumes of acetone and ether may not be acceptable, and disk electrodes with electrolyte paste are preferable. Needle electrodes should never be used.

2.3 (MTR 2.3) It is a matter of individual preference whether or not a reduced array is routinely acceptable for neonates. Some electroencephalographers prefer the full 10–20 array; others prefer a reduced array. It is generally agreed that a reduced array is acceptable in premature infants with small heads or where, as in neonatal intensive care units, time or other circumstances may not allow application of the full array.

The following electrodes are suggested as a minimum reduced array: Fp1, Fp2, C3, Cz, C4, T3, T4, O1, O2, A1, and A2. If a baby's earlobes are too small, mastoid leads may be substituted and can be designated M1 and M2. Acceptable alternative frontal placements in the reduced array are Fp3 and Fp4 instead of Fp1 and Fp2. Fp3 and Fp4 are halfway between the Fp1 and F3, and the Fp2 and F4, positions, respectively. (Note that the use of Fp3 and Fp4 makes for unequal inter-electrode distances in scalp–scalp montages.)

549

Determining electrode sites by measurement is just as important in infants and children as in adults. Deviation from this principle is permissible only in circumstances in which it is impossible or clinically undesirable to manipulate the child's head to make the measurements. If an electrode placement must be modified due to intravenous lines, pressure bolts, scalp hematomas, and the like, the homologous contralateral electrode placement should be similarly modified. If no measurements are made, the technologist should note this on the recording.

2.4 (MTR 2.4) Electrode impedances of less than 5 kohms can be obtained regularly, although higher impedances may be allowed in order to avoid excessive manipulation or excessive abrasion of tender skin. It is most important that marked differences in impedances among electrodes be avoided.

2.5 (MTR 3.1) In neonates in whom 2 or more channels must be devoted to polygraphic variables, the following montages are recommended:

Channel	A	B	C
1	Fp1-F3	Fp1-A1	Fp1-C3
2	F3-C3	Fp2-A2	C3-O1
3	C3-P3	F3-A1	Fp1-T3
4	Fp2-F4	F4-A2	T3-O1
5	F4-C4	C3-A1	Fp2-C4
6	C4-P4	C4-A2	C4-O2
7	F7-T3	P3-A1	Fp2-T4
8	T3-T5	P4-A2	T4-O2
9	T5-O1	O1-A1	T3-C3
10	F8-T4	O2-A2	C3-Cz
11	T4-T6	T3-A1	Cz-C4
12	T6-O2	T4-A2	C4-T4

These are based on the assumption that a 16-channel instrument is used with 4 channels devoted to polygraphic variables, leaving 12 channels for EEG. Montages A and B are for full 10–20 System electrode arrays; Montage C for the reduced array.

In Montages B and C, Fp3 and Fp4 may be substituted for Fp1 and Fp2, and M1 and M2 may be substituted for A1 and A2.

It is not implied that the above montages are the only ones that can be used. Rather, they should be considered standard montages, and at least one of them should be used for at least a portion of a neonate's EEG recording in all laboratories, to provide some standardization among laboratories. Since Montage C includes the midline, it can be particularly helpful when recording premature infants. In any case, Cz should always be included because positive "rolandic" sharp waves (a common pathologic finding) may occur only at Cz in this population. Various other montages can be devised for special purposes. Even a montage combining referential and scalp–scalp derivations is acceptable for neonatal EEGs.

The use of a single montage throughout a recording of a neonate may be, and often is, sufficient, and is preferred in many laboratories. It is not implied, however, that a single montage is always adequate. Even in laboratories preferring single montages, additional montages should be used when the need arises, for example, to better delineate unifocal abnormalities.

For recording polygraphic variables, the following derivations are recommended: (1) For eye movements (EOG): use E1-A1 and E2-A1 or E2-A1 and E1-A2. (2) For submental EMG: two electrodes under the chin, each 1–2 cm on either side of the midline. (3) For EKG, lead 1 (right arm–left arm) is preferred. If submental EMG is being recorded and if only heart rate is of interest, the EKG channel can often be omitted because the R wave is usually visible in the EMG channel.

2.6 (MTR 3.2) Before recording the EEGs of inpatients, especially those in so precarious a condition that the recording must be done at bedside, the technician should consult with the nursing staff concerning the patient's condition and any limitations on recording procedures.

The baby's gestational age at birth and conceptional age (gestational age at birth plus time since birth) on the day of recording, stated in weeks, are absolutely essential to interpretation and must be included, together with chronological age since birth, in the information available to the electrocephalographer. All other available relevant clinical information (including concentration of blood gases, serum electrolyte values, and current medications) should be noted for the electroencephalographer's use.

2.7 (MTR 3.4) In young infants' EEGs, the most appropriate sensitivity is usually 7 μV/mm, but adjustments up or down are more often needed than in the case of older patients. At least a portion of the recording should be run at a sensitivity adequate to display low-voltage fast activity. The low-frequency filter setting should be between 0.3 and 0.6 Hz (–3dB) (time constants of 0.27–0.53 s), not the commonly used 1 Hz (0.16 s).

For EOG, a sensitivity of 7 μV/mm and the same time constant as for the concomitantly recorded EEG derivations are recommended. For respirogram, amplification should be adjusted to yield a clearly visible vertical deflection, and a low-frequency filter setting of 0.3–0.6 Hz, but not direct current (DC), should be used. For the submental EMG recording, a sensitivity of 3 μV/mm, a low-frequency filter setting of about 5 Hz (time constant of about 0.03 s), and a high-frequency filter setting of 70 Hz should be employed.

2.8 (MTR 3.9, 3.12) If possible, it is advantageous to schedule the EEG at feeding time and arrange to feed the child after the electrodes have been applied, but before beginning the recording, as babies tend to sleep after feedings.

Allow for extra recording time for the EEGs of neonates. Time is commonly lost due to a greater number of movement and other physiologic artifacts during wakefulness, and extra time is usually needed in order to obtain sufficient recording to permit evaluation of stages of the wake–sleep cycle and other states.

Except when the EEG is grossly abnormal, 20- or 30-min recordings are usually insufficient. In those neonates in whom patterns appear to be invariant, it may be necessary to obtain at least 60 min of recording to demonstrate that the tracings are not likely to change. In the rest, adequate sampling of both major sleep states is important. The initial sleep state in the neonate is usually active sleep, which may last a very short time or continue for many minutes. An adequate sleep tracing must include a full episode of quiet sleep.

It is never necessary or desirable to use sedation to obtain a sleep recording in a neonate.

Repetitive photic stimulation is rarely, if ever, clinically useful in neonates, and is not recommended.

2.9 (MTR 3.13) The child's condition, including head and eyelid position, should be clearly indicated at the beginning of every montage. Continuous observations by the technologist, with frequent notations on the recording, are particularly important when recording from neonates.

In stuporous or comatose patients and in those showing invariant EEG patterns of any kind, visual, auditory, and somatosensory stimuli should be applied systematically during recording, but only toward the end of the recording period, lest normal sleep cycles be disrupted or unexpected arousal-produced artifact render the tracings unreadable thereafter. The stimuli and the patient's clinical responses or failure to respond should be noted on the recording paper as near as possible to their point of occurrence.

REFERENCE

1. Jasper HH. The ten-twenty electrode system of the International Federation. *Electroencephalogr. Clin. Neurophysiol.* 1958;10:371–3.

INTRODUCTION

EEG studies for the determination of cerebral death are no longer confined to major laboratories. Many small hospitals have intensive care units and EEG facilities. The need for minimal standard guidelines has thus increased.

The first (1970) edition of Minimum Technical Standards for EEG Recording in Suspected Cerebral Death reflected the state of the art and the technique of the late 1960s. Substantially improved EEG instrumentation is now available, and many laboratories have had years of experience in this area. Equally important, there is now a much larger number of competent EEG technologists. Finally, the EEG results of a collaborative study of cerebral death that was being planned in 1970 have been published (1).

The survey in the late 1960s by the American EEG Society's Ad Hoc Committee on EEG Criteria for the Determination of Cerebral Death revealed that, of 2,650 cases of coma with presumably "isoelectric" EEGs, only three whose records satisfied the committee's criteria showed any recovery of cerebral function. These three had suffered from massive overdoses of nervous system depressants, two from barbiturates, and one from meprobamate. Many of the reported "isoelectric" records were, on review, either low-voltage records or obtained with techniques inadequate to bring out low-voltage activity. That is, inadequate technique alone gave the graphs the appearance of being "flat". It should be pointed out, however, that this study did not include children. Hence, the comparable data on which to base recommendations for this young age group do not exist at present. The 1970 com-

This material originally appeared in *J. Clin. Neurophysiol.* 1986;3(2):144–9.

mittee recommended dropping nonphysiologic terms such as "isoelectric" or "linear" (the word "flat" should likewise not be used) and renaming the state "electrocerebral silence". Subsequently, "electrocerebral inactivity" was the term recommended in the Glossary of the International Federation of Societies for EEG and Clinical Neurophysiology (2).

The current Guideline includes an updating of the criteria for electrocerebral inactivity, reflecting what has been learned since the first appearance of these standards (1–6).

At the present time, telephone transmission of EEG cannot be used for determination of electrocerebral silence in the diagnosis of brain death because of the inherent and unpredictable electrical noise present in telephone networks relative to the very low signal in the electrocerebral silence recording (see also Guideline Six: Recommendations for Telephone Transmission of EEGs).

DEFINITION

Electrocerebral inactivity (ECI) or electrocerebral silence (ECS) is defined as no EEG activity over 2 μV when recording from scalp electrode pairs 10 or more cm apart with inter-electrode impedances under 10,000 ohms, but over 100 ohms.

Ten guidelines for EEG recordings in cases of suspected cerebral death, with the rationale for each, are set forth with explanatory comments.

1. A Minimum of Eight Scalp Electrodes Should Be Utilized

The major brain areas must be covered to be certain that absence of activity is not a focal phenomenon. The use of a single-channel instrument such as is sometimes used for EEG monitoring of anesthetic levels is therefore unacceptable for the purpose of determining ECS. The frontal, central, occipital, and temporal areas are recommended as the minimal required coverage. A grounding electrode should be added. However, for recordings in intensive care units, a ground electrode should *not* be used if grounding from other electrical equipment is already attached to the patient.

Since, prior to the recording, one does not know whether an ECS record will be obtained, it is desirable to use a full set of scalp electrodes on the initial examination, as defined in Guideline One: Minimum Technical Requirements for Performing Clinical Electroencephalography, Section 2.3. In any event, the initial study should not use less than the routine coverage standard for the particular clinical laboratory. A full set of electrodes includes midline placements (Fz, Cz, Pz); these are useful for the detection of residual low-voltage physiologic activity and are relatively free from artifact. Since the EEGs of patients with suspected ECS actually may have EEG abnormalities other than ECS, the use of more complete, rather than less complete, electrode coverage is often essential.

2. Inter-Electrode Impedances Should Be Under 10,000 Ohms But Over 100 Ohms

2.1 Unmatched electrode impedances may distort the EEG. When one electrode has a relatively high impedance compared to the second electrode of the pair, the amplifier becomes unbalanced and is prone to amplify extraneous signals unduly. This may result in the occurrence of 60-Hz interference or other artifacts. Situations characterized by low-voltage electrocerebral activity and high instrument sensitivity demand especially scrupulous electrode application.

2.2 There is a marked dropoff of potentials with impedances below 100 ohms and, of course, no potential at 0 ohms. Such an occurrence could be one possible reason for a false ECI record. A test of inter-electrode impedances to assure that they are of adequate magnitude thus should be performed during the recording.

556

When fixed arrays of electrodes ("electrode cap" or similar devices) are utilized, it is essential that excess jelly does not spread from one electrode to another, creating a shunt or short circuit, which would attenuate the signal.

Stable, low-impedance electrodes are absolutely essential for all bedside (i.e., away from the laboratory) studies.

2.3 Although not recommended for general use, needle electrodes have been used effectively in suspected ECI recordings. The greater impedance they may have is offset by a greater probability of similar values among different electrodes, so that the likelihood that artifact will occur in the record is not increased. (See also Guideline One: Minimum Technical Requirements for Performing Clinical Electroencephalography, Section 2.2.)

3. The Integrity of the Entire Recording System Should Be Tested

Ordinary instrumental calibration tests the operation of the amplifiers and writer units, but it does not exclude the possibility of shunting or an open circuit at the electrodes, electrode board, cable, or input of the machine. If, after recording on one montage at increased amplification, an EEG suggesting ECS is found, the integrity of the system may be tested by touching each electrode of the montage gently with a pencil point or cotton swab to create an artifact potential on the record. This test verifies that the electrode board is connected to the machine; records made with the electrode board inadvertently not connected can sometimes resemble low-amplitude EEG activity. The test further proves that the selector switch settngs match the electrode placements.

4. Inter-Electrode Distances Should Be at Least 10 Centimeters

In the International 10–20 System, the average adult inter-electrode distances are between 6 and 6.5 cm. A record taken with average inter-electrode distances at ordinary sensitivity may suggest ECS; however, if it were recorded using longer inter-electrode distances, cerebral potentials might be seen in the tracing. Hence, with longitudinal or transverse bipolar montages, some double distance electrode linkages are recommended (e.g., Fp1-C3, F3-P3, C3-O1, etc.).

Ear reference recording is almost invariably too contaminated by EKG to be useful, but a Cz reference may be satisfactory. In one study (1), the best montage was: Fp2-C4, C4-O2, Fp1-C3, C3-O1, T4-Cz, Cz-T3, with one-channel EKG and one-channel noncephalic (hand). Occipital leads, however, are more difficult to attach in immobilized patients and are particularly susceptible to movement artifact induced by artificial respirators. A montage that includes F7-T5, F8-T6, F3-P3, F4-P4 and Fz-Pz may therefore yield a better record.

None of the foregoing should imply that the usual preselected laboratory montages could not also be used.

5. Sensitivity Must Be Increased from 7 μV/mm to at Least 2 μV/mm *for at Least 30 Minutes* of the Recording, with Inclusion of Appropriate Calibrations

5.1 This is undoubtedly the most important and the most often overlooked parameter. One has only to realize that at a sensitivity of 7 μV/mm a signal of 2 μV cannot be seen because the average ink line is ¼ mm in width, i.e., about the size of the signal one desires to see. Obviously, the criterion voltage of 2 μV will deflect the pen only 1 mm at a sensitivity of 2 μV/mm. Such a signal should be visible at 2 μV/mm, and more certainly so at a sensitivity of 1.5 or 1 μV/mm. However, very slow activity with gradual wave slopes still may be difficult to see. Contemporary equipment permits extended recording at a sensitivity of 1.5 or 1 μV/mm. This 50–100% increase in sensitivity will allow a more confident assessment of the presence, or the absence, of a 2-μV signal.

5.2 Adequate and appropriate calibration procedures are essential. It is good practice to calibrate with a signal near the size or value of the EEG signal that has been recorded; thus, for electrocerebral silence, a calibration of 2 or 5 μV is appropriate. A 50-μV calibration signal at a sensitivity of 2 or 1 $\mu V/mm$ is useless, since the pens block. The inherent noise level of the recording system also should be noted.

5.3 Self-limited periods of ECI of up to 20 min may occur in low-voltage records (7), and, therefore, a single recording should be at least 30 min long to be certain that intermittent low-voltage cerebral activity is not missed.

6. Filter Settings Should Be Appropriate for the Assessment of Electrocerebral Silence

In order to avoid attenuation of low-voltage fast or slow activity, whenever possible, high-frequency filters should not be set below a high-frequency setting of 30 Hz, and low-frequency filters should not be set above a low-frequency setting of 1 Hz.

It is well known that short time constants attenuate slow potentials. In the situation approaching ECS, there may be potentials in the theta and delta ranges, so every effort should be made to avoid attenuation of these low frequencies. However, it has been demonstrated that a low-frequency setting of 1 Hz is adequate for the determination of ECI (1,7). There need be no hesitation in the use of the 60-Hz notch filter.

7. Additional Monitoring Techniques Should Be Employed When Necessary

The EEG record is a composite of true brain waves, other physiologic signals, and artifacts (either internal or external to the machine, and of mechanical, electromagnetic, and/or electrostatic origin). When the sensitivity is increased, such artifacts are accentuated and therefore must be identified in order to accurately assess whether EEG is present. It should be emphasized that the best insurance against many artifacts is a stable, low-impedance electrode system.

The *Atlas of Electronencephalography in Coma and Cerebral Death* should be consulted for information about a wide range of artifacts (1).

7.1 Since one rarely sees an ECI record without varying amounts of EKG artifact, an EKG monitor is essential.

7.2 If respiration artifact cannot be eliminated, the artifact must be documented by specific technician notation on the record or be monitored by transducer. Briefly disconnecting the respirator will allow definitive identification of the artifact.

7.3 Frequently, an additional monitor is needed for other artifact emanating from the patient or for artifact induced from the surroundings. The most convenient for this purpose is a pair of electrodes on the dorsum of the hand separated by about 6–7 cm.

7.4 It is now clear that some EMG contamination can persist in patients with ECI recordings. If EMG potentials are of such amplitude as to obscure the tracing, it may be necessary to reduce or eliminate them by use of a neuromuscular blocking agent such as pancuronium bromide (Pavulon) or succinylcholine (Anectine). This procedure should be performed under the direction of an anesthesiologist or other physician familiar with the use of the drug.

7.5 Machine noise and external interference may be conveniently checked by a "dummy patient", i.e., a 10,000-ohm resistor between input terminal 1 (G1) and input terminal 2 (G2) of one channel.

7.6 Even with good technique, however, an EEG recorded at the increased sensitivities required above can at times leave the electroencephalographer who interprets the recordings in considerable difficulty. An attempt must be made to determine what portion of the record results from noncerebral physiologic signals, or nonphysiologic artifacts, including the ongoing noise level of the complete system in the particular ICU as indicated, for example, by a recording from the hand. An estimate must then be made of whether or not the remaining activity exceeds 2 μV in amplitude. When this cannot be done with confidence, the EEG report must indicate the uncertainty, and the record cannot be classified as demonstrating ECI (see Section 10).

8. There Should Be No EEG Reactivity to Intense Somatosensory, Auditory, or Visual Stimuli

In the collaborative study there was no instance of stimulus-related activity in routine recordings of patients with ECS (1,5,6). Any apparent EEG activity resulting from the above stimuli or any others (airway suctioning and other nursing procedures can be potent stimuli) must be carefully distinguished from noncerebral physiologic signals and from nonphysiologic artifacts. For example, an electroretinogram can still persist in response to photic stimulation when there is ECS. Stimulation may be of help also in documenting the degree of reactivity of records found not to be characterized by ECS.

9. Recordings Should Be Made Only by a Qualified Technologist

Great skill is essential in recording cases of suspected ECS. The recordings are frequently made under difficult circumstances and include many possible sources for artifact. Elimination of most artifact and identification of all others can be accomplished by a qualified technologist.

Qualifications for a competent EEG technologist for ECS recordings include the requirement of supervised instruction in the techniques of recording in ICU settings. The technologist should work under the direction of a qualified electroencephalographer (see Guidelines Four and Five).

10. A Repeat EEG Should Be Performed If There Is Doubt About ECS

In the Collaborative Study of Cerebral Death (1,5,6), there were no patients who survived for more than a short period after an EEG showed ECS, provided that overdose of depressant drugs was excluded. This finding confirmed the results of the earlier survey, which were summarized in the Introduction. It is evident, therefore, that a single EEG showing ECS is a highly reliable procedure for the determination of cortical death. (For other guidelines to assist physicians in the determination of brain death, see the References.)

In the event that technical or other difficulties lead to uncertainty in the evaluation of the question of ECS, the entire procedure should be repeated after an interval, for example, after 6 h (see Section 7).

REFERENCES

1. Bennett DR, Hughes, JR, Korein J, Merlis JK, Suter C. *An atlas of electroencephalography in coma and cerebral death*. New York: Raven Press, 1976.
2. Chatrian GE, Bergamini L, Dondey M, Klass DW, Lennox-Buchthal M, Petersen I. A glossary of terms most commonly used by clinical electroencephalographers. *Electroencephalogr. Clin. Neurophysiol.* 1974;37:538–48.
3. Chatrian GE. Electrophysiologic evaluation of brain death: a critical appraisal. In: Aminoff MJ, ed. *Electrodiagnosis in clinical neurology*. New York: Churchill Livingstone, 1980.
4. The Medical Consultants on the Diagnosis of Death to the President's Commission for the Study of Ethical Problems in Medicine and Biomedical and Behavioral Research. Guidelines for the determination of death. *JAMA* 1981;246:2184–6.
5. The NINCDS Collaborative Study of Brain Death. NINCDS Monograph No. 24, NIH Publication No. 81-2286, December 1980.
6. Walker AE. *Cerebral death*. Baltimore: Urban & Schwarzenberg, 1981.
7. Jorgensen, EO. Requirements for recording the EEG at high sensitivity in suspected brain death. *Electroencephalgr. Clin. Neurophysiol.* 1974;36:65–9.

1. Minimal Qualifications of a Clinical Electroencephalographer

These standards are proposed for individuals entering the EEG field after 1978. Many highly competent electroencephalographers who entered the field before 1978 and currently interpret EEGs do not meet the requirements listed below.

1.1 The clinical electroencephalographer should be a physician with board eligibility or certification in neurology, pediatric neurology, neurosurgery, or psychiatry.

1.2 Training should meet the minimal requirements for examination by the American Board of Qualitification in EEG. Currently, these include board eligibility or certification in neurology, neurosurgery, or psychiatry and a minimum of 12 months supervised experience in EEG during or following the residency, of which at least 3 months must include full-time training in EEG and clinical neurophysiology.

2. Qualifications of EEG Technologists and Technicians

2.1 The qualifications of EEG technologists shall be those set forth in Guideline Five: Recommended Job Descriptions for Electroencephalographic Technologists.

2.2 In no case should a technician with less than 6 months of supervised clinical experience, following formal training, operate independently or in an unsupervised capacity.

This material originally appeared in *J. Clin. Neurophysiol.* 1986;3(2):150–1.

3. Laboratory Organization

3.1 Hospital laboratories should meet accreditation requirements of the American EEG Society's Committee on Laboratory Accreditation (1).

3.2 The chief electroncephalographer shall have the primary responsibility for the overall operations and policies of the laboratory. The policies of the laboratory should be documented in a policy and procedures manual. Under the supervision of the EEG laboratory director, the chief EEG technologist shall be responsible for the daily operation of the laboratory. The chief technologist, together with the laboratory director, shall maintain the highest standards of EEG technical practice.

3.4 All EEGs should be analyzed by, and official reports, including clinical interpretations, provided by, a qualified electroencephalographer. Under no circumstances should a technologist, however well qualified and experienced, have primary responsibility for clinical interpretation of EEGs.

Qualified technologists, however, should be able to give a descriptive technical report of the record.

3.4. Records should be maintained in an orderly manner and should be available for review by the patient's referring physician and other qualified persons.

4. Equipment

Technical standards recommended by the American EEG Society Instrumentation Committee and the International Federation of Societies for EEG and Clinical Neurophysiology should form the basis for selection of clinical EEG equipment.

4.1 Basic recording equipment should conform to the recommendations of Guideline One: Minimum Technical Requirements for Performing Clinical Electroencephalography.

REFERENCE

1. American Electroencephalographic Society. Guidelines for laboratory accreditation. *J. Clin. Neurophysiol.* 1986;3:85–92.

INTRODUCTION

These job descriptions are intended for directors of EEG laboratories and to provide guidelines for federal and state agencies and hospital administrations concerned
with classification of personnel.

1. Electroencephalographic Technologist I

1.1 Summary and distinguishing characteristics

An EEG Technologist I conducts EEG examinations under the general supervision of the senior staff.

The technologist in this class is responsible for the preparation of the patient, the
conduct of various EEG examinations, and the collection of information pertinent
to the interpretation of the tests.

1.2 Examples of duties

1.2.1 Performs standard EEG recording (wake and sleep, nasopharyngeal, bedside, isolation, and electrocerebral inactivity evaluations).

1.2.2 Summarizes the patient's neurologic status and clinical history from the
chart, patient, or other knowledgeable persons. Explains the recording procedure
to the patient and any family members present.

1.2.3 Adapts methods and instrumentation to obtain optimal results based on
history, clinical observations, and EEG findings.

This material originally appeared in *J. Clin. Neurophysiol.* 1986:3(2):152–4.

1.2.4 Provides appropriate patient care and detailed observations of clinical manifestations during seizures and other patient emergency situations.

1.2.5 Insures electrical safety of the patient at all times.

1.2.6 Keeps equipment in clean operating condition. Performs maintenance and minor repair of laboratory equipment and reports the need for major repairs.

1.2.7 Participates in conferences, technical meetings, and other educational activities.

1.2.8 Performs other related duties as required.

1.3 Educational and professional qualifications

1.3.1 Successful completion of an educational program for EEG technologists accredited by the AMA Committee on Allied Health Education and Accreditation, or equivalent training.

1.4 Personal qualifications

1.4.1 Maturity. The ability to establish good rapport with patients, public, and staff.

1.4.2 Capacity to deal with severely ill patients.

2. Electroencephalographic Technologist II

2.1 Summary and distinguishing characteristics

An EEG Technologist II performs standard and complex EEG recordings under minimum supervision. Has developed expertise in other electrophysiologic studies.

The technologist in this class is responsible for obtaining standard as well as special procedure EEG recordings, is able to monitor additional physiologic phenomena by means of appropriate techniques and instrumentation, may provide training, and may participate in research.

2.2 Examples of duties

2.2.1 Performs all the duties of an EEG Technologist I.

2.2.2 Records computer-averaged electrical responses to visual, auditory, somatosensory, or other stimuli. Determines during averaging that recordings are of adequate technical quality.

2.2.3 Records EEGs from neonates including those in the neonatal intensive care unit.

2.2.4 Carries out EEG or evoked potential monitoring procedures during surgery.

2.2.5 Records polysomnograms.

2.2.6 Performs CCTV-EEG recordings.

2.2.7 Performs ambulatory EEG recordings.

2.2.8 Sends and receives telephone transmission EEG recordings (see Guideline Six: Recommendations for Telephone Transmission of EEGs).

2.2.9 Participates in conferences, technical meetings, and other educational activities. Serves as inservice training instructor for junior staff, technologist trainees, and other medical personnel.

2.2.10 Performs other related duties as required.

2.3 Educational and professional qualifications

2.3.1 One-year experience at the Technologist I level. Certification by the American Board of Registration of Electroencephalographic Technologists, or its equivalent.

2.4 Personal qualifications

2.4.1 The qualifications of an Electroencephalographic Technologist I (see Section 1.4, above).

2.4.2 Independent judgment and initiative.

3. Electroencephalographic Technologist III

3.1 Summary and distinguishing characteristics

An EEG Technologist III is qualified to serve as a chief technologist and to supervise the technical operation and training activities of the laboratory.

The person in this class is distinguished by a high degree of sophistication in the field of EEG technology, is responsible for the technical operation of laboratories performing clinical or research work, directs related clerical activity, and supervises, plans, and helps develop training activities.

3.2 Examples of duties

3.2.1 Supervises, plans, and reviews the work of the technical staff and performs their duties when required. When necessary, takes corrective action or suggests technical innovations.

3.2.2 Plans laboratory schedules and assigns priorities according to the workload and clinical urgency.

3.2.3 Supervises or performs particularly difficult or unusual procedures.

3.2.4 Assumes the role of laboratory administrator, as required.

3.2.5 Arranges for the maintenance and repair of equipment.

3.2.6 Takes part in the recruiting, selection, and evaluation of technical staff.

3.2.7 Organizes and participates in conferences, technical meetings, and other educational activities.

3.2.8 Performs other related duties as required.

3.3 Educational and professional qualifications

3.3.1 Certification by the American Board of Registration of Electroencephalographic Technologists, or the equivalent.

3.2.2 Three years of experience in EEG technology at the Technologist II level.

3.4 Personal qualifications

3.4.1 The qualifications of an EEG Technologist II (see Section 2.4, above).

3.4.2 High degree of leadership and organizational and teaching talents.

GUIDELINE SIX: RECOMMENDATIONS FOR TELEPHONE TRANSMISSION OF EEGs

1. Basic Standards

The basic standards and technical specifications for clinical EEG, defined in Guideline One: Minimum Technical Requirements for Performing Clinical Electroencephalography, and Guideline Four: Standards of Practice in Clinical Electroencephalography, should be followed in the transmission, interpretation, and preservation of clinical EEGs by telephone (1–5). Within these specifications, recordings at the transmitting and receiving sites should be essentially identical.

1.1 Manufacturers should provide frequency response, noise, and cross-talk data under operating conditions, so that consumers can make intelligent comparisons. Periodic checks of equipment at both the transmitting and the receiving laboratories should be carried out.

1.2 "Fail-safe" indication of difficulties due to line losses or other transmission or receiving problems should be included in the transmitting–receiving system itself. (Assistance from telephone companies with general information concerning the identification of artifacts generated within the telephone systems could be most helpful.)

This material originally appeared in *J. Clin. Neurophysiol.* 1986;3(2):155–7.

1.3 Signal checks of equipment at both the transmitting and receiving laboratories should be introduced preceding and following each recording, i.e., prior to the initial calibration and subsequent to the final calibration.

1.4 The identification appearing on the original (transmitted) and the received record should be adequate to identify the latter as being a copy of the former. Identification should include patient ID, all calibrations, and changes in instrument controls and montages.

1.5 The EEG should be recorded both at the transmitting and receiving end of the circuit, so that the technologists can correlate EEG events with behavior changes or activities of the patient and can determine whether artifacts are present. The preferable method of transmission is to utilize a paper record at both the transmitting and receiving end. Whether paper or alternate methods are used, equipment at both ends should permit simultaneous real-time review of the activities from all recorded channels, should permit re-assessment of the activity recorded over the previous minutes of the recording, and should allow comparison of different segments of the record.

Relevant patient behavior and activity should be noted (see Guideline One: Minimum Technical Requirements for Performing Clinical Electroencephalography). Voice or other signaling capabilities should be incorporated in the telephone–EEG system, from transmitting to receiving stations, to identify EEG-clinical correlations as they occur, with minimal interference with the EEG record. Such on-line correlation will assist in avoiding misinterpretation (e.g., muscle artifact being regarded as spikes, etc.). The use of a standard code for transmitting such information should be required.

1.6 The EEG at both ends should be stored (whether on paper or utilizing an alternate method such as tape or disk). The EEG at the transmitting site should be available when necessary for backup comparison and, to ensure quality control, recordings from both ends should be compared regularly.

2. Technologist Qualifications

The statements set forth in Guideline Five: Recommended Job Descriptions for Electroencephalographic Technologists are reaffirmed for telephone transmission of EEGs. These standards define the basic level of competence of the EEG technologists at the transmitting and at the receiving sites. Under no circumstances should the technologist at the transmitting laboratory be less qualified than one who works independently under a laboratory director who is based outside of a hospital. Indeed, the responsibilities falling upon the EEG technologist staffing a telephone transmitting laboratory are greater than those of a technologist working under relatively direct supervision in a hospital or office laboratory.

2.1 The technologist at the transmitting laboratory, because of its remoteness from the receiving center, should be well trained, especially in telephone transmission EEG, irrespective of any limited utilization because of size of referral load. This technologist should also be acquainted with the receiving laboratory. In view of the isolation of the transmitting laboratory, provisions for continued education and updating of information are essential to maintaining the skill of the transmitting technologist.

2.2 Technologists staffing a receiving facility should be skilled and experienced, should be specifically trained in telephone transmission EEG, and should particularly be familiar with the recognition of artifacts that are peculiar to this technology. A program of continuing education should be available for the technologist at the receiving laboratory.

2.3 A qualified electroencephalographer should interpret the received EEG and supervise the technologists at both the transmitting and receiving ends (see Guideline Four).

3. Ethical Considerations

Provided that all of the above and previously approved procedures are followed, no ethical problem in the use of telephone systems for expediting interpretation of EEGs should arise.

If the procedures in this and in previously adopted Guidelines are not followed, and if users are not aware of the characteristics of ancillary equipment used in telephone transmission of EEGs, the installation of a telephone transmission system may well cause a degradation of the quality of practice of clinical electroencephalography.

4. Brain Death

At the present time, telephone transmission of EEG cannot be used for determination of electrocerebral silence in the diagnosis of brain death because of the inherent and unpredictable electrical noise present in telephone networks relative to the very low signal amplitudes in the EEG recording itself in this situation (see Guideline Three: Minimum Technical Standards for EEG Recording in Suspected Cerebral Death).

REFERENCES

1. Barlow JS, Kamp A, Morton HB, Ripoche A, Shipton H. EEG instrumentation standards: Report of the Committee on EEG Instrumentation Standards of the International Federation of Societies for Electroencephalography and Clinical Neurophysiology. III. EEG telephone (telephone transmission of EEG data). *Electroencephalogr. Clin. Neurophysiol.* 1974;37:552.
2. Bennett DR, Gardner RM. A model for the telephone transmission of six-channel electroencephalograms. *Electroencephalogr. Clin. Neurophysiol.* 1970;29:404–8.
3. Committee on Standards of Clinical Practice of EEG and EMG. Telephone Transmission. In: *International Federation of Societies for Electroencephalography and Clinical Neurophysiology: Recommendations for the Practice of Clinical Neurophysiology.* Amsterdam: Elsevier, 1983:52–3.
4. Frost Jr JD, Barlow JS. Telephone transmission of EEGs–practical aspects. In: Frost Jr JD, Barlow JS, eds. *Graphic and magnetic-tape recording of bioelectrical phenomena.* Amsterdam: Elsevier, 1976:3B20–3. (*Handbook of electroencephalography and clinical neurophysiology*, vol 3, part B).

5. Roy OZ. Biotelemetry and telephone transmission. In: Broughton RJ, ed. *Acquisition of bioelectrical data: collection and amplification*. Amsterdam: Elsevier, 1976:3A46–66. (*Handbook of electroencephalography and clinical neurophysiology*, vol 3, part A).

GUIDELINE SEVEN: A PROPOSAL FOR STANDARD MONTAGES TO BE USED IN CLINICAL EEG

INTRODUCTION

A great diversity of montages exists among different EEG laboratories, and many of these montages fail to display the EEG adequately or are inordinately complex. Moreover, this diversity impedes interchange of information among electroencephalographers, to the ultimate detriment of patients.

Recognizing the need for improving this aspect of EEG practice, the montages listed in this Guideline are recommended for standard use by clinical laboratories. This proposal should not be construed as an attempt to limit the total number of montages used by any EEG laboratory. Indeed, depending on individual recording circumstances, additional montages may be necessary for an adequate EEG examination and for the solution of particular problems. The proposed montages are intended to constitute a basic minimum, not a maximum, for general-purpose use. If these recommendations are adopted widely, communication among electroencephalographers should be facilitated.

Further, the proposed montages are not designed for special purposes such as for neonatal EEGs, recording with nasopharyngeal or sphenoidal leads, all-night sleep recordings, or for verification of electrocerebral inactivity.

This material originally appeared in *J. Clin. Neurophysiol.* 1986:3(2):158–65.

1. Montage Designations

1.1 The class of montage is designated as follows: longitudinal bipolar (LB), transverse bipolar (TB), or referential (R).

1.2 The numeral to the left of the point indicates the number of channels. Montages are designed for four types of instruments: 8, 10, 16, and 18 channels.

1.3 The numeral 2 or 3 to the right of the point indicates an alternative montage of the same class for a particular size of instrument (e.g., LB-16.2 and LB-16.3 are alternatives for LB-16.1). The number of alternatives has been limited to a maximum of three.

1.4 A small letter to the right of the point (for 8- and 10-channel instruments) indicates a montage that is to be used in conjunction with at least one other for adequate area coverage (e.g., R-10.1a and R-10.b).

2. Recommendations Governing Selection of the Proposed Montages with Explanatory Notes

2.1 The Committee *reaffirms* the statements pertaining to montages set forth previously in the Guidelines of the American EEG Society and that are paraphrased as follows:

TABLE 1. *Number of montages recommended[a]*

No. channels per instrument	Longitudinal bipolar	Transverse bipolar	Referential	Total
18	1 (3)	1 (2)	1 (3)	3
16	1 (3)	1 (3)	1 (3)	3
10	2 (6)	3 (3)	2 (4)	7
8	2 (2)	3 (3)	2 (4)	7

[a]Figures in parentheses refer to the number of alternative montages proposed.

(a) that no less than 8 channels of simultaneous recording be used, and that a larger number of channels be encouraged,

(b) that the full 21 electrode placements of the 10–20 System be used,

(c) that both bipolar and referential montages be used,

(d) that the electrode connections for each channel be clearly indicated at the beginning of each montage,

(e) that the pattern of electrode connections be made as simple as possible and that montages should be easily comprehended,

(f) that the electrode connections (bipolar) preferentially should run in straight (unbroken) lines and the interelectrode distances kept equal,

(g) that tracings from the more anterior electrodes be placed above those from the more posterior electrodes on the recording page, and

(h) that it is very desirable to have some of the montages comparable for all EEG laboratories.

2.2 The Committee recommends a "left above right" order of derivations, i.e., on the recording page left-sided leads should be placed above right-sided leads for either alternating pairs of derivations or blocks of derivations.

This recommendation coincides with the prevailing practice of the vast majority of EEG laboratories in North America and by laboratories in some, but not all, other countries.

2.3 A maximum number of electrodes should be represented in each montage, within limitations imposed by the number of recording channels, to ensure adequate coverage of head areas.

2.4 Three classes of montage should be represented in each recording: longitudinal bipolar (LB), transverse bipolar (TB), and referential (R).

2.5 For 16- and 18-channel recording, one montage from each of the three classes will be needed. For 8- and 10-channel recording, seven montages (2 LB, 3 TB, and 2 R) will be needed (see Table 1).

For adequate mapping of electrical fields, additional montages may need to be devised that include LB and TB chains recorded simultaneously.

In the montages listed for R recording, leads on the mandibular angles may be substituted for the leads on the earlobes if the change is duly noted.

Potential pitfalls in referential recording are numerous, and caution should be exercised if unwanted activity appears in a reference lead. In such instances, another reference should be chosen and the change should be clearly noted in the recording.

2.6 A logical order of arrangement should prevail in each montage and in comparable montages designed for instruments of different sizes.

Recognizing the fact that experienced electroencephalographers differ for valid reasons in their approach to the display of EEG activity, alternative sets of montages have been included in the recommendations. Further details about the principles of montage design and the different preferences by members of this Committee have been published (*Am. J. EEG Technol.,* 17:Nos. 1 and 2, 1977).

In general, the LB.1 and the R.1 series consist of leads grouped in anatomical proximity and extending sequentially across the head from the left to the right. In this system, hemispheric differences are readily appreciated. In the LB.2 and LB.3 series, blocks of homologous derivations are compared (LB.2 extending from the midline sagittal region laterally, LB.3 extending from lateral regions medially). In the R.2 and R.3 series, homologous derivations are juxtaposed in adjacent channels to facilitate comparison of localized regions (R.2 extending from the midline sagittal region laterally and R.3 extending from the lateral regions medially). The alternative montages in the TB series depend, in part, on the extent of polar coverage.

Minor modifications of the recommended montages may be instituted during part of the recording, especially for monitoring other physiologic variables, if the modifications do not infringe upon the principles set forth in these Recommendations.

Longitudinal Bipolar Montages

Channel No.	LB-18.1	LB-18.2	LB-18.3
1	FP1-F7	Fz-Cz	Fp1-F7
2	F7-T3	Cz-Pz	F7-T3
3	T3-T5	Fp1-F3	T3-T5
4	T5-O1	F3-C3	T5-O1
5	Fp1-F3	C3-P3	Fp2-F8
6	F3-C3	P3-O1	F8-T4
7	C3-P3	Fp2-F4	T4-T6
8	P3-O1	F4-C4	T6-O2
9	Fz-Cz	C4-P4	Fp1-F3
10	Cz-Pz	P4-O2	F3-C3
11	Fp2-F4	Fp1-F7	C3-P3
12	F4-C4	F7-T3	P3-O1
13	C4-P4	T3-T5	Fp2-F4
14	P4-O2	T5-O1	F4-C4
15	Fp2-F8	Fp2-F8	C4-P4
16	F8-T4	F8-T4	P4-O2
17	T4-T6	T4-T6	Fz-Cz
18	T6-O2	T6-O2	Cz-Pz

Channel No.	LB-16.1	LB-16.2	LB-16.3
1	Fp1-F7	Fp1-F3	Fp1-F7
2	F7-T3	F3-C3	F7-T3
3	T3-T5	C3-P3	T3-T5
4	T5-O1	P3-O1	T5-O1
5	Fp1-F3	Fp2-F4	Fp2-F8
6	F3-C3	F4-C4	F8-T4
7	C3-P3	C4-P4	T4-T6
8	P3-O1	P4-O2	T6-O2
9	Fp2-F4	Fp1-F7	Fp1-F3
10	F4-C4	F7-T3	F3-C3
11	C4-P4	T3-T5	C3-P3
12	P4-O2	T5-O1	P3-O1

577

Longitudinal Bipolar Montages *(continued)*

Channel No.	LB-16.1	LB-16.2	LB-16.3
13	Fp2-F8	Fp2-F8	Fp2-F4
14	F8-T4	F8-T4	F4-C4
15	T4-T6	T4-T6	C4-P4
16	T6-O2	T6-O2	P4-O2

Channel No.	LB-10.1a	LB-10.1b	LB-10.2a	LB-10.2b	LB-10.3a	LB-10.3b
1	Fp1-F7	Fp1-F3	Fz-Cz	Fz-Cz	Fp1-F7	Fp1-F3
2	F7-T3	F3-C3	Cz-Pz	Cz-Pz	F7-T3	F3-C3
3	T3-T5	C3-P3	Fp1-F3	Fp1-F7	T3-T5	C3-P3
4	T5-O1	P3-O1	F3-C3	F7-T3	T5-O1	P3-O1
5	Fz-Cz	Fz-Cz	C3-P3	T3-T5	Fp2-F8	Fp2-F4
6	Cz-Pz	Cz-Pz	P3-O1	T5-O1	F8-T4	F4-C4
7	Fp2-F8	Fp2-F4	Fp2-F4	Fp2-F8	T4-T6	C4-P4
8	F8-T4	F4-C4	F4-C4	F8-T4	T6-O2	P4-O2
9	T4-T6	C4-P4	C4-P4	T4-T6	Fz-Cz	Fz-Cz
10	T6-O2	P4-O2	P4-O2	T6-O2	Cz-Pz	Cz-Pz

Channel No.	LB-8.1a	LB-8.1b
1	Fp1-F3	Fp1-F7
2	F3-C3	F7-T3
3	C3-P3	T3-T5
4	P3-O1	T5-O1
5	Fp2-F4	Fp2-F8
6	F4-C4	F8-T4
7	C4-P4	T4-T6
8	P4-O2	T6-O2

Transverse Bipolar Montages

Channel No.	TB-18.1	TB-18.2
1	F7-Fp1	Fp1-Fp2
2	Fp1-Fp2	F7-F3
3	Fp2-F8	F3-Fz
4	F7-F3	Fz-F4
5	F3-Fz	F4-F8
6	Fz-F4	A1-T3
7	F4-F8	T3-C3
8	T3-C3	C3-Cz
9	C3-Cz	Cz-C4
10	Cz-C4	C4-T4
11	C4-T4	T4-A2
12	T5-P3	T5-P3
13	P3-Pz	P3-Pz
14	Pz-p4	Pz-P4
15	P4-T6	P4-T6
16	T5-O1	O1-O2
17	O1-O2	Fz-Cz
18	O2-T6	Cz-Pz

Channel No.	TB-16.1	TB-16.2	TB-16.3
1	F7-Fp1	Fp1-Fp2	F7-Fp1
2	Fp1-Fp2	F7-F3	Fp2-F8
3	Fp2-F8	F3-Fz	F7-F3
4	F7-F3	Fz-F4	F3-Fz
5	F3-Fz	F4-F8	Fz-F4
6	Fz-F4	A1-T3	F4-F8
7	F4-F8	T3-C3	T3-C3
8	T3-C3	C3-Cz	C3-Cz
9	C3-Cz	Cz-C4	Cz-C4
10	Cz-C4	C4-T4	C4-T4

Transverse Bipolar Montages *(continued)*

Channel No.	*TB-16.1*	*TB-16.2*	*TB-16.3*
11	C4-T4	T4-A2	T5-P3
12	T5-P3	T5-P3	P3-Pz
13	P3-Pz	P3-Pz	Pz-P4
14	Pz-P4	Pz-P4	P4-T6
15	P4-T6	P4-T6	T5-O1
16	O1-O2	O1-O2	O2-T6

Channel No.	*TB-10.1a*	*TB-10.1b*	*TB-10.1c*
1	F7-Fp1	F7-F3	A1-T3
2	Fp1-Fp2	F3-Fz	T3-C3
3	Fp2-F8	Fz-F4	C3-Cz
4	T3-C3	F4-F8	Cz-C4
5	C3-Cz	A1-T3	C4-T4
6	Cz-C4	T3-C3	T4-A2
7	C4-T4	C3-Cz	T5-P3
8	T5-O1	Cz-C4	P3-Pz
9	O1-O2	C4-T4	Pz-P4
10	O2-T6	T4-A2	P4-T6

Channel No.	*TB-8.1a*	*TB-8.1b*	*TB-8.1c*
1	F7-Fp1	F7-F3	T3-C3
2	Fp1-Fp2	F3-Fz	C3-Cz
3	Fp2-F8	Fz-F4	Cz-C4
4	C3-Cz	F4-F8	C4-T4
5	Cz-C4	T3-C3	T5-P3
6	T5-O1	C3-Cz	P3-Pz
7	O1-O2	Cz-C4	Pz-P4
8	O2-T6	C4-T4	P4-T6

Referential Montages

Channel No.	R-18.1	R-18.2	R-18.3
1	F7-A1	Fz-A1	F7-A1
2	T3-A1	Pz-A2	F8-A2
3	T5-A1	Fp1-A1	T3-A1
4	Fp1-A1	Fp2-A2	T4-A2
5	F3-A1	F3-A1	T5-A1
6	C3-A1	F4-A2	T6-A2
7	P3-A1	C3-A1	Fp1-A1
8	O1-A1	C4-A2	Fp2-A2
9	Fz-A1	P3-A1	F3-A1
10	Pz-A2	P4-A2	F4-A2
11	Fp2-A2	O1-A1	C3-A1
12	F4-A2	O2-A2	C4-A2
13	C4-A2	F7-A1	P3-A1
14	P4-A2	F8-A2	P4-A2
15	O2-A2	T3-A1	O1-A2
16	F8-A2	T4-A2	O2-A2
17	T4-A2	T5-A1	Fz-A1
18	T6-A2	T6-A2	Pz-A2

Channel No.	R-16.1	R-16.2	R-16.3
1	F7-A1	Fp1-A1	F7-A1
2	T3-A1	Fp2-A2	F8-A2
3	T5-A1	F3-A1	T3-A1
4	Fp1-A1	F4-A2	T4-A2
5	F3-A1	C3-A1	T5-A1
6	C3-A1	C4-A2	T6-A2
7	P3-A1	P3-A1	Fp1-A1
8	O1-A1	P4-A2	Fp2-A2
9	Fp2-A2	O1-A1	F3-A1
10	F4-A2	O2-A2	F4-A2
11	C4-A2	F7-A1	C3-A1
12	P4-A2	F8-A2	C4-A2

Referential Montages *(continued)*

Channel No.	R-16.1	R-16.2	R-16.3
13	O2-A2	T3-A1	P3-A1
14	F8-A2	T4-A2	P4-A2
15	T4-A2	T5-A1	O1-A1
16	T6-A2	T6-A2	O2-A2

Channel No.	R-10.1a	R-10.1b	R-10.2a	R-10.2b
1	Fp1-A1	Fp1-A1	Fp1-A1	Fp1-A1
2	F3-A1	F7-A1	Fp2-A2	Fp2-A2
3	C3-A1	T3-A1	F3-A1	F7-A1
4	P3-A1	T5-A1	F4-A2	F8-A2
5	O1-A1	O1-A1	C3-A1	T3-A1
6	Fp2-A2	Fp2-A2	C4-A2	T4-A2
7	F4-A2	F8-A2	P3-A1	T5-A1
8	C4-A2	T4-A2	P4-A2	T6-A2
9	P4-A2	T6-A2	O1-A1	O1-A1
10	O2-A2	O2-A2	O2-A2	O2-A2

Channel No.	R-8.1a	R-8.1b	R-8.2a	R-8.2b
1	F3-A1	Fp1-A1	F3-A1	Fp1-A1
2	C3-A1	F7-A1	F4-A2	Fp2-A2
3	P3-A1	T3-A1	C4-A1	F7-A1
4	O1-A1	T5-A1	C4-A2	F8-A2
5	F4-A2	Fp2-A2	P3-A1	T3-A1
6	C4-A2	F8-A2	P4-A2	T4-A2
7	P4-A2	T4-A2	O1-A1	T5-A1
8	O2-A2	T6-A2	O2-A2	T6-A2

These guidelines are not meant to represent rigid rules but only a general guide for reporting EEGs. They are intended to apply to standard EEG recordings rather than to special procedures. When reporting on more specialized types of records (e.g., neonatal records, records for suspected electrocerebral silence), description of technical details should be more complete than in the case of standard recordings. However, if the technique used is the one recommended for those special procedures in the "Guidelines in EEG" (American EEG Society, 1980), a sentence to that effect should be sufficient (Guidelines 3, "Minimum Technical Requirements for Performing Clinical EEG" (MTR); 4, "Minimum Technical Standards for EEG Recording in Suspected Cerebral Death;" and 6, "Minimal Technical Standards for Pediatric Electroencephalography").

1. *The printed forms for reporting EEGs should provide for a minimum of information about the patient, which could be copied from the Basic Data Sheet (MTR, Sec. 6.1) by the person who types the report. It should be, therefore, unnecessary for the electroencephalographer to repeat in the report the age, sex, etc., of the patient. However, in order to avoid confusion, the name of the patient and the EEG identification number should be included.*

2. *The report of an EEG should consist of three principal parts: (A) Introduction, (B) Description of the record, and (C) Interpretation, including (a) impression regarding its normality or degree of abnormality, and (b) correlation of the EEG findings with the clinical picture.*

3. **Introduction.** *The introduction should start with a statement of the kind of preparation the patient had, if any, for the recording session.* The initial sentence should state whether the patient received any medication or other preparation, such

as sleep deprivation, as well as the patient's state of consciousness at the onset of the record. If the patient was fasting, this should be stated.

If the printed form used for the report does not provide a space for the regular medication the patient is receiving, as distinguished from medication given specifically for the recording, any medication that could influence the EEG should be included in the electroencephalographer's report.

If the number of electrodes used is not the standard 21 of the 10–20 system or if montitoring of other physiological parameters is used, this should be stated in the introduction. Reporting the total recording time is also advisable if for some special reason this is significantly shorter or longer than recommended in the American EEG Society Guidelines (MTR, Sec. 7.1).

4. **Description.** *The description of the EEG should include all the characteristics of the record, both normal and abnormal, presented in an objective way, avoiding, as much as possible, judgment about their significance.*

The aim is to produce a complete and objective report that would allow another electroencephalographer to arrive at a conclusion concerning the normality or degree of abnormality of the record from the written report, without the benefit of looking at the EEG. This conclusion could conceivably be different from that of the original interpreter, since it is by necessity a subjective one.

The decription should start with the background activity,[1] beginning with the dominant activity, its frequency, quantity (persistent, intermittent), location, amplitude, symmetry or asymmetry, and whether it is rhythmic or irregular. The

---

This material originally appeared in *J. Clin. Neurophysiol.* 1984;1(2):219–22.

[1] The term "background activity" is used here as defined by the International Federation of Societies of EEG and Clinical Neurophysiology Committee on Terminology (Chatrian GE, et al: A glossary of terms most commonly used by clinical electroencephalographers. *Electroencephalogr. Clin. Neurophysiol.* 1974; 37:538–48).

frequency should be given preferably in Hertz or cycles per second. For the purpose of standardizing the report, while recognizing that any decision on this point must be arbitrary, it is recommended that the amplitude of this activity be determined in derivations employing adjacent scalp electrodes placed according to the 10–20 system. It is desirable but not mandatory that the estimated mean amplitude be given in microvolts. This will obviate the need for defining terms such as "low," "medium," and "high."

Enumeration of nondominant activities with their frequency, quantity, amplitude, location, symmetry or asymmetry, and rhythmicity or lack of it should follow, using the same units as for the dominant frequency.

Response to opening and closing eyes as well as to purposeful movement of the extremities when appropriate, should then be described. The response should be described as symmetric or asymmetric, complete or incomplete, sustained or unsustained.

Abnormal records, infants' records, or records limited to sleep may not have clearly dominant frequencies. In those cases, the different activities with their amplitude, frequency, etc., should be described, in any other. When the record shows a marked interhemispheric asymmetry, the characteristics of each hemisphere should be described separately (i.e., dominant, nondominant frequency, etc., of one hemisphere first, followed by those of the other).

The description of the background activity should be followed by description of the abnormalities that do not form part of this background activity. This should include a description of the type (spikes, sharp waves, slow waves), distribution (diffuse or focal), topography or location, symmetry, synchrony (intra- and interhemispheric), amplitude, timing (continuous, intermittent, episodic, or paraoxysmal), and quantity of the abnormal patterns. Quantity has to be expressed in a subjective fashion, since in clinical, unaided interpretation of the EEG, no exact quantities or ratios can be given.

When the abnormality is episodic, attention should be given to the presence or absence of periodicity[2] between episodes and to the rhythmicity or irregularity of the pattern within each episode. The range of duration of the episodes should be given.

In the description of activation procedures, a statement should be included pertaining to their quality (e.g., good, fair, or poor hyperventilation, duration of sleep, and stages attained). The type of photic stimulation used (i.e., stepwise or glissando) should be stated and the range of frequencies given. Effects of hyperventilation and photic stimulation should be described, including normal and abnormal responses. If hyperventilation or photic stimulation are not done, the reason for this omission should be given. If referring clinicians know that these procedures are used routinely, they may expect results even if they have not been specifically requested.

There is no point in including in the description the absence of certain characteristics, except for the lack of normal features, such as low voltage fast frequencies, sleep spindles, etc. Phrases such as ''No focal abnormality'' or ''No epileptiform abnormality'' have a place in the impression when the clinician has asked for it either explicitly or implicitly in the request form. They have no place in the description.

Artifacts should be mentioned only when they are questionable and could represent cerebral activity, when they are unusual or excessive (eye movements, muscle) and interfere with the interpretation of the record, or when they may provide valuable diagnostic information (e.g., myokymia, nystagmus, etc.).

5. **Interpretation.**

   (a) Impression. *The impression is the interpreter's subjective statement about the normality or abnormality of the record.* The description of the record is directed

---

[2] For definition of ''periodic'' see Chatrian GE, et al. quoted in footnote 1. Acceptance 2 applies in this instance.

primarily to the electroencephalographer who writes it for review at a later date, or to another expert, and should be detailed and objective. The impression, on the other hand, is primarily written for the referring clinician and should, therefore, be as succinct as possible. Most clinicians know that their information will not significantly increase by reading the detailed description, and hence limit themselves to reading the impression. If this is too long and seemingly irrelevant to the clinical picture, the clinician will lose interest and the report of the record becomes less useful.

If the record is considered abnormal, it is desirable to grade the abnormality in order to facilitate comparison between successive records for the person who receives the report. Since this part of the report is largely subjective, the grading will vary from laboratory to laboratory, but the different grades should be properly defined and the definitions consistently adhered to in any given laboratory.

After the statement regarding normality or degree of abnormality of the record, the reasons upon which the conclusion is based should be briefly listed. When dealing with several types of abnormal features, the list should be limited to the two or three main ones; the most characteristic of the record. If all the abnormalities are enumerated again in the impression, the more important ones become diluted and emphasis is lost. If previous EEGs are available, comparison with previous tracings should be included.

(b) Clinical Correlation. *The clinical correlation should be an attempt to explain how the EEG findings for (or do not fit) the total clinical picture. This explanation should vary, depending on whom it is addressed to. More careful wording is necessary if the recipient is not versed in EEG or neurology.*

If an EEG is abnormal it is *indicative* of cerebral dysfunction, since EEG is a manifestation of cerebral function. However, the phrase "cerebral dysfunction" may sound too strong to some and it should be used only when the abnormality is more than mild and when enough clinical information is available to make the statement realistic within the clinical context. Otherwise, a sentence like, "The record indicates minor irregularities in cerebral function," may be appropriate.

Certain types of EEG patterns are *suggestive* of more or less specific clinical entities; a delta focus may suggest a structural lesion in the proper clinical context; certain types of spikes or sharp waves suggest potential epileptogenesis. If the EEG abnormality fits the clinical information containing the diagnosis or the suspicion of the presence of a given condition, it may be stated that the EEG finding is *consistent* with or supportive of the diagnosis.

In EEG reports, the term "compatible with" is frequently found. Strictly speaking, any EEG is compatible with practically any clinical picture. Therefore, the term is not helpful and should not be used.

In cases in which the EEG is strongly suggestive of a certain condition that is not mentioned in the clinical history, it is prudent to mention the fact that such EEG abnormalities are frequently found in association with the clinical condition but are not necessarily indicative of it.

An EEG can be said to be *diagnostic* of a certain condition only in the rare cases in which there is a clinical manifestation present at the time of the recording of an EEG and the record shows an electrical abnormality known to be generally associated with the specific clinical manifestation. Such a case would be one in which a patient presents a typical absence concomitant with a bilaterally synchronous 3/s spike and wave burst.

In situations in which the diagnostic clinical impression seems at odds with the EEG findings, some possible reasons for the apparent discrepancy should be offered in the EEG report. These reasons should be presented cautiously, trying to avoid any impression of criticism of the clinical diagnosis, or to appear apologetic for an apparent failure of the EEG as a supplemental diagnostic test.

If an EEG is abnormal but the abnormal features could be produced, at least in part, by medication or other therapeutic interventions such as recent electroconvulsive treatment, it should be so stated.

Under no circumstances should the electroencephalographer suggest changes in medication or other clinical approaches. However, the clinical correlation statement could be followed by a recommendation pertaining to further EEGs with different added procedures, e.g., "In view of the clinical picture a sleep record could be useful," or "Since the record was taken shortly after a clinical seizure, a follow-up EEG may be helpful in determining whether the slow wave focus present in this record is of permanent or of only transitory nature."

A normal record does not, in general, require further explanation. However, when the clinical information suggests a serious question between two conditions, such as hysteria and epilepsy, a statement should be added that might prevent the clinician from jumping to a wrong conclusion. Such a statement could be: "A normal record does not rule out a convulsive disorder. If the clinical picture warrants, a recording with (some type of activation) may be helpful."

Appendix III

CLINICAL AND ELECTROENCEPHALIC CLASSIFICATION OF EPILEPTIC SEIZURES:
DEFINITION OF TERMS

Each seizure type will be described so that the criteria used will not be in doubt.

Partial seizures

The fundamental distinction between simple partial seizures and complex partial seizures is the presence or the impairment of the fully conscious state.

Operationally in the context of this classification, *consciousness* refers to the degree of awareness and/or responsiveness of the patient to externally applied stimuli. *Responsiveness* refers to the ability of the patient to carry out simple commands or willed movements and *awareness* refers to the patient's contact with events during the period in question and its recall. A person aware and unresponsive will be able to recount the events that occurred during an attack and his inability to respond by movement or speech. In this context, unresponsiveness is other than the result of paralysis, aphasia or apraxia.

(A) Partial seizures

(1) *With motor signs.* Any portion of the body may be involved in focal seizure activity depending on the site of origin of the attack in the motor strip. Focal motor seizures may remain strictly focal or they may spread to contiguous cortical areas producing a sequential involvement of body parts in an epileptic 'march'. The seizure is then known as a Jacksonian seizure. Consciousness is usually preserved; however, the discharge may spread to those structures whose participation is likely

---

Adapted from *Epilepsia*, 1981, 22: 489–501. © 1981 The International League Against Epilepsy.

to result in loss of consciousness and generalized convulsive movements. Other focal motor attacks may be versive with head turning to one side, usually contraversive to the discharge. If speech is involved, this is either in the form of speech arrest or occasionally vocalization. Occasionally a partial dysphasia is seen in the form of epileptic pallilalia with involuntary repetition of a syllable or phrase.

Following focal seizure activity, there may be a localized paralysis in the previously involved region. This is known as Todd's paralysis and may last from minutes to hours.

When focal motor seizure activity is continuous it is known as epilepsia partialis continua.

(2) *Seizures with autonomic symptoms* such as vomiting, pallor, flushing, sweating, piloerection, pupil dilatation, boborygmi, and incontinence may occur as simple partial seizures.

(3) *With somatosensory or special sensory symptoms.* Somatosensory seizures arise from those areas of cortex subserving sensory function, and they are usually described as pins-and-needles or a feeling of numbness. Occasionally a disorder of proprioception or spatial perception occurs. Like motor seizures, somatosensory seizures also may march and also may spread at any time to become complex partial or generalized tonic-clonic seizures as in A.1 of Table 16.1. Special sensory seizures include visual seizures varying in elaborateness and depending on whether the primary or association areas are involved, from flashing lights to structured visual hallucinatory phenomena, including persons, scenes, etc. (see A.4.f., Table 16.1). Like visual seizures, auditory seizures may also run the gamut from crude auditory sensations to such highly integrated functions as music (see A.4.f., Table 16.1). Olfactory sensations, usually in the form of unpleasant odors, may occur.

Gustatory sensations may be pleasant or odious taste hallucinations. They vary in elaboration from crude (salty, sour, sweet, bitter) to sophisticated. They are frequently described as 'metallic'.

TABLE 16.1
Proposal for revised seizure classification*

I. Partial (focal, local) seizures

Partial seizures can be classified into one of the following three fundamental groups:

A. Simple partial seizures
B. Complex partial seizures
    1. With impairment of consciousness at onset
    2. Simple partial onset followed by impairment of consciousness
C. Partial seizures evolving to generalized tonic-clonic convulsions (GTC)
    1. Simple evolving to GTC
    2. Complex evolving to GTC (including those with simple partial onset)

Clinical seizure type	EEG seizure type	EEG interictal expression
A. *Simple partial seizures* (consciousness not impaired)	Local contralateral discharge starting over the corresponding area of cortical representation (not always recorded on the scalp)	Local contralateral discharge
1. With motor signs (a) Focal motor without march (b) Focal motor with march (Jacksonian) (c) Versive (d) Postural (e) Phonatory (vocalization or arrest of speech)		
2. With somatosensory or special-sensory symptoms (simple hallucinations, e.g., tingling, light flashes, buzzing) (a) Somatosensory (b) Visual (c) Auditory (d) Olfactory (e) Gustatory (f) Vertiginous		

* Adapted from Epilepsia, 22: 498–501, 1981.

TABLE 16.1 *(continued)*

Clinical seizure type	EEG seizure type	EEG interictal expression

3. With autonomic symptoms or signs (including epigastric sensation, pallor, sweating, flushing, piloerection and pupillary dilatation)

4. With psychic symptoms (disturbance of higher cerebral function). These symptoms rarely occur without impairment of consciousness and are much more commonly experienced as complex partial seizures
   (a) Dysphasic
   (b) Dysmnesic (e.g., déjà-vu)
   (c) Cognitive (e.g., dreamy states, distortions of time sense)
   (d) Affective (fear, anger, etc.)
   (e) Illusions (e.g., macropsia)
   (f) Structured hallucinations (e.g., music, scenes)

Clinical seizure type	EEG seizure type	EEG interictal expression

B. *Complex partial seizures* (with impairment of consciousness; may sometimes begin with simple symptomatology)
 1. Simple partial onset followed by impairment of consciousness
   (a) With simple partial features (A.1.–A.4.) followed by impaired consciousness
   (b) With automatisms
 2. With impairment of consciousness at onset
   (a) With impairment of consciousness only
   (b) With automatisms
	Unilateral or frequently bilateral discharge, diffuse or focal in temporal or frontotemporal regions	Unilateral or bilateral generally asynchronous focus; usually in the temporal or frontal regions

TABLE 16.1 *(continued)*

Clinical seizure type	EEG seizure type	EEG interictal expression
C. *Partial seizures evolving to secondarily generalized seizures* (This may be generalized tonic-clonic, tonic, or clonic) 1. Simple partial seizures (A) evolving to generalized seizures 2. Complex partial seizures (B) evolving to generalized seizures 3. Simple partial seizures evolving to complex partial seizures evolving to generalized seizures	Above discharges become secondarily and rapidly generalized	

II. Generalized seizures (convulsive or nonconvulsive)

Clinical seizure type	EEG seizure type	EEG interictal expression
A. 1. *Absence seizures*	Usually regular and symmetrical 3 Hz but may be 2–4 Hz spike-and-slow-wave complexes and may have multiple spike-and-slow-wave complexes. Abnormalities are bilateral	Background activity usually normal although paroxysmal activity (such as spikes or spike-and-slow-wave complexes) may occur. This activity is usually regular and symmetrical
(a) Impairment of consciousness only (b) With mild clonic components (c) With atonic components		

595

TABLE 16.1 *(continued)*

Clinical seizure type	EEG seizure type	EEG interictal expression
(d) With tonic components (e) With automatisms (f) With autonomic components (b through f may be used alone or in combination)		
2. *Atypical absence*	EEG more heterogeneous; may include irregular spike-and-slow-wave complexes, fast activity or other paroxysmal activity. Abnormalities are bilateral but often irregular and asymmetrical	Background usually abnormal; paroxysmal activity (such as spikes or spike-and-slow-wave complexes) frequently irregular and asymmetrical
May have: (a) Changes in tone that are more pronounced than in A.1 (b) Onset and/or cessation that is not abrupt		
B. *Myoclonic seizures* Myoclonic jerks (single or multiple)	Polyspike and wave, or sometimes spike and wave or sharp and slow waves	Same as ictal
C. *Clonic seizures*	Fast activity (10 c/sec or more) and slow waves; occasional spike-and-wave patterns	Spike-and-wave or polyspike-and-wave discharges
D. *Tonic seizures*	Low voltage, fast activity or a fast rhythm of 9–10 c/sec or more decreasing in frequency	More or less rhythmic discharges of sharp and slow waves, sometimes asymmetri-

TABLE 16.1 *(continued)*

Clinical seizure type	EEG seizure type	EEG interictal expression
	and increasing in amplitude	cal. Background is often abnormal for age
E. *Tonic-clonic seizures*	Rhythm at 10 or more c/sec decreasing in frequency and increasing in amplitude during tonic phase, interrupted by slow waves during clonic phase	Polyspike and waves or spike and wave, or, sometimes, sharp and slow wave discharges
F. *Atonic seizures* (Astatic) (combinations of the above may occur, e.g., B and F, B and D)	Polyspikes and wave or flattening or low-voltage fast activity	Polyspikes and slow wave

III. Unclassified epileptic seizures

Includes all seizures that cannot be classified because of inadequate or incomplete data and some that defy classification in hitherto described categories. This includes some neonatal seizures, e.g., rhythmic eye movements, chewing, and swimming movements.

IV. Addendum

Repeated epileptic seizures occur under a variety of circumstances:

1. as fortuitous attacks, coming unexpectedly and without any apparent provocation; 2. as cyclic attacks, at more or less regular intervals (e.g., in relation to the menstrual cycle, or the sleep-waking cycle); 3. as attacks provoked by: (a) nonsensory factors (fatigue, alcohol, emotion, etc.), or (b) sensory factors, sometimes referred to as 'reflex seizures'.

Prolonged or repetitive seizures (status epilepticus). The term 'status epilepticus' is used whenever a seizure persists for a sufficient length of time or is repeated frequently enough that recovery between attacks does not occur. Status epilepticus may be divided into partial (e.g., Jacksonian), or generalized (e.g., absence status or tonic-clonic status). When very localized motor status occurs, it is referred to as epilepsia partialis continua.

Vertiginous symptoms include sensations of falling in space, floating, as well as totatory vertigo in a horizontal or vertical plane.

(4) *With psychic symptoms* (disturbance of higher cerebral function). These usually occur with impairment of consciousness (i.e., complex partial seizures).

(a) *Dysphasia.* This was referred to earlier.

(b) *Dysmnesic symptoms.* A distorted memory experience such as distortion of the time sense, a dreamy state, a flashback, or a sensation as if a naive experience had been experienced before, known as déjà vu, or as if a previously experienced sensation had not been experienced, known as jamais-vu, may occur. When this refers to auditory experiences these are known as déjà-entendu or jamais-entendu. Occasionally as a form of forced thinking, the patient may experience a rapid recollection of episodes from his past life, known as panoramic vision.

(c) *Cognitive disturbances* may be experienced. These include dreamy states; distortions of the time sense; sensations of unreality, detachment, or depersonalization.

(d) *With affective symptomatology.* Sensation of extreme pleasure or displeasure, as well as fear and intense depression with feelings of unworthiness and rejection may be experienced during seizures. Unlike those of psychiatrically induced depression, these symptoms tend to come in attacks lasting for a few minutes. Anger or rage is occasionally experienced, but unlike temper tantrums, epileptic anger is apparently unprovoked, and abates rapidly. Fear or terror is the most frequent symptom; it is sudden in onset, usually unprovoked, and may lead to running away. Associated with the terror, there are frequently objective signs of autonomic activity, including pupil dilatation, pallor, flushing, piloerection, palpitation, and hypertension.

Epileptic or gelastic seizure laughter should not, strictly speaking, be classed as an affective symptom because the laughter is usually without affect and hollow. Like other forms of pathological laughter it is often unassociated with true mirth.

(e) *Illusions.*   These take the form of distorted perceptions in which objects may appear deformed. Polyoptic illusions such as monocular diplopia, distortions of size (macropsia or micropsia) or of distance may occur. Similarly, distortions of sound, including microacusia and macroacusia, may be experienced. Depersonalization, as if the person were outside his body, may occur. Altered perception of size or weight of a limb may be noted.

(f) *Structured hallucinations.*   Hallucinations may occur as manifestations or perceptions without a corresponding external stimulus and may affect somatosensory, visual, auditory, olfactory, or gustatory senses. If the seizure arises from the primary receptive area, the hallucination would tend to be rather primitive. In the case of vision, flashing lights may be seen; in the case of auditory perception, rushing noises may occur. With more elaborate seizures involving visual or auditory association areas with participation of mobilized memory traces, formed hallucinations occur and these may take the form of scenery, persons, spoken sentences, or music. The character of these perceptions may be normal or distorted.

(B) Seizures with complex symptomatology

Automatisms.   These may occur during both complex partial and absence seizures. In the *Dictionary of Epilepsy* (Gastaut, 1973), automatisms are described as more or less coordinated adapted (eupractic or dyspractic) involuntary motor activity occurring during the state of clouding of consciousness either in the course of, or after an epileptic seizure, and usually followed by amnesia for the event. The automatism may be simply a continuation of an activity that was going on when the seizure occurred, or, conversely, a new activity developed in association with the ictal impairment of consciousness. Usually, the activity is commonplace in nature, often provoked by the subject's environment, or by his sensations during the seizure; exceptionally, fragmentary, primitive, infantile, or antisocial behavior is seen. From a symptomatological point of view the following are distinguished: (a) eating automatisms (chewing, swallowing); (b) automatisms of mimicry, expressing the subject's emotional state (usually of fear) during the seizure; (c) gestural automatisms, crude or elaborate; directed toward either the subject or his environment; (d) ambulatory automatisms; (e) verbal automatisms.

Automatisms may also occur as a postictal phenomenon, particularly following tonic-clonic seizures, and are usually associated with confusion.

Ambulatory seizures again may occur either as prolonged automatisms of absence, particularly prolonged absence continuing, or of complex partial seizures. In the latter, a patient may occasionally continue to drive a car, although may contravene traffic light regulations.

There seems to be little doubt that automatisms are a common feature of different types of epilepsy. While they do not lend themselves to simple anatomic interpretation, they appear to have in common a discharge involving various areas of the limbic system. Crude and elaborate automatisms do occur in patients with absence as well as complex partial seizures. The EEG is of cardinal localizational importance here.

Drowsiness or somnolence implies a sleep state from which the patient can be aroused to make appropriate motor and verbal responses. In stupor, the patient may make some spontaneous movement and can be aroused by painful or other vigorously applied stimuli to make avoidance movements. The patient in confusion makes inappropriate responses to his environment and is disoriented as regards place or time or person.

Aura. The aura is that portion of the seizure which occurs before consciousness is lost and for which memory is retained afterwards. It may be that, as in simple partial seizures, the aura is the whole seizure. Where consciousness is subsequently lost, the aura is, in fact, the signal symptom of a complex partial seizure.

An aura is a retrospective term which is described after the seizure is ended.

Generalized seizures

(A) *Absence seizures*

The hallmark of the absence attack is a sudden onset, interruption of ongoing activities, a blank stare, possibly a brief upward rotation of the eyes. If the patient is speaking, speech is slowed or interrupted; if walking, he stands transfixed; if eating, the food will stop on its way to the mouth. Usually the patient will be unresponsive when spoken to. In some, attacks are aborted when the patient is spoken to. The attack lasts from a few seconds to half a minute and evaporates as rapidly as it commenced.

(1) *Absence with impairment of consciousness only.* The above description fits the description of absence simple in which no other activities take place during the attack.

(2) *Absence with mild clonic components.* Here the onset of the attack is indistinguishable from the above, but clonic movements may occur in the eyelids, at the corner of the mouth, or in other muscle groups which may vary in severity from almost imperceptible movements to generalized myoclonic jerks. Objects held in the hand may be dropped.

(3) *Absence with atonic components.* Here there may be a diminution in tone of muscles subserving posture as well as in the limbs leading to drooping of the head, occasionally slumping of the trunk, dropping of the arms, and relaxation of the grip. Rarely, tone is sufficiently diminished to cause this person to fall.

(4) *Absence with tonic components.* Here during the attack tonic muscular contraction may occur, leading to increase in muscle tone which may affect the extensor muscles or the flexor muscles symmetrically or asymmetrically. If the patient is stan-

ding the head may be drawn backward and the trunk may arch. This may lead to retropulsion. The head may tonically draw to one or another side.

(5) *Absence with automatisms.* (See also prior discussion on automatisms.) Purposeful or quasipurposeful movements occurring in the absence of awareness during an absence attack are frequent and may range from lip licking and swallowing to clothes fumbling or aimless walking. If spoken to the patient may grunt or turn to the spoken voice and when touched or tickled may rub the site. Automatisms are quite elaborate and may consist of combinations of the above-described movements or may be so simple as to be missed by casual observation. Mixed forms of absence frequently occur.

(B) *Tonic-clonic seizures*

The most frequently encountered of the generalized seizures are the generalized tonic-clonic seizures, often known as grand mal. Some patients experience a vague ill-described warning, but the majority lose consciousness without any premonitory symptoms. There is a sudden sharp tonic contraction of muscles, and when this involves the respiratory muscles there is stridor, a cry or moan, and the patient falls to the ground in the tonic state, occasionally injuring himself in falling. He lies rigid, and during this stage tonic contraction inhibits respiration and cyanosis may occur. The tongue may be bitted and urine may be passed involuntarily. This tonic stage then gives way to clonic convulsive movements lasting for a variable period of time. During this stage small gusts of grunting respiration may occur between the convulsive movements, but usually the patient remains cyanotic and saliva may froth from the mouth. At the end of this stage, deep respiration occurs and all the muscles relax, after which the patient remains unconscious for a variable period of time and often awakes feeling stiff and sore all over. He then frequently goes into a deep sleep and when he awakens feels quite well apart from soreness and frequently headache.

Generalized tonic-clonic convulsions may occur in childhood and in adult life; they are not as frequent as absence seizures, but vary from one a day to one every three months and occasionally to one every few years.

Very short attacks without postictal drowsiness may occur on occasion.

Myoclonic seizures

Myoclonic jerks (single or multiple) are sudden, brief, shock-like contractions which may be generalized or confined to the face and trunk or to one or more extremities or even to individual muscles or groups of muscles. Myoclonic jerks may be rapidly repetitive or relatively isolated. They may occur predominantly around the hours of going to sleep or awakening from sleep. They may be exacerbated by volitional movement (action myoclonus). At times they may be regularly repetitive.

Many instances of myoclonic jerks and action myoclonus are not classified as epileptic seizures. The myoclonic jerks of myoclonus due to spinal cord disease, dyssynergia cerebellaris myoclonica, subcortical segmental myoclonus, paramyoclonus multiplex, and opsoclonus-myoclonus syndrome must be distinguished from epileptic seizures.

Clonic seizures

Generalized convulsive seizures occasionally lack a tonic component and are characterized by repetitive clonic jerks. As the frequency diminishes the amplitude of the jerks do not. The postictal phase is usually short. Some generalized convulsive seizures commence with a clonic phase passing into a tonic phase, as described below, leading to a 'clonic-tonic-clonic' seizure.

Tonic seizures

To quote Gowers, a tonic seizure is 'a rigid, violent muscular contraction, fixing the limbs in some strained position. There is usually deviation of the eyes and of the head toward one side, and this may amount to rotation involving the whole body (sometimes actually causing the patient to turn around, even two or three times). The features are distorted; the color of the face, unchanged at first, rapidly becomes pale and then flushed and ultimately livid as the fixation of the chest by the spasms stops the movements of respiration. The eyes are open or closed; the conjunctiva is insensitive; the pupils dilate widely as cyanosis comes on. As the spasm continues, it commonly changes in its relative intensity in different parts, causing slight alterations in the position of the limbs'.

Tonic axial seizures with extension of head, neck, and trunk may also occur.

Atonic seizures

A sudden diminution in muscle tone occurs which may be fragmentary, leading to a head drop with slackening of the jaw, the dropping of a limb or a loss of all muscle tone leading to a slumping to the ground. When these attacks are extremely brief they are known as 'drop attacks'. If consciousness is lost, this loss is extremely brief. The sudden loss of postural tone in the head and trunk may lead to injury by projecting objects. The face is particularly subject to injury. In the case of more prolonged atonic attacks, the slumping may be progressive in a rhythmic, successive relaxation manner.

(So-called drop attacks may be seen in conditions other than epilepsy, such as brainstem ischemia and narcolepsy cataplexy syndrome.)

Unclassified epileptic seizures

This category includes all seizures that cannot be classified because of inadequate or incomplete data and includes some seizures that by their natures defy classification in the previously defined broad categories. Many seizures occurring in the infant (e.g., rhythmic eye movements, chewing, swimming movements, jittering, and apnea) will be classified here until such time as further experience with video-tape

604

confirmation and electroencephalographic characterization entitles them to subtyping in the extant classification.

Epilepsia partialis continua

Under this name have been described cases of simple partial seizures with focal motor signs without a march, usually consisting of clonic spasms, which remain confined to the part of the body in which they originate, but which persist with little or no intermission for hours or days at a stretch. Consciousness is usually preserved, but postictal weakness is frequently evident.

Postictal paralysis (Todd's paralysis)

This category refers to the transient paralysis that may occur following some partial epileptic seizures with focal motor components or with somatosensory symptoms. Postictal paralysis has been ascribed to neuronal exhaustion due to the increased metabolic activity of the discharging focus, but it may also be attributable to increased inhibition in the region of the focus, which may account for its appearance in non-motor somatosensory seizures.

REFERENCES

Gastaut, H. (1970) Clinical and electroencephalographic classification of epileptic seizures. Epilepsia 11: 102.
Gastaut, H. (1973) Definitions. In: Dictionary of Epilepsy. Part I. World Health Organization, Geneva.
Jackson, J.H. (1931) In: Taylor, J.A. (Ed.), Selected Writings of J. Hughlings Jackson, Vol. I: On Epilepsy and Epileptiform Convulsions. Hodder and Staughton, London.

Appendix IV

GUIDELINES FOR STANDARD ELECTRODE POSITION NOMENCLATURE

as proposed by The American EEG Society

Electrode Position Nomenclature Committee: Dr. Frank Sharbrough, Chairman; Dr. Gian-Emilio Chatrian; Dr. Ronald P. Lesser; Dr. Hans Lüders; Dr. Marc Nuwer; Dr. Terrence W. Picton

INTRODUCTION

These guidelines propose a method for combining a slight modification of the '10–20 System' with a slight modification of a strict combinatorial rule which allows for an extension of the present 10–20 System to designate the 10% electrode positions which are currently unnamed.

The content of this report has the following sections:

1. Desirable characteristics of an alphanumeric nomenclature.
2. Head diagram of proposed modified combinatorial nomenclature.
3. Explanation of the 10–20 nomenclature changes within the modified combinatorial system.
4. Explanation of the deviation from a strict combinatorial nomenclature in the modified system proposed herein.

1. DESIRABLE CHARACTERISTICS OF AN ALPHANUMERIC NOMENCLATURE

   I: The alphabetical part should consist preferably of one but no more than two letters.

  II: The letters should be derived from names of underlying lobes of the brain or other anatomic landmarks.

 III: The complete alphanumeric term should serve as a system of coordinates locating the designated electrode according to the following rules:

   1. Each letter should appear on only one coronal line. (In standard 10–20 terminology, the only outstanding exception to this rule are the 'T' (temporal) names which appear on both the central and parietal coronal lines. For reasons explained in section 3, this exception is replaced by a more consistent terminology within the nomenclature recommended by the Committee. For emphasis, this modification is displayed on the head diagram in section 2 with white lettering on a black background.)

   2. Each number should designate a sagittal line so the same postscripted number identifies all positions lying on that sagittal line. (Again, the only outstanding exception to this rule in the current 10–20 System is in the 'T' numbering. For example, this results in the F7, T3, and T5 designations all appearing on a single sagittal line. This exception is also eliminated within the recommended nomenclature. Once more for emphasis, this modification is displayed in the head diagram in section 2 with white lettering on a black background.)

In the diagram below, the modifications of the current 10–20 terminology, instituted for reasons explained in section 3, are emphasized by displaying them with white lettering on a black background.

MODIFIED COMBINATORIAL NOMENCLATURE

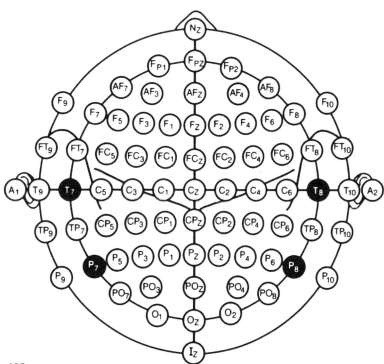

3. EXPLANATION OF THE MODIFICATION OF THE 10–20 NOMENCLATURE WITHIN THE MODIFIED COMBINATORIAL NOMENCLATURE

The modified combinatorial terminology replaces the inconsistent T3/T4 and T5/T6 terms with the consistent T7/T8 and P7/P8. The head diagrams in section 2 emphasize consistency of the terms T7/T8 and P7/P8 by showing them with white lettering on black circles. The value of this becomes evident when inspecting the head diagram which shows that, except for Fp1/Fp2 and 01/02, all electrode positions along the same sagittal line have the same postscripted number and that all electrodes designated by the same letter(s) lie on the same coronal line. Thus, the alphanumeric nomenclature for each electrode specifies its coordinate location within the ten–twenty grid system. Once this is done, the positions *10% inferior* to the standard frontotemporal electrodes are easily designated as F9/F10, T9/T10, and P9/P10, respectively.

As indicated above, the straightforward designation of an electrode's coordinate localization by its nomenclature requires replacement of the inconsistent T3/4 by T7/8, which is a readily understandable modification. A more radical modification replaces T5/6 by P7/8. However, even with this more radical departure, P can easily be recognized as representing Parietal when it is associated with a postscripted number with a value of 6 or less, whereas it can be readily recognized as implying Posterior Temporal if P is associated with a number with a value of 7 or greater.

However, even though T7/8 and P7/8 in the head diagram *emphasize the internally consistent logic* of the system, it would clearly be *an acceptable alternative* to continue to use T3/4 and T5/6 without detracting from the logic of the remaining system.

4. EXPLANATION OF THE DEVIATION FROM A STRICT COMBINATORIAL NOMENCLATURE IN THE MODIFIED SYSTEM PROPOSED HEREIN

The current 10–20 system does not name electrode positions forming the four 10% intermediate coronal lines lying between the five standard coronal lines containing currently named electrode positions. The strict combinatorial system designates the currently unnamed positions by combining the names or letters for the two standard electrode positons that surround a currently undesignated 10% intermediate electrode position.

Thus, positions in the second intermediate coronal line are designated as either the Fronto-Temporal positions (FT) or the Fronto-Central positions (FC), depending on their location as noted in the head diagram.

The electrode positions in the third intermediate coronal line are designated as Temporal-Posterior temporal (TP) or Centro-Parietal (CP) as noted in the figure.

The positions in the fourth and final intermediate coronal line are designated as Posterior temporo-Occipital (PO) or Parieto-Occipital (PO).

The *only proposed deviation* from the strict combinatorial rule discussed above is in naming the first intermediate transverse positions as Anterior Frontal (AF) electrodes rather than Frontopolar-Frontal electrodes. The latter terminology would designate the electrodes with either three letters (FpF) or the same two letters (FF). Since both of these letter designations are undesirable (the first because it uses three letters and the second because it uses the same letter twice), the Committee proposes using the readily understandable Anterior Frontal (AF) designation displayed in the preceding figure.

Once the above letters are assigned to the currently unnamed 10% intermediate positions, then their alphanumeric designation is completed by postscripting the letters assigned to an electrode by the number designating the sagittal line upon which the electrode lies. For example, in the figure AF3, FC3, CP3, and PO3, all lie on the same sagittal line designated by the number 3.

611

When this is done, each new alphanumeric designation not only is directly related to a slight modification of the currently accepted 10–20 terminology but serves as an internally consistent coordinate system which locates each newly designated electrode position at the intersection of a specified coronal (identified by the prefixed letter) and sagittal (identified by the postfixed number) line.

5. EXTENSION OF COMBINATORIAL NOMENCLATURE TO POSITIONS INFERIOR TO THOSE DEMONSTRATED IN THE FIGURES

Positions posterior to electrodes displayed in the ninth and tenth rows would be designated as PO9 (10% inferior to PO7), PO10 (10% inferior to PO8), O9 (10% inferior to O1), and O10 (10% inferior to O2). Electrodes 10% inferior to the ninth row would be designated with the postscripted number 11 (F11, FT11, T11, TP11, P11, PO11, O11) and those 10% inferior to the tenth row would be designated with a postscripted number 12 (F12, FT12, T12, TP12, P12, and O12).

Index of subjects

Readers may also refer to the Glossary of terms most commonly used by clinical electroencephalographers, pp. 519–535.

Italic numbers: the corresponding keyword (or chain of keywords) refers to a headline.

Abnormal
  amount of generalized slow wave in normal
    subjects, 426
  amplitude, 271, 275
    definition, 271
    of alpha rhythm, 495
  asymmetries, 463
  brain function and EEG, *161*
  EEG, *see* EEG abnormalities
  frequency of alpha rhythm, *493*
  posterior sharp waves, 114
  reactivity of the alpha rhythm, 499
  response to hyperventilation, 253
  response to photic stimulation, 261
  slowing of the alpha rhythm, 493
  slow wave patterns, 274
  timing and incidence of sleep patterns, 505
Abscess, *see* Brain abscess
Absence
  atonic, 295
  atypical, 287, 295
  automatic, 295
  complex absence attacks, 295
  mixed forms, 296
  myoclonic, 295
  of alpha rhythm, 488
  of spikes and sharp waves during ictal patterns,
    381
  retropulsive, 295

seizures, 286, 294, 601
simple absence attacks, 295
status, 295
typical, 295
with atonic components, 601
with automatisms, 602
with impairment of consciousness only, 601
with mild clonic components, 601
with tonic components, 601
Absolute
  band amplitude, 135
  peak frequency, 135, 137
Action potential, 8–10
Activation procedures, *251*
  auditory stimuli, 263
  convulsant drugs, *264*
  hyperventilation, *see* Hyperventilation
  patterned visual stimuli, 263
  pentylenetetrazol, *264*
  photic stimulation, 92, 257, 512
  photometrazol test, 264
  reading, 263
  sleep, *255*
  tactile stimulation, 264
Active reference electrode, 72
Activité moyenne, 185, 186
  also referred to as Low voltage irregular pattern
Acute
  alcoholic intoxication, 432

alcohol withdrawal syndrome, 432
focal epileptiform activity, 314
intermittent porphyria, 349, 451
Adolescence, *200*
  alpha rhythms, 200, 204
  cerebral abnormalities, 344
  EEG patterns, 200
  focal epileptiform patterns, 310
  generalized epileptiform activity, 344
  low voltage patterns, 207
  sleep stages, 205
  slow waves, 200
Adults
  of 20–60 years of age
    EEG abnormalities, *225, 238*
    normal EEG, *213*
    sleep EEG, *229*
  over 60 years of age
    EEG abnormalities, *249*
    normal EEG, *243*
    sleep EEG, *247*
Adversive seizures, 292
Agenesis of the corpus callosum, 207, 208
Agyria, 317, 348
Aicardi's syndrome, 207
AIDS dementia complex, 437
Akinetic seizures, 296
Alcohol withdrawal syndrome, 432
Alcoholic intoxication, 432

Aliasing, 129
All-night sleep recording, 236
Alpha
  blocking
    and blindness, 499
    bilateral failure, 499
    unilateral failure in normal subjects, 499
      also referred to as Bancaud's phenomenon
  coma
    pattern, 500–502
    posterior dominant, 501
  frequency band, 168, 196
  rhythm
    absence or decrease of, *488*
    asymmetry, 411, 464, *472*
    attenuation, slowing and disorganization,
      427, 449
    bilateral
      decrease in amplitude, 495, 496
      increase in frequency, 495, 497
    clinical significance of abnormal frequency,
      495
    failure of blocking, 498
    frontal localization, 501
    generalized
      alpha activity, 501
      decrease or absence, *488*
    ictal discharges and slowing of, 497
    in children and adolescents, 200, 204
    in coma or seizure, 227, *501*
    increase, following eye closure, 215
      also referred to as Squeak phenomenon
    non-specific slowing, 497
    normal attenuation, 488
    of abnormal amplitude, 495
    of abnormal frequency, *493*, 495
    of abnormal reactivity, 499

  of adults of 20–60 years of age, *213*
  of adults over 60 years of age, *243*
  paradoxical alpha rhythm, 217, 218
  physiological significance, 219
  postictal slowing, 497
  reactivity in aging, 244, 245
  seizures and EEG activity of alpha frequency,
    501
  selective decrease, 465
  unilateral decrease in frequency, 495
  wave form of alpha activity in adults, 213
  variant
    fast, 217, 219
    slow, 202, 217, 225
  waves, 384
Alternating
  montages, 77
  seizures, 298
Alzheimer's disease, 246, 278
  and alpha rhythm of abnormal frequency, 496
  and epileptiform activity, 316
  and generalized changes in amplitude of EEG,
    484
  and slow waves, 413, 428, 450
Amaurotic familial idiocy, 430
Ambulatory EEG cassette recording, *150*
American EEG Society Guidelines,
  Appendix II, 537
Amount of EEG pattern, 172
Amphetamines, 239
Amplifier
  offset, 140
  technical background, 3, *43*
  see also Filters
Amplification, 45, 50
Amplitude of the EEG, *168*
  abnormalities, 271, 275

  and distance between cortex and recording
    electrodes, 482
  as descriptor of EEG activity, *168*
  asymmetries of, 169, *459*, 466
  changes
    and degenerative diseases, 459, 473, 483
    and encephalopathies, 467, 484
    and infectious diseases, 471, 488
    and Jakob-Creutzfeldt disease, 484
    and psychiatric diseases, 472, 488
    and subdural hematomas, 467, 472, 487
    generalized, 275, *477*, 482, 486
      and Alzheimer's disease, 484
      mechanisms causing, *482*
    lateralized, *459*
    local, *459*, 465
      asymmetry, 275
      mechanisms causing, *465*
      underlying lesions, 465
    of sleep patterns, *490*
    of specific EEG patterns, 481
  decrease
    flattening of the EEG, 193, 488
    generalized
      of alpha rhythm, *488*
      of EEG activity, 346, 383, 483
    ictal, 471, 487
    local, 313, 346, 449, 465
      of background activity, 346
    of all types of activity, 463
    of specific patterns, 481
    pattern of electrocerebral silence, 480
    postictal depression of, 471, 488
    sudden loss of amplitude, 384
    sudden transient decrease, 339
    see also Low voltage EEG
  high and low amplitude EEG patterns

associated EEG abnormalities, *482*
clinical significance, *481*
description, *479*
symmetrical, *477*
underlying mechanisms, *482*
increase, 464, 466
  generalized, of beta rhythm, *489*
  high voltage slow wave pattern, 190, 208
  of beta rhythm, 483
  of EEG patterns, 479, 483
  of specific patterns, 481
of EEG waves, 168
of the alpha rhythm, 216, 245
relative band amplitude, 135
spectrum, 135, 136
see also High voltage
  Interhemispheric asymmetry
Anachronism, 176
Analog to digital conversion, *128*
Analysis methods, *127*
Anoxia, 208, 484
  postanoxic encephalopathy, 350, 434, 454, 485
Anterior slow dysrhythmia, 185, 190, 191, 208
  also referred to as Monorhythmic frontal
    slowing
Antidepressant medications, 239
Anxiety reactions, 489
Aphasic seizures, 291, 322
Apnea, 177
Arceau rhythm, *see* Mu rhythm
Arrhythmical repetitive waves, 166
Artifacts, *105*
  and suspected cerebral death, 102, 560
  automated detection, 145
  cardioballistographic, 113
  definition, 5, 18
  dental filling, 117

detection, 145
dissimilar metals, 117
electrocardiogram, 114, 141
electrode, 118, 121, 360
eye movement, 108, 109, 111, 223
failure to reject, 48
from the equipment, *121*
from the patient, *105*
from the recording electrodes, *121*
from the recording machine, 124
galvanic skin response, 116, 120
glossokinetic, 117, 123
heart beat, 83, 115
hiccough, 360
interference, *119*
intravenous drip, 117
lateral rectus spike, 109
lid flutter, 111
monitoring of extracerebral activity, *80*, 110
movement, 113
muscle, 112
oropharyngeal movement, 117
palatal myoclonus, 117, 122, 123
paper stop, 118
perspiration, 116
pulse wave, 115
respiratory, 84
rhythmic, 360
60 Hz electrical interference, 118
spike-like, 117
sucking, 360
tongue movement, 117
tremor, 113
Ascending reticular activating system, 16
Astatic seizures, 288
Asymmetry, *see* Interhemispheric asymmetry
Asynchronous

generalized slow waves, *421*
  abnormal amount of, 426
  and abnormal frequency of alpha rhythm,
    495
  and bisynchrounous slow waves, 449
  and focal slow waves, 409
  and generalized epileptiform activity, 346
  associated EEG abnormalities, *427*
  clinical significance, 274, *426*
  description, *421*
  ictal, 436
  in normal subjects, *426*
  interhemispheric asymmetry, 462
  normal patterns, 426
  postictal, 436
  underlying mechanisms, *427*
waves, definition, 172
Asynchrony
  during the neonatal period and infancy, 208
  of sleep activity, 473
Atonic
  absences, 295
  seizures, 288, 297, 298, 604
Atypical
  absences, 287, 295
  spike-and-wave complexes, 335
Auditory
  seizures, 291
  stimuli, 263
Augmenting response, 13
Aura, 600
Automated
  artifact detection, 145
  feature extraction, 128
Automatic absences, 295
Automatisms, 293, 599, 602
Autonomic absences, 296

Average reference electrode, 42, 72
Averaging of evoked potentials, 146, 148

Background activity
  descriptors of, 511
  during hyperventilation, 255
  during wakefulness, 194
  interhemispheric asymmetry, 461
  local decrease in amplitude, 346
Bancaud's phenomenon, 499
Barbiturates, 221, 432, 433, 485, 489
Basilar artery migraine, 318
Beilschowsky–Jansky form of ceroid
  lipofuscinosis, 317
Benign
  bilateral epileptiform pattern, 344
  childhood epilepsy with centrotemporal spikes,
    321
    also referred to as Rolandic epilepsy
  epileptiform transients, 76
    of sleep, 390, 395
  intracranial hypertension, 451, 455
    also referred to as Pseudotumor cerebri
  see also Subclinical
Benzodiazepines, 221, 489
Beta
  coma pattern, 501, 503
  frequency band, 168, 203, 219
    and seizures, 501
  rhythms
    generalized increase, *489*
    ictal and interictal, 473
    in adults of 20–60 years of age, *219*
    in adults over 60 years of age, *245*
    in coma and seizures, *501*
    interhemispheric asymmetry, 411, 464, *472*,
      473

normal prominence, 489
  of high amplitude, 483
  persistence, 221
  physiological significance, 221
  posterior, *see* Alpha variant, fast
  reactivity, 219
  widespread, 219
  waves, 384
Bias potentials, 30, 31
Bilateral
  benign epileptiform pattern, 344
  failure of alpha blocking, 499
  independent PLEDs, 371
  massive epileptic myoclonus, 296
  pacemaker for bilateral discharges, 17
  synchrony, 17, 171
    primary, 311
    secondary, 311, 313, 346
Bilaterally synchronous
  generalized slow waves, 495
  periodic lateralized epileptiform discharges,
    see BIPLEDs
  slow waves, *441*
    and focal slow waves, 409, 410
    and generalized asynchronous slow waves,
      427
    clinical correlations, 274, 448
    description, 445, 446
  slow wave pattern description, *443*
  waves, 171
  see also Slow waves
Biocalibration, 43, 91
Biphasic discharge, 339
BIPLEDS, 371
Bipolar montages, *see* Montages
Bisynchronous, *see* Bilaterally synchronous
Blindness

and alpha blocking, 499
  occipital spikes, 397
Blinking, 109
Block montages, 77
Blood
  oxygen saturation, 85
  pressure monitoring, 85
Body temperature monitoring, 85
Brain
  abscess, 278, 323, 419, 471, 473
  death, *see* Cerebral death
  functions and normal EEG, 159, 161
  stem
    lesions, 16, 278
    reticular formation, 16, 347
  surgery, 417, 473
  tumors
    and asymmetries of amplitude, 471, 473
    and epileptiform patterns, 350
    and generalized decrease in amplitude of
      EEG, 487
    and slow waves, 436
    diagnostic value of the EEG, 278
    infratentorial, 455, 497
    pseudotumor cerebri, 451, 455
    supratentorial, 319, 417, 455, 497
Bursts
  fourteen and 6 Hz positive, 205, 388, 391
  suppression-burst pattern, 207, 377, 378
  theta, 183

Cable telemetry, 152
Calibration, *42*
  biocalibration, 43, 91
  guidelines for calibration, 539
  technical standards, 90
Carbon monoxide, 433

Cardioballistographic artifact, 113
Carotid artery occlusion, 416
Cell membrane properties, 9
Central apnea, 177
Centrencephalic
  discharges, 17
  seizures, 346
Centroid, 137
Centrotemporal spikes, 321
Cerebellar
  diseases and lesions, 278
  dyssynergia cerebellaris myoclonica, 348
  fit, 384, 388
Cerebral
  abnormalities
    in adults and adolescents, 344
      underlying focal epileptiform patterns, 310
      generalized epileptiform activity, 344
  blood flow reduction, 278
    see also Stroke
  cortex, 8, 11
  death
    definition, 555
    EEG inactivity, 99, 206, 555
    guidelines for EEG recording, 554
      for telephone transmission of EEG, 99, 572
    pattern of electrocerebral silence, 480
    suspected cerebral death
      and artifacts, 102, 560
      and filtering, 101
      decrease in amplitude of all types of
        activity, 487
      diagnostic value of the EEG, 278
      electrode impedance and placement, 100
      monitoring techniques, 101
      sensitivity of amplifiers, 101, 558
      stimulation of the patient, 102

infarction
  hemispheric infarct, 472
  multiple cerebral infarcts, 415, 435
  see also Stroke
lesions
  and focal slow waves, 406, 407
  cerebellar, 278
  of the brain stem, 16, 278
  perinatal, 414
lipidoses, 317
potential rejection, 49
trauma
  abnormal frequency of alpha rhythm, 496
  and bilaterally synchronous slow waves, 454
  and EEG asymmetries, 468, 473
  and generalized decrease in amplitude of
    EEG, 487
  and generalized epileptiform activity, 350
  early posttraumatic seizures, 318
  late traumatic epilepsy, 319
  posttraumatic epilepsy, 319
  progressive traumatic encephalopathy,
    417, 435, 455
  traumatic seizures, 318
  see also Cerebral lesions
  see also Head injury
Cerebrovascular diseases
  and alpha rhythm of abnormal frequency, 496
  and asymmetries of amplitude, 467, 473
  and epileptiform patterns, 317, 350
  and generalized decrease in amplitude, 485
  and slow waves, 415, 433, 453
  see also Infarction
    Ischemia
    Hematoma
    Hemorrhage
    Migraine

Stroke
Ceroid lipofuscinosis, 321
  see also Beilschowsky–Jansky form
Channel selector switches, 41
Childhood
  benign epilepsy with centrotemporal spikes, 321
  epilepsy with occipital paroxysms, 322
Children
  alpha rhythm, 200, 204
  guidelines for pediatric EEG, 546
  low voltage patterns, 207
  normal EEG, 200
  sleep stages, 205
  slow waves, 200
  standards for pediatric recordings, 96, 546
  see also Infants
Chloral hydrate, 93
Chlorpromazine, 490
Chorea, see Huntington's chorea
  Sydenham's chorea
Chorioretinal lacunae, 207
Chronic
  epileptogenic lesions, 310
  focal epileptiform activity, 315
  headaches, 278
  withdrawal from chronic use of drugs, 349
Classification
  of generalized seizures, 595, 601
  of partial seizures, 591, 593
  of seizures, 281, 283, 284, 290, 591
  unclassified seizures, 288, 289, 296
Clinical
  significance of
    alpha rhythm of abnormal frequency, 495
    asymmetries, 463
    EEG abnormalities, 271
    epileptiform activity, 273

focal epileptiform activity, *307*
focal slow waves, *406*
generalized asynchronous slow waves, *426*
generalized decrease in amplitude of EEG, *483*
generalized epileptiform activity, *339*
high and low amplitude patterns, *481*
slow waves, 274
see also Disorders causing
Clip electrode, 22, 24
Clonic
component in absence, 601
seizures, 287, 296, 603
Closed circuit TV and EEG recording, 151
Coherence functions, 150
Collodian, 88
Coma
alpha coma pattern, 500–502
alpha rhythm in, 227
Atlas of EEG in, 560
beta coma pattern, 501, 503
diagnostic value of the EEG, 277
sleep EEG in comatose patients, 505
spindle coma pattern, 16, 501, 503
theta coma pattern, 501, 503
Comb rhythm, *see* Mu rhythm
Common mode
amplification, 47
rejection, 45
Complex
absence attacks, 295
partial seizures, 285, 289, 292
seizures, 599
Complexes
K, 411
multiple spike, 164
periodic, 370, 373, 383, 427

polyspike, 164, 305
pseudoperiodic, 373
repetitive spike-and-wave, 305
sharp-and-slow-wave, 164, 303, 338
slow spike-and-wave
description, 164, 335, 338
in neonates and infants, 356, 363, 366, 368
spike-and-wave, 164, 303, 333, 335, 338
three Hz spike-and-wave, 332–334, 338, 343
typical spike-and-wave, 333, 343
Compressed spectral array, 142–144
Computer
assisted signal analysis, *127*, 133
averaging of evoked potentials, 146
digitized signal, 130
Conceptual age, 176
Conduction of neuronal potentials
see Volume conduction
Cone waves, 197, 205
Congenital encephalopathies, 430
Continuous
focal irregular delta activity, 411
slow wave pattern, 190, 208
also referred to as High voltage slow pattern
Contraversive seizures, 291
Contusion, *see* Head trauma *and* Cerebral trauma
Convulsant drugs, *264*
Convulsions, 282
hemiconvulsions, hemiplegia and epilepsy syndrome, 323
see also Seizures
Corpus callosum, 207
Cortex to electrode distance, 482
Corticoreticular theory, 347
Costovertebral anomalies, 207
Cranial defects, 468, 470
Cross-correlation, 150

Ctenoids, 391
Curvilinear distortion, 61

Death, *see* Cerebral death
Definition of
abnormal amplitude EEG, 271
artifacts, 5, 18
asynchronous waves, 172
cerebral death, *555*
epilepsy, 282
normal EEG, *157*
seizures, *281*
Degenerative, developmental, and demyelinating diseases
and alpha rhythm of abnormal frequency, 496
and changes in amplitude of EEG, 466, 473, 483
and epileptiform patterns, 316, 348
and slow waves, 413, 428, 430, 450
Déjà-entendu, vu, vécu, 293
Delirium tremens, 432
Delta
brush pattern, 178, 181, 184
frequency band, 168, 208
rhythm
abnormal posterior sharp waves, 114
continuous focal irregular activity, 411
diffuse pattern, 208
frontal intermittent, 411, 442, 443
monorhythmic frontal, 190, 191, 447
occipital intermittent, 447
also referred to as Monorhythmic frontal delta
Rythmes à distance
Projected slow waves
waves, 383, 406
Dementia, 246, 316, 413, 428, 484

see also Alzheimer's disease

Dental filling artifacts, 117

Depolarization, 10–11

Depth
EEG, 18
electrode, 27

Description of
asymmetries, *459*, 511
EEG abnormalities, 511
EEG activity, *163*
EEG record, *509*
instrument settings, general standards, 96
local epileptiform patterns, *300*
local slow wave pattern, *403*
montages, general standards, 95
normal background, 511
sleep EEG abnormalities, 512
see also Amplitude
Distribution
Frequency
Glossary of terms, Appendix I, 519
Persistence
Phase
Reactivity
Repetition
Timing
Wave form

Desynchronization of the EEG, 16, 483

Development of the normal EEG, 175

Deviations from normal EEG patterns in adults, 227

Diagnostic
of epilepsy, 255
of seizures, 262, 277
value of the EEG, *276*, 515
in suspected cerebral death, 278

Differential amplification, 3, 44–47, 48

Diffuse
delta pattern, 208
EEG activity, 169

Digital filtering, 145

Digitized signal, 130

Diphasic waves, 163

Dipole, 75
horizontal, 75, 76
parallel generator, 75, 76

Discrimination, 43, 45, 47

Disorders causing
asymmetries of amplitude, *466*
bilateral increase in the alpha frequency, 497
bisynchronous slow waves, 447, *450*
decrease in frequency of alpha, 496
focal
epileptiform activity, *316*
slow waves, *413*
generalized
asynchronous slow waves, *428*
decrease in amplitude of EEG activity, *483*
epileptiform activity, *348*

Distribution
of electrical activity, *169*
of local epileptiform activity, 303

Dreaming, 234

Dreamy state, 293

Drowsiness, 195, 239, 600
mini-blinks, 231
slow lateral eye movements, 204, 231
small fast irregular eye movements, 231, 233
small fast rhythmic eye movements, 231, 233
see also Paroxysmal hypnogogic hypersychrony

Duration of local epileptiform activity, 303

Dysmaturity, 176

Dysphasia, 598

Dyssynergia cerebellaris myoclonica, 348

Early posttraumatic seizures, 318
also referred to as Traumatic seizures

EEG abnormalities, *271*
associated with
alpha rhythm of abnormal frequency, 495
asymmetries, *464*
bisynchronous slow waves, *449*
focal epileptiform patterns, *311*
focal slow waves, *409*
generalized asynchronous slow waves, *427*
generalized epileptiform activity, *345*
high and low amplitude, *482*
asymmetric patterns, *459*
definition of the abnormal EEG, *271*
description, *269*, 511
deviations from normal patterns, 276, *493*
diagnostic value of the EEG, *276*
during sleep, *238*, 512
during the neonatal period and infancy, *205*
epileptiform activity, 272, *300*, 330
immature patterns, 176, *506*
in adults of 20–60 years of age, 225
in adults over 60 years of age, 249
of low amplitude in normal subjects, 481
pathological and clinical correlates, *272*
slow waves, 274, *403*, *421*, *443*
symmetric patterns of high and low amplitude, *477*

EEG
activity, descriptors, *163*
at different ages, 160
epochs, 138
equipment, *537*
inactivity, 99, 206, 555
also referred to as Silence
see also Cerebral death
interpretation, 514

machine, 3, 4, *39*
    artifacts, 124
    input board, *40*
    paper transport, 63
    writing unit, *60*
    see also Amplifiers
        Calibration
        Filters
    normal EEG, *see* Normal EEG
    patterns, 163
    report, *509*, 516, *583*
    rhythmical EEG activity, 12, *13*-16
    summary, *513*
    technologists and technicians, *563*, *565*, *571*
    writing EEG reports, 516, *583*
EEG recording
    all-night sleep recording, 237
    ambulatory EEG cassette recording, *150*
    analysis methods, *127*
    clinical EEG record, *87*
    for EEG recording in suspected cerebral death, 554, 572
    guidelines, *537*, *540*, 554
    in suspected cerebral death, 99, *554*, 572
    neonatal EEG procedures, 177
    signal storage, *131*
    simultaneous video monitoring, *151*
    sleep EEG, 92, 255, 544
    strategy, 5, *67*, 77
    technical standards, *see* Standards
    telephone transmission, *103*
    with scalp electrodes, *16*
    see also Montages
        Pediatric EEG recording
Electrical field, 69–71, 130
Electrical interference, 119
    in suspected cerebral death, 102

Electrocardiogram artifact, 114, 141
Electrocerebral activity, *see* EEG
Electrocerebral inactivity
    see Cerebral death
Electrocorticogram, 17
Electrodecremental
    pattern, 365
    seizure, 383, 487
Electrodes
    application methods, *21*
    artifacts from the recording electrodes, 121
    clip, 22, 24
    depth, 27
    electrical properties, 27
    electrocorticographic, 26
    epidural, 26
    for pediatric recordings, 96
    guidelines, *538*
    impedance, 28, 29, 89
        for suspected cerebral death, 100
        imbalance, 48
    master selector switch, 41
    materials, 29
    metal disc and cup, 22, 23
    nasopharyngeal, 22, 23, 25
    needle, 22, 24
    nonpolarizable, 31
    placement, *31*
        alphanumeric nomenclature, *608*
        for pediatric recordings, 97
        for suspected cerebral death, 100
        general standards, 96, *607*, 608
        International 10–20 system, 31, 32, 78, 89
        modification of the 10–20 nomenclature, *610*
        modified combinatorial nomenclature, 34, *609*
    polarization, 30, 31

pop, 118, 121, 360
recording, 3, *21*
    distance between cortex and, 482
    electrical properties, *27*
reference, 71, 79
    active, 72
    average, 42, 72
resistance, 29
scalp, *16*, 17, 21
shapes, *21*
sphenoidal, 26
subdural, 26
true anterior temporal, 36
types, 88
see also Interelectrode
    Montage
Electrographic seizure, 303
Electrostatic interference, 119
Embolism
    air, 435, 487
    fat, 435
    see also Stroke
Encephalitis
    and generalized and synchronous abnormal patterns, 436, 488
    and localized or asynchronous abnormal EEG patterns, 323, 419, 471
    diagnostic value of the EEG, 278
    Herpes simplex, 324
    leukoencephalitis, 471
    subacute sclerosing panencephalitis, 324, 375, 377, 437
Encephalopathies
    hepatic, 432, 485
    toxic and metabolic
        and alpha rhythm of abnormal frequency, 496

620

and changes in amplitude of EEG, 467, 484
and epileptiform patterns, 317, 349
and slow waves, 414, 430, 431, 452
and triphasic waves, 163, 377, 380, 411, 446
clinical correlations, 277
Encoches frontales, 185, 190, 191
also referred to as Frontal sharp waves
Epidural electrode, 26
Epidural hematoma, 454
Epilepsia partialis continua, 283, 289, 605
Epilepsy
  and generalized epileptiform activity, 339
  childhood
    benign, with centrotemporal spikes, 321
    with occipital paroxysms, 322
  definition, 282
  diagnosis, 255
  hemiconvulsions, hemiplegia and epilepsy
    syndrome, 323
  idiopathic, 350
  Lafora's inclusion body, 348
  reading, 263, 264
  reflex, 283
  Rolandic, 76
  tactile stimulation and, 264
  television, 263
  traumatic, 319
  Unverricht–Lundborg's myoclonus, 348
  without epileptiform activity, 344
  see also Absence
    Convulsions
    Epileptiform
    Infantile spasm
    Myoclonus
    Seizures
Epileptic
  acquired aphasia, 322

drop attacks 297
  also referred to as Brief atonic seizures
myoclonus, 296
neuron, 314
neuronal aggregate, 314
seizures, *see* Seizures
Epileptiform
  activity, 165, 271, 272
    and asynchronous generalized slow waves,
    346
    and cerebral trauma, 350
    and underlying cerebral abnormalities, 344
    associated with seizures, 339
    basic patterns, 273
    clinical significance, 273, 307, *339*
    descriptors, 300, 320, 511
    during sleep, 255
    generalized, 330, 339, 345, 346, 348
    in neonates and infants, 309
    in patients with seizure history, 307
    in subjects without seizure history, 309
    local, 300, 303, 305, 314–316
    pathological and clinical correlates, 273
    unilateral, 313
    without seizures, 344
  discharges, periodic lateralized, 370, 374
  patterns, 164–166
    description, *300, 330*
    ictal patterns without spikes and sharp waves,
    381
    induced by hyperventilation, 254
    infantile and juvenile, 356
    focal, in adolescents, 310
      and associated EEG abnormalities, 311
      and underlying cerebral abnormalities, 310
      descriptors, 300
    generalized, *329*, 333, 338

    descriptors, *330*
    localized, *299*
    periodic complexes, *370*
    special patterns, *355*
    without proven relation to seizures, *384*
    pseudoepileptogenic patterns, *384*
    spikes, 76
    spikes-and-sharp-waves, 300
    transients, 76
    see also Seizures
      Spikes
Epileptogenic focus, 255, 303
Ethical considerations for telephone transmission
  of EEGs, *571*
Ethosuximide, 310
Evoked potential averaging, 146
Excessive daytime drowsiness, 239
Excitatory postsynaptic potential, 8, 10
Extracerebral activity, *80*, 110
Eye closure, increase in alpha activity, 215
  shut eye waves, 201
Eye movements, 81
  artifacts, 108, 109, 111, 223
  during sleep, 231
  lateral rectus spike, 109
  mini-blinks, 231
  rapid, 195, 234
  slow lateral, 204, 231
  small fast irregular, 231
  small fast rhythmic, 231, 233
Eye position monitoring, 85

Failure to reject artifacts, 48
Fast
  alpha variant, 217, 219
  Fourier transform, 134
  small irregular eye movements, 231

waves, 168, 339
Feature extraction, 128, 144
Febrile seizures, 349
Fever, *see* Hyperthermia
Field of EEG potentials, 73
Filters, *51*
    digital filtering, 145
    for pediatric recordings, 98
    for suspected cerebral death, 101
    frequency, 3
    guidelines for filtering, 542
    high frequency, 51, 58, 90
    low frequency, 51, 53, 90, 542
    notch, 51, 542
    60 Hz, 59, 542
        also referred to as Notch filter
FIRDA, 411, 442, 443
First night effect, 237
Flattening of the EEG, 193, 488
    see also Low voltage patterns
        Cerebral death
Focal
    EEG activity, 170
    epileptiform activity, *300*
        acute, 314
        and bisynchronous slow waves, 449
        and seizures, 307
        associated with asymmetries, 465
        associated with generalized epileptiform
            activity, 345
        chronic, 315
        clinical significance, 273, *307*
        description, *300*
        in adults and adolescents, 310
        in neonates and infants, 309, 311
        in normal subjects, 321
        interictal, 300, 301, 314

        underlying mechanisms, *314*
        underlying specific disorders, *316*
        without known underlying diseases, 321
    ictal discharge, 306
    irregular delta activity, 406, 411
    seizures, *see* Partial seizures
    sharp transients, 311
    sharp waves, 170, 304, 411
    slow waves, *403*
        and asymmetries, 464
        and bisynchronous slow waves, 449
        and cerebral lesions, 406, 407
        and generalized epileptiform patterns, 346
        and seizure disorders, 418
        associated EEG abnormalities, 409
        clinical significance, *406*
        descriptors, 170
        irregular arrhythmical, 406
        localizing value, 408
        underlying cerebral lesion, 406, 407
        underlying specific disorders, *413*
    spikes, 411, 412
    see also Local
        Multifocal
        Partial seizures
Focus
    epileptogenic, 255, 303
    mirror, 316
    secondary, 315
    sharp wave, 303
    slow wave, 404, 405
    spike, 303
    see also Epileptogenic lesion
Forced thinking, 293
Fourteen and 6 Hz positive spikes, 205, 391
    also referred to as Ctenoids
Frequency, *167*

    abnormality of alpha rhythm, 493, 495, 497
    absolute peak, 135, 137
    alpha band, 168, 196
    beta band, 168, 203, 219
    delta band, 168, 208
    domain, 134, 140
    filters, *see* Filters
    limits of low, 57
    mean peak, 135, 137
    of repetitive waves, 167
    spectral edge, 135, 137
    theta band, 168
Frontal
    alpha rhythm, 501
    beta rhythm, 219
    encoches frontales, 185, 190, 191
    intermittent rhythmical delta, (FIRDA),
        411, 442, 443
    monorhythmic delta, 190, 191, 447
    monorhythmic slowing, 185, 208
    sharp transients in infants, 184, 191
    sharp waves, 185, 190

Gain of amplifiers, 50
Galvanic skin responses, 85, 116, 120
Generalized
    abnormal patterns, and encephalitis, 436, 488
    alpha activity, 501
        decrease, 488
    asynchronous slow waves, *421*
        abnormal patterns, 426
        and asymmetries, 462, 465
        and other EEG abnormalities, *427*
        and seizures, 436
        clinical significance, 274, *426*
        normal patterns, 426
        underlying mechanisms, *427*

beta activity increase, 489
bisynchronous slow waves, 346, 465
changes in amplitude, 275, *477*, 482, 486
decrease in amplitude of EEG activity, 346, 383
   and cerebral trauma, 487
   or absence of alpha rhythm, 488
   underlying specific disorders, *483*
epileptiform activity, *329*, 427
   and cerebral trauma, 350
   and thalamus, 347
   associated with asymmetries, 465
   association with other EEG abnormalities, *345*
   clinical significance, 273, *339*
   corticoreticular theory, 347
   description, *330*
   ictal, 338
   in adolescents, 344
   in normal subjects, 350
   interictal, 311, 333
   underlying mechanisms, *346*
   underlying specific disorders, *348*
   widespread lasting structural damage, 345
   without known underlying diseases, 350
flattening, 193
paroxysmal fast activity, 335
periodic complexes, 375
seizures
   classification, 286, *294*, 595, 601
   primarily generalized seizure disorder, 262
   secondarily generalized seizures, 286, 294
   see also Absence
      Akinetic seizures
      Atonic seizures
      Bilateral massive epileptic myoclonus
      Clonic seizures
      Grand mal seizures

      Infantile spasm
      Petit mal seizures
      Tonic seizures
slow waves
   clinical significance, 426
   during hyperventilation, 251
   in infants, 193
   sporadic generalized slow waves, *246*
Generators of the EEG, 7, 8, 75
   dipole, 75
   see also Pacemaker
      Source of the EEG
Gestational age, 176
Glossokinetic artifact, 117, 123
Grand mal seizures, 299
Ground, 42
   connection to the patient, 49
   recordings, 49
Guidelines
   for calibration, 540
   for electrodes, 539
   for EEG recording, *537*
   for EEG recording in suspected cerebral death, *554*, 572
   for filtering, 542
   for hyperventilation, 544
   for montages, 540
   for pediatric EEG, *546*
   for practice in clinical EEG, *563*
   for sensitivity of the EEG equipment, 541
   for standard electrode position nomenclature, *607*
   for standard montages, *573*
   for telephone transmission of EEGs, *569*, 572
   for writing EEG reports, 516, 583
   job descriptions for EEG technologists, *565*
   standard montages to be used in clinical EEG,

   573
Gustatory seizures, 291

Hallucinations, 293, 599
Haloperidol, 433
Headache, *see* Migraine
Head injury, 278, 417, 435, 454, 468, 473, 487, 496
   see also Cerebral trauma
Heart beat artifact, 83, 115
   cardioballistographic artifact, 113
   electrocardiogram artifact, 114, 141
   in suspected cerebral death, 102
Hematoma
   epidural, 454
   subdural
      and abnormal EEG patterns, 278
      and changes in amplitude of EEG, 467, 472, 487
      and epileptiform patterns, 318
      and slow waves, 416, 432, 435, 454
      in neonatal period and infancy, 209
   subgaleal, 468
   see also Stroke
Hemiconvulsions, hemiplegia and epilepsy syndrome, 323
Hemispherectomy, 417, 468
Hemispheric infarct, 472
   see also Interhemispheric asymmetry
Hemorrhage, *see* Stroke
Hepatic encephalopathy, 432, 485
Hereditary predisposition, 347
Herpes simplex encephalitis, 324
HHE syndrome, 323
High amplitude, *see* Amplitude
High frequency filter, 51, 58, 90
High voltage slow wave pattern, 190, 208

Holoprosencephaly, 317, 348, 414, 466
Horizontal dipole, 75, 76
Huntington's chorea, 278, 429, 483
Hydrocephalus, 208, 317, 414, 429
    normal pressure, 414
Hyperthermia, 436, 456, 485, 497
    febrile seizures, 349
Hyperthyroidism, 489, 497
Hyperventilation, 92, 95, *251–253*, 511
    abnormal responses, 253
    and epileptiform patterns, 254
    and slow waves, 254
    asymmetric response, 254, 255
    asymmetry of background activity, 255
    guidelines, 544
    incidence and intensity, 253
    in Moya Moya disease, 254, 454
    prolonged response, 254
    see also Activation procedures
Hypnogogic hypersynchrony, 195, 204
    paroxysmal, 392, 393, 397
Hypnotics, 490
Hypoglycemia, 116, 253, 254, 445
Hypoparathyroidism, 485, 490
Hypothermia, 484
Hypothyroidism, 485, 490
Hypsarrhythmia, 335, 356, 362, *363–365*, 383
    modified, 365

Ictal
    asynchronous generalized slow waves, 436
    beta rhythms, 473
    bisynchronous slow waves, 456
    decrease in amplitude of EEG, *see*
        Electrodecremental seizure
    discharges and alpha rhythm slowing, 497
    focal epileptiform discharges, 306, 314

generalized asynchronous slow waves, 436
generalized epileptiform patterns, 338
generalized slow waves, 383
local epileptiform activity, 300, 305
local slow waves, 383
patterns, 165
    associated with hypsarrhythmia, 365
    in premature and full-term infants, 358
    without spikes and sharp waves, *381, 382*
    see also Interictal
        Postictal
Idiopathic epilepsy, 350
Illusions, 598
Immature EEG patterns, *506*
Impedance of electrodes, *see* Electrodes
Infantile spasm, 207, 296, 364–366
Infants
    epileptiform activity, 309
    epileptiform patterns, 356
    focal epileptiform patterns, 309, 311
    from full term to 3 months of age, *191*
    from 3 months to 12 months of age, *193*
    from premature to the age of 19 years, *175*
    frontal sharp transients, 191
    ictal patterns, 358
    major EEG abnormalities, *200*
    multifocal independent spikes, *363*
    neonatal normal EEG, *175*
    normal EEG patterns, 192
    of 38 to 42 weeks of age, 185
    patterns of hypsarrhythmia, *363*
    sleep EEG, 188, 189
    sleep stages, 195, 197, 205
    slow spike-and-wave discharges, *363*
    see also Childhood
        Children
        Pediatric EEG recording

Premature
Infarction, *see* Stroke
Infectious diseases
    and alpha rhythm of abnormal frequency, 497
    and changes in amplitude of EEG, 471, 488
    and epileptiform patterns, 323, 351
    and periodic patterns
        PLEDs, 370, 371
        subacute sclerosing panencephalitis, 324, 375,
            377, 437
    and slow waves, 419, 436, 456
Infratentorial tumors, 455, 497
Inhibitory
    motor seizures, 291
    postnaptic potential, 8, 10
Input
    board, *40*
    selector switches, *41*
Instrumental phase reversal, 69
Intensive care unit monitoring, 144
Interelectrode
    distances, 72, 90
        for suspected cerebral death, 101, 557
    impedance, 556
Interference, *119*
Interhemispheric
    asymmetry, *459*
        associated EEG abnormalities, *464*
        clinical significance, *463*
        description, *459*
        during hyperventilation, 255
        during neonatal period and infancy, 208, 309
        in adults over 60 years of age, 249
        of alpha rhythm, 411, 464, *472*
        of asynchronous generalized slow waves, 462
        of background activity, 461, 463
        of beta rhythm, 411, 464, *472*, 473

of generalized asynchronous slow waves, 462
of K complexes, 411
of mu rhythm, 411, *472*, 473
of seizure disorders, 471
of sleep spindles, 411
of vertex waves, 411
underlying mechanisms, *465*
underlying specific disorders, *466*
see also Hemiconvulsion
    Lateralized
    Local
    Unilateral
synchrony, 181
see also Bilateral synchrony
    Bilaterally synchronous
    Generalized bisynchronous
    Synchronous waves
Interictal
  beta rhythms, 473
  bisynchronous slow waves, 456
  epileptiform activity, 165
  focal epileptiform activity, 300, 301, 314
  generalized asynchronous slow waves, 436
  generalized epileptiform patterns, 311, 333
  specific localized epileptiform patterns, 303
Intermittent
  rhythmic delta activity
    frontal, 411, 442, 443
    occipital, 447
  spikes, 335
  temporal slow waves, 246
International Classification of Seizures, 591
International 10–20 system, 31, 32, 78, 89
Intoxication, 433, 485
  see also Alcohol
    Encephalopathies
Intracranial hemorrhage, *see* Stroke

Intraventricular hemorrhage, *see* Stroke
Ischemic attack, 282, 415, 433, 453, 467
Isoelectric pattern, 206
  also referred to as Electrocerebral inactivity
Isopotential lines, 75

Jacksonian seizures, 291
Jakob–Creutzfeldt disease, 278
  and changes in amplitude of EEG, 484
  and epileptiform patterns, 316, 348, 375
  and slow waves, 414, 429
Jamais vu, 293

Kappa rhythm, *224*
K complexes, 198, 231, 234
Kindling phenomenon, 316
Kleine–Levin syndrome, 457
Korsakoff's psychosis, 432
Krabbe's disease, 430

Labelling and editing
  the EEG record, 93
  the pediatric EEG record, 98
Lacunar state, 435
Lafora's inclusion body epilepsy, 348
Lambda waves, 194, *223*, 225
Landau–Kleffner syndrome of acquired epileptic
  aphasia, 322
Late traumatic epilepsy, 319
Lateral
  rectus spike, 109
  slow eye movements, 204, 231
Lateralized
  changes in amplitude, 459
  EEG activity, 170
  periodic epileptiform discharges, 370, 374
    also referred to as PLEDs

Length of the EEG recording, 91, 98
Lennox–Gastaut syndrome, 363, 367
Lesions
  brain stem, 16, 278
  cerebellar, 278
  chronic epileptogenic, 310
  underlying
    bisynchronous slow waves, 447
    focal slow waves, 406
    local changes in amplitude, 465
  see also Cerebral lesions
    Cerebral trauma
Leukodystrophies, 430
Leukoencephalitis, 471
Leukoencephalopathy, 419, 437, 471, 488
Limits of low frequency, 57
Lithium intoxication, 377
Local
  abnormal EEG patterns and encephalitis,
    323, 419, 471
  amplitude abnormalities, 313, 346, 449, 465
  asymmetry, 275
  changes in amplitude, 459, 465
  decrease in amplitude of background activity,
    346
  epileptiform activity
    clinical correlations, 314–316
    description, *300*, 301, 303, 305
    patterns, *299*
  ictal slow waves, 383
  reduction of amplitude, 313, 346
  slow waves, 274, 313, 383, 403
  specific ictal epileptiform patterns, 305
  specific interictal epileptiform patterns, 303
  see also Focal
    Partial
    Unilateral

Localized, *see* Local
Localizing value of focal slow waves, 408
Longitudinal bipolar montages, 79, 89
Low
    frequency filter, 51, 53, 57, 90, 542
    voltage
        associated EEG abnormalities, 482
        clinical significance, 481
        fast activity, 225, 384
        in adults of 20–60 years of age, *225*
        in adults over 60 years of age, 249
        in children and adolescents, 207, 481

Master electrode selector switch, 41
Mean
    peak frequency, 135, 137
    sleep latency, 239
Mechanisms causing
    alpha rhythm of abnormal frequency, 495
    bisynchronous slow waves, *450*
    focal
        epileptiform activity, *314*
        slow waves, *413*
    generalized
        asynchronous slow waves, *427*
        changes in amplitude, *482*
        epileptiform activity, *346*
    local changes in amplitude, *465*
Meningitis, 323, 419, 436, 456, 488
Mental retardation, 365
Mesencephalic reticular formation, 14
Metabolic encephalopathies, *see* Encephalopathies
Metachromatic leukodystrophy, 430
Metal disc and cup electrode, 22, 23
Microcephaly, 484
Microgyria, 317, 348
Midbrain strokes, 434

Migraine attack, 278, 416, 435, 468, 472
Mini-blinks, 231
Minimum technical standards, *see* Guidelines
Mirror focus, 316
Modified '10–20' system, 34, 36
Monitoring
    of extracerebral activity, *80*
    techniques for suspected cerebral death, 101
Monorhythmic
    frontal delta, 190, 191, 447
    frontal slowing, 185, 208
Montages, *76*, *573*
    alternating, 77
    bipolar, *69*
        longitudinal, 79, 89, 577
        transverse, 79, 89, 578
    block, 77
    for monitoring of extracerebral activity, *80*
    for pediatric recordings, 97
    general standards, 89, 95
    guidelines for, 540, *573*
    referential, 70, 71, 78, 79, 89, 580
    reformatting, 145
    specific, *76*, 77
    standard, in clinical EEG, 573
    transverse bipolar, 578
Movement
    artifacts, *see* Artifacts
    monitoring, 84
    of eyes, *see* Eye movements
Moya Moya disease, 254, 454
  in children, 454
Multichannel recording, *67*
Multifocal
    independent spikes, 356, *363*, 367, 372
    progressive leukoencephalopathy, 419, 437, 471, 488

sharp transients, 183, 185, 190, 191, 355
Multiple
    cerebral infarcts, 415, 435
    sclerosis, 414, 430, 452, 467, 484
    sleep latency test, 239
    spike complexes, 164
    spike-and-slow-wave complexes, 164
    see also Polyspike
Multiplexed signal, 152
Mu rhythm
    and focal slow waves, 411
    asymmetry, *472*, 473
    in childhood and adolescence, 201, 204
    of adults of 20–60 years of age, *222*
    also referred to as Arceau rhythm
        Comb rhythm
        Wicket rhythm
Muscle
    activity monitoring, 84
    artifacts, *see* Artifacts
    tone during sleep, 236
Myoclonic
    absences, 295
    jerks, 296
        also referred to as Bilateral massive
            epileptic myoclonus
    seizures, 287, 603
    see also Photomyoclonic response
Myoclonus
    bilateral massive epileptic, 296
    epileptic, 296
    palatal, 117, 123
    Ramsay Hunt's syndrome, 348
    Unverricht–Lundborg's disease, 348
Myotonic dystrophy, 496

Narcolepsy, 239

Nasopharyngeal electrode, 22, 23, 25
Needle electrode, 22, 24
Negative vertex spike, 193
Neonatal
    asynchrony of EEG, 208
    EEG, *175*, *548*
    EEG abnormalities, *205*
    EEG recording procedures, 177
    epileptiform activity, 309, 311
    premature newborns, 208
    seizures, *355*, 357
    status epilepticus, 359
Neuromuscular blocking agents, 560
Neurosurgery, 455
Nonpolarizable electrodes, 31
Nonspecific thalamic nuclei, 13
Normal
    asymmetries, 463
    attenuation of alpha rhythm, 488
    background EEG, descriptors, 511
    EEG, *157*
        above the age of 60 years, 159
        definition, *157*
        development, 175
        deviations from, 227, 276, 511
        from premature to the age of 19 years, *175*
        of adults, 160, 214, 220
        of adults of 20–60 years of age, *213*
        of adults over 60 years of age, *243*
        of children and infants, 192, 200
        patterns
            asynchronous generalized slow waves, 426
            generalized asynchronous slow waves, 426
            in full-term infants, 192
            in prematurity, 180
        relation to brain function, *159*, *161*
        up to the age of 19 years, 160, 175, 199, 200

full-term infant, sleep EEG, 188, 189
posterior theta rhythms, *224*
pressure hydrocephalus, 414, 429
prominence of beta rhythms, 489
sleep EEG of adults over 20 years, *229*
transients in prematurity, 182
Notch filter, 51, 542
Notched pattern, 392
Number of recording channels
    general standards, 89
    for pediatric recordings, 97
Nyquist theorem, 129

Obstructive apnea, 177
Occipital
    intermittent rhythmic delta activity, 447
    paroxysms in childhood epilepsy, 322
    positive sharp transients of sleep, 205, 229, 233
    rhythms, 194
    spikes of blind subjects, 397
Occult seizures, 361
    also referred to as Subclinical seizures
Olfactory seizures, 291
Operative room monitoring, 144
Optic neuritis, 317
Oropharyngeal movement artifacts, 117
Oversampling a signal, 129
'O' waves, 197
    also referred to as Cone waves

Pacemaker
    for bilateral discharges, 17
    thalamic pacemaker cells, 13, 14
    theory, 12, 15
Pachygyria, 317
Paget's disease, 466
Palatal myoclonus, 117, 123

Paper speed, 91
Paper transport, 63
Paradoxical
    alpha rhythm, 217, 218
    sleep, 234
    slow wave response on alerting stimuli, 504, 505
Parallel generator, 75, 76
Parkinson's disease, 278, 428, 450
Paroxysmal
    childhood epilepsy with occipital paroxysms, 322
    depolarizing shift, 314
    discharges, 166
    generalized fast activity, 335
    hypnogogic hypersynchrony, 392, 393, 397
    pattern, 207, 208
    photoparoxysmal response, 262
    see also Epileptiform activity
        Epileptiform patterns
        Spikes
Partial seizures
    classification, 283, 286, *290*, 591, 593
    complex, 285, 289, 292
    epilepsia partialis continua, 283, 289, 605
    secondarily generalized, 294
    simple, 283, 284, 289
    with affective symptoms, 293, 598
    with autonomic symptoms, 292, 592
    with cognitive symptoms, 292, 598
    with complex symptoms, 292
        see also Automatisms
            Déjà entendu, vécu, vu
            Dreamy state
            Forced thinking
            Jamais vu
    with dysmnesic symptoms, 598
    with elementary symptoms, 290

see also Adversive seizures
  Aphasic seizures
  Auditory seizures
  Contraversive seizures
  Focal motor seizures
  Gustatory seizures
  Inhibitory motor seizures
  Jacksonian seizures
  Olfactory seizures
  Phonatory seizures
  Postural seizures
  Somatosensory seizures
  Versive seizures
  Vertiginous seizures
  Visual seizures
with motor symptoms, 291, 591
with psychic symptoms, 293, 598
with sensory and somatosensory symptoms, 291, 592
see also Focal
Pattern visual stimuli, 263
Pediatric EEG recordings
  electrodes, 96, 97
  filters, 98
  guidelines, 546
  labelling and editing the record, 98
  length of the recording, 98
  montages, 97
  number of recording channels, 97
  standards, 96
Pelizaeus–Merzbacher's disease, 430
Pen alignment and misalignments, 61, 62
Pentylenetetrazol, 264
Perinatal cerebral damage, 414
Periodic
  complexes, 370, 373, 383, 427
  generalized complexes, 375

generalized sharp waves, 375, 376
lateralized epileptiform discharges, 370, 371, 374
  also referred to as PLEDs
sharp waves, 482
slow waves, 383, 482
suppression-burst pattern, 207, 377, 378
triphasic wave pattern, 163, 377, 380, 411, 446
see also Multifocal independent spikes
  Pseudoperiodic
Periventricular leukomalacia, 208
Persistence of a wave or pattern, 172
Perspiration artifact, 116
Petit mal
  seizures, 294
    see also Absence
  status, 338
  typical, 295
  variant, 295, 366
Phantom spike-wave, see Six Hz spike-and-wave discharges
Phase
  instrumental vs. true, 69
  relation between waves, 170
  reversal, 69, 171
Phenothiazines, 433
Phenylketonuria, 430, 489
Phonatory seizures, 291
Photic
  driving, 257, 259
  stimulation, 92, 256, 257, 261, 512
  stimulation for pediatric recordings, 98
Photoconvulsive response, see Photoparoxysmal response
Photometrazol test, 264
Photomyoclonic response, see Photomyogenic response

Photomyogenic response, 258, 261
Photoparoxysmal response, 260, 262
Pick's disease, 428
PLEDS, 370, 371
Polarity of the signal, 45
Polymorphic delta waves, 406
Polyphasic waves, 163
Polyspike
  and sharp waves, 335
  and-slow-wave complexes, 164, 305
  and-wave discharges, 338
  complexes, 164, 305
  see also Multiple spike
Porencephalic cysts, 207
Porencephaly, 317, 414, 466
Positive
  bursts, 388
  fourteen and 6 Hz positive bursts, 205, 391
  occipital sharp transients of sleep, 205, 229, 233
  sharp transients of sleep, 205, 229, 233
  sharp waves in neonates, 208, 357
  spikes, 391
Postanoxic encephalopathy, see Anoxia
Postanoxic myoclonus, 350
Posterior
  alpha coma pattern, 501
  beta rhythm, 219, 221
  dominant alpha coma pattern, 501
  fast alpha variant, 217, 219
  sharp waves, 114
  slow waves of youth, 202
  theta rhythms, 224
Postictal
  asynchronous generalized slow waves, 436
  bisynchronous slow waves, 456
  depression of amplitude, 471, 488
  paralysis, 282, 605

slowing of the alpha rhythm, 497
Postsynaptic potential, 8, 9
Posttraumatic epilepsy, 319
also referred to as Late traumatic epilepsy
Postural seizures, 291
Potentials generated at distant sites, 18
Power, 135
Power spectrum, 132, 134
Premature
  infants, 175, 178
    frontal sharp transients, 184
    ictal patterns, 358
    of less than 29 weeks of age, 179
    of 29 to 31 weeks of age, 181
    of 32 to 34 weeks of age, 183
    of 34 to 37 weeks of age, 183
    sleep EEG, 181, 183
  newborns, 208
Presenile dementia, *see* Dementia
Primarily generalized seizure disorder, 262
Primary
  bilateral synchrony, 311
  reading epilepsy, 263
Progressive
  multifocal leukoencephalopathy, 419, 437, 471, 488
  supranuclear palsy, 429, 452, 490
  traumatic encephalopathy, 417, 435, 455
Projected
  rhythms, 17
  slow waves, 447
Prominence of an EEG pattern, 172
Pseudo-epileptogenic patterns, 323, 344, *384*, 386
  see also fourteen and six per second positive
    spikes, 386, 391
      paroxysmal hypnogogic hypersynchrony,
        386, 392

six Hz 'phantom' spike and slow waves,
  381, 386
small sharp spikes, 386, 395
  also referred to as SSS, benign epileptiform
    transients of sleep; BETS
subclinical rhythmic EEG discharge of adults
  (SREDA), 386, 397, 398
wicket spikes, 386, 395
Pseudohypoparathyroidism, 485
Pseudoperiodic complexes, 373
Pseudotumor cerebri, 455
Psychiatric diseases
  and abnormal EEG patterns, 278
  and changes in amplitude of EEG, 472, 488
  and epileptiform patterns, 282, 324, 352
  and slow waves, 419, 437, 456
Psychogalvanic skin response, 116
Psychomotor variant, 391
Pulse wave artifacts, 115
Pyramidal cells, 11

Qualifications of
  a clinical electroencephalographer, *563*
  EEG technologists and technicians, 561, *563*,
    565, *571*
Quantitative EEG analysis, 127, 133
Quiet sleep in neonates, 181

Ramsay Hunt's syndrome, 348
Rapid eye movements, *see* Sleep stage REM
Rauwolfia derivatives, 433
Reactivity of EEG patterns, *173*
  alpha rhythm and aging, 244, 245
  Bancaud's phenomenon, 499
Reading and reading epilepsy, 263, 264
Recording
  ambulatory EEG cassette, *150*

EEG with scalp electrodes, *16*
electrodes, *21*
methods, 127
multichannel, *67*
strategy, 5, *67*, 77
see also Electrodes
  EEG recording
Recruiting response, 13
Reference electrode, 71, 79
  active, 72
  average, 42, 72
Referential montages, 70, 71, 78, 79, 89
Reflex epilepsy, 283
Regular waves, 163
Rejection
  of cerebral potentials, 49
  ratio, 47
Relative band amplitude, 135
REM stage of sleep, *see* Sleep REM stage
Renal encephalopathy, 485
Repetitive
  spike-and-wave complexes, 305
  waves, 166
Respiratory artifacts, 84
  in suspected cerebral death, 102
Respiratory monitoring, 177
Resting
  potential, 7–9
  wakefulness, 200
Retropulsive absences, 295
Rhythm
  see Kappa rhythm
    Mu rhythm
    Occipital rhythms
    Projected rhythms
Rhythmic
  artifacts, 360

bisynchronous slow waves at 3 Hz, 383
EEG activity, 12, 13–16
midtemporal discharges, 389, 391, 397
repetitive waves, 166
slow waves, 225, 383
subclinical EEG discharge of adults, 394, 396, 397
see also Monorhythmic
Riley–Day's familial dysautonomia, 348
Rolandic spikes, 320, 321
Rythmes à distance, 447

Safety of the patient, 40
Sampling rate, 129
Sawtooth waves, in REM sleep, 234
Scalp
edema, 468
electrodes, 16, 17, 21
Schilder's disease, 414
Schizophrenia, 456
Secondarily generalized seizures, 286, 294
Secondary
bilateral synchrony, 311, 315, 346
focus, 315
reading epilepsy, 264
Sedatives, 489
Seesaw seizures, 296
Seizures
absence, 286, 294, 601
adversive, 292
akinetic, 298
alternating, 298
and alpha rhythm, 227, 501
and beta frequency band, 501
and EEG activity of alpha, beta and theta frequency, 501
and focal epileptiform activity, 307

and focal slow waves, 418
and generalized asynchronous slow waves, 436
and generalized epileptiform activity, 339
aphasic, 291, 322
associated epileptiform activity, 339
atonic, 292, 297, 298, 604
centrencephalic, 346
classification, *see* Classification
complex, 599
complex partial, 285, 289, 292
definitions, 281
diagnosis, 262, 277
electrodecremental, 383, 487
electrographic, 303
febrile, 349
generalized, *see* Generalized seizures
grand mal, 297
Jacksonian, 291
myoclonic, 287, 603
neonatal, *355*, 357
occult, 361
partial, *see* Partial seizures
patients with seizure history, 307
patterns, 165
petit mal, 294
also referred to as Absence
secondarily generalized, 286, 294
seesaw, 298
simple partial, 283, 284, 289
subclinical, 165, 303, 361
subjects without seizure history, 309
tonic, 288, 297, 603
tonic-clonic, 288, 297, 602
also referred to as Grand mal seizures
traumatic and posttraumatic, 318
unclassified, 288, 289, *298*, 604
versive, 291

with complex symptomatology, 599
without epileptiform activity, 344
without relations to epileptiform patterns, 384
see also Ictal
Interictal
Postictal
Status epilepticus
Senile dementia, *see* Dementia
Sensitivity of amplifiers
for pediatric recordings, 97
for suspected cerebral death, 101, 558
guidelines, 541
technical background, 50, 90
Sharp-and-slow-wave complexes, 164, 303, 338
Sharp
transients, 164, 190
focal, 311
frontal, in infants, 184, 191
multifocal, 183, 185, 190, 191, 355
positive, of sleep, 205, 229, 233
vertex, 198, *223*, 225, 230
waves, 164
abnormal posterior, 114
description, 303
focal, 170, 304, 411
frontal, 185, 190
periodic, 375, 376, 482
positive, 208, 357
rhythmic midtemporal discharges, 389, 391, 397
also referred to as Psychomotor variant
see also Epileptiform activity
Spikes and sharp waves
Shut eye waves, 201
Signal
analysis with computer, *127*, *133*
averaging, 146–149

comparisons, 150
digitized, 130
feature extraction, 128, 144
multiplexed, 152
storage, *131*
Silence, *see* Cerebral death
Simple
   absence attacks, 295
   partial seizures, 283, 284, 289
Sinusoidal waves, 163
Six Hz 'phantom' spike and slow waves, 385, 387
Six Hz spike-and-wave discharges, 385, 387
Sixty Hz filter, 59, 542
Skin potential, 116
Skull defect, 111, 468–470
Sleep
   abnormal, 255
   all-night recording, 236
   apnea, 238
   as activation procedure, *255*
   asymmetry and asynchrony of EEG activity,
      473
   benign epileptiform transients of, 390, 395
   cycles, 236, *237*, 238
   deprivation, 255
   EEG
      in comatose patients, 505
      in normal full-term infant, 188, 189
      of adults over 20 years, *229*
      of adults over 60 years of age, *247*
      of premature infants, 181, 183
      recording, 92, 255, 544
      transitional or indeterminate sleep, 183
   EEG abnormalities, *238*
      abnormal timing and incidence of sleep
         patterns, 505
      disorders of sleep cycles, 238, 505

reduction of REM sleep, 505
      short latency of sleep onset, 238, 505
      sleep onset REM periods, 238, 505
   epileptiform activity during, 255
   eye movements during, 231
   mean latency, 239
   multiple latency test, 239
   muscle tone during, 236
   occipital positive sharp transients, 205, 229, 233
   onset, 241, 242
   onset REM periods (SOREMP), 238, 239
   paroxysmal hypnogogic hypersynchrony,
      190, 239, 392, 393, 397
   patterns
      abnormal timing and incidence, *505*
      changes in amplitude, *490*
      major abnormalities, *238*
   REM stage of, 195, 234, 235, 247
      also referred to as Paradoxical sleep
   spikes and sharp waves during, 238
   spindles
      generation, 13, 16
      in adults, 231, 234
      in infants, 193, 198
      interhemispheric asymmetry, 411
   stages
      in adults, *231*, 235
      in children and adolescents, 205
      in infants, 195, 197, 205
   see also Drowsiness
      Narcolepsy
Slow
   alpha variant, 202, 217, 225
   anterior dysrhythmia, 185, 190, 191, 208
   lateral eye movements, 204, 231
   spike-and-wave complexes, 164, 356, *363*, 366,
      368

description, 335, 338
   spike-and-wave pattern, 366, 368
      also referred to as Petit mal variant
waves, 168, *403*, 421, 441
   abnormal amount in normal subjects, 426
   and hyperventilation, 254
   asynchronous generalized, 274, *421*, 462
      and epileptiform activity, 346
      and seizures, 436
      clinical significance, *426*, 427, 428
      in normal subjects, 350
      of low voltage, 482
   bilaterally synchronous, 274, *441*
      and local slow waves, 409, 410
      clinical significance, 346, *447*, 448, 450
      description, *443*, 445, 446
      paroxysmal bisynchronous, 444
      underlying mechanisms, *450*
   clinical correlations, 274
   continuous pattern, 190, 208
   focal, *406*, 407, 409, 413
      and seizures, 418
      localizing value, 408
   focus, 404, 405
   ictal
      asynchronous generalized, 436
      bisynchronous, 456
      discharges and alpha rhythm slowing, 497
      generalized, 383
      local, 383
   in adults, 227
   in adults over 60 years of age, 249
   in children and adolescents, 200
   in periodic complexes, 383
   in sleep EEG of adults, 229
   interhemispheric asymmetry, 462
   interictal

bisynchronous, 456
generalized asynchronous, 436
intermittent temporal, *246*
irregular arrhythmical focal, 406
also referred to as Polymorphic delta waves
local, 274, 313, 383, *403*
of high voltage, 190, 208
paradoxical response on alerting stimuli,
504, 505
pathological and clinical correlates, 274
periodic, 383, 482
posterior, of youth, 202
postictal, 436, 456
projected, 447
rhythmic, 225, 383
sporadic, *246*, 248
Slowing
monorhythmic frontal, 185, 208
of the alpha rhythm, 427, 449, 493, 497
Small fast irregular eye movements, 231, 233
Small fast rhythmic eye movements, 231, 233
Small sharp spikes, 76, 390, 395
also referred to as SSS or benign epileptiform
transients of sleep (BETS)
Small sharp spike pattern, 76, 390, 395
Somatosensory seizures, 291
Somnolence, 600
Source of the EEG, 3, *7*, 17, 75
Special procedures, 93
Specific thalamic nuclei, 13
Spectral
averaging, 138
edge frequency, 135, 137
Sphenoidal electrode, 26
Spike
centrotemporal, in benign childhood epilepsy,
321

description, 164, 303
epileptiform spikes, 76
focal spikes, 411, 412
focus, 303
fourteen and six per second positive, 205, 391
also referred to as Ctenoids
lateral rectus, 109
multifocal independent, 356, 363, 367, 372
multiple spike complexes, 164
negative vertex, 193
occipital, of blind subjects, 397
small sharp spike pattern, 76, 390, 395
Wicket, 164, 395
see also Epileptiform activity
Spikes and sharp waves
during sleep, 238
epileptiform, 300
ictal patterns without, *381*, 382
in EEG of adults, 225
in EEG of adults over 60 years of age, 249
Spike-and-wave
complexes, 164, 303, 333, 335, 338
slow, 164, 335, 338, 356, 366, 368
three Hz, 332–334, 338, 343
typical, 333, 343
Spike-like artifacts, 117
Spindle, 166
coma pattern, 16, 501, 503
sleep spindles
generation, 13, 16
in adults, 231, 234
in infants, 193, 198
interhemispheric asymmetry, 411
Spindle-like activity, 13
Spinocerebellar degenerations, 278
Sporadic slow waves, *246*, 248
Squeak phenomenon, 215

Stages of sleep, *see* Sleep
Standards
EEG equipment, 564
EEG laboratory organization, *564*
for EEG recording, *88*, 90
for pediatric recordings, *96*, *546*
in cases of suspected cerebral death, *99*, 554,
572
instrument settings, 96
job description for EEG technologists, *565*
montages, 89, 95, 573
number of recording channels, 89
of practice in clinical EEG, *563*
placement of electrodes, 96, *607*, 608
qualification of clinical
electroencephalographer, *563*
qualification of EEG technologists, *563*, *571*
telephone transmission of EEGs, *103*, *569*
see also Guidelines
Status epilepticus, 282, 289
Stimulation
of the patient with suspected cerebral death,
102
tactile stimulation and epilepsy, 264
see also Activation procedures
Stokes–Adams attack, 433
Stroke
and epileptiform patterns, 317, 318, 350
and interhemispheric symmetry, 467
and slow waves, 415, 434, 435, 453
diagnostic value of the EEG, 278
hemispheric infarct, 472
Moya Moya disease, 254, 454
multiple cerebral infarcts, 415, 435
subarachnoid hemorrhage, 416, 454, 468
thrombophlebitis, 323, 471
Sturge–Weber syndrome, 317, 348, 466

Subacute sclerosing panencephalitis, 324, 375, 377, 437
Subarachnoid hemorrhage, 416, 454, 468
Subclinical
  rhythmic EEG discharge of adults, 394, 396, 397
  seizures, 165, 303, 361
Subdural
  electrode, 26
  hematomas, 209, 278
    and changes in amplitude of EEG, 467, 472, 487
    and epileptiform activity, 318
    and slow waves, 416, 432, 435, 454
Subgaleal hematoma, 468
Suppression–burst pattern, 207, 377, 378
Supratentorial brain tumor, 319, 417, 455, 497
Suspected cerebral death, see Cerebral death
Sydenham's chorea, 324, 437, 456
Symmetrically high and low amplitude EEG, 477
Synaptic potentials, 8, 9
Synchronous, see Bilaterally synchronous
Syncope, 282, 433, 485

Tactile stimulation and epilepsy, 264
Technical
  background of EEG recording, 1
  requirements, 5
  standards, see Standards
Telephone transmission of EEGs, 103, 569
Television epilepsy, 263
Ten–twenty International System, 31–37
Terminology, Appendix I, 519
Testing the integrity of the recording system, 100
Thalamic
  inhibitory interneurons, 15
  nuclei, 13

pacemaker cells, 13, 14
Thalamocortical relay neuron, 12, 15
Thalamus and generalized epileptiform activity, 347
Theta
  bursts, 183
  coma pattern, 501, 503
  frequency band, 168
  in coma and seizures, 501
  normal posterior, 224
  waves, 383
Three-dimensional plotting, 73
Three Hz spike-and-wave complexes, 332–334, 338, 343
  also referred to as Typical spike-and-wave complex
Thrombophlebitis, 323, 471
Time
  constant, 55, 90
  domain, 133, 140
Timing of waves, 171
Todd's paralysis, 282, 605
Tongue movement artifacts, 117
Tonic
  absence, 601
  seizures, 288, 297, 603
Tonic–clonic seizures, 288, 289, 297, 340–342, 602
  also referred to as Grand mal seizures
Topographic mapping, 136, 139
Toxic
  agents, 433
  encephalopathies, see Encephalopathies
Tracé
  alternant, 179, 185, 189–191, 193
  discontinu, 179, 183, 185
Tranquilizers, 489
Transients

benign epileptiform, 76
  of sleep, 390, 395
  description, 163
  focal sharp, 311
  normal, in prematurity, 182
  sharp, 164, 190
    frontal, in full-term infants, 191
      in premature infants, 182, 184
    multifocal, 183, 185, 190, 191, 355
    occipital positive, of sleep, 205, 229, 233
    vertex, 198, 223, 225, 230
Transverse bipolar montages, 79, 89
Traumatic seizures, 318
Tricyclic antidepressants, 433, 490
Triphasic wave pattern, 163, 377, 380, 411, 446
True
  anterior temporal electrodes, 36
  phase reversal, 69
Tuberous sclerosis, 316, 414, 430
Tumors, see Brain tumors
Typical
  petit mal absence, 295
  spike-and-wave complexes, 333, 343

Unclassified seizures, 288, 289, 298
Unilateral
  cerebral lesions, 499
  decrease in frequency of alpha, 495, 496
  failure of alpha blocking, 499
    also referred to as Bancaud's phenomenon
  seizures, 298
Unverricht–Lundborg's myoclonus epilepsy, 348
Uremia, 490

Versive seizures, 291
Vertebro-basilar insufficiency, 487
  see also Ischemia

Vertex
  sharp transients, 198, *223*, 225, 230
  waves, 205
Vertiginous seizures, 291
Video monitoring, *151*
Visual
  evoked potentials, 194, 257
  seizures, 291
  see also Photic stimulation
Volume conduction, 18
V waves, 198, *223*, 230
  also referred to as Vertex sharp transients

Wakefulness, 194, 231, 232
Wave form, *163*
  of alpha activity in adults, 213
  of local epileptiform activity, 301
Wavelength, 167
Wernicke's encephalopathy, 432
West syndrome, 365
Wicket
  rhythm, 222

  spikes, 164, 395
Widespread
  asynchronous slow waves, 409
  beta rhythm, 219
  EEG activity, 169
Wilson's disease, 278, 431
Withdrawal from chronic use of drugs, 349
Writing EEG reports, 516, *583*
Writing unit, *60*